Health Insurance Is a Family Matter

Committee on the Consequences of Uninsurance

Board on Health Care Services

INSTITUTE OF MEDICINE
OF THE NATIONAL ACADEMIES

THE NATIONAL ACADEMIES PRESS
Washington, D.C.
www.nap.edu

THE NATIONAL ACADEMIES PRESS · 500 Fifth Street, N.W. · Washington, DC 20001

NOTICE: The project that is the subject of this report was approved by the Governing Board of the National Research Council, whose members are drawn from the councils of the National Academy of Sciences, the National Academy of Engineering, and the Institute of Medicine. The members of the committee responsible for the report were chosen for their special competences and with regard for appropriate balance.

Support for this project was provided by The Robert Wood Johnson Foundation. The views presented in this report are those of the Institute of Medicine Committee on the Consequences of Uninsurance and are not necessarily those of the funding agencies.

International Standard Book Number 0-309-08518-7

Library of Congress Control Number 2002111131

Additional copies of this report are available for sale from the National Academies Press, 500 Fifth Street, N.W., Box 285, Washington, D.C. 20055. Call (800) 624-6242 or (202) 334-3313 (in the Washington metropolitan area); Internet, http://www.nap.edu.

For more information about the Institute of Medicine, visit the IOM home page at **www.iom.edu.**

"Knowing is not enough; we must apply.
Willing is not enough; we must do."
—Goethe

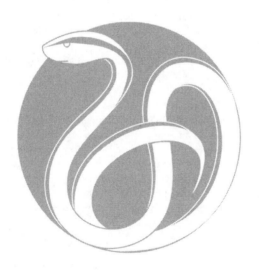

INSTITUTE OF MEDICINE

Shaping the Future for Health

THE NATIONAL ACADEMIES
Advisers to the Nation on Science, Engineering, and Medicine

The **National Academy of Sciences** is a private, nonprofit, self-perpetuating society of distinguished scholars engaged in scientific and engineering research, dedicated to the furtherance of science and technology and to their use for the general welfare. Upon the authority of the charter granted to it by the Congress in 1863, the Academy has a mandate that requires it to advise the federal government on scientific and technical matters. Dr. Bruce M. Alberts is president of the National Academy of Sciences.

The **National Academy of Engineering** was established in 1964, under the charter of the National Academy of Sciences, as a parallel organization of outstanding engineers. It is autonomous in its administration and in the selection of its members, sharing with the National Academy of Sciences the responsibility for advising the federal government. The National Academy of Engineering also sponsors engineering programs aimed at meeting national needs, encourages education and research, and recognizes the superior achievements of engineers. Dr. Wm. A. Wulf is president of the National Academy of Engineering.

The **Institute of Medicine** was established in 1970 by the National Academy of Sciences to secure the services of eminent members of appropriate professions in the examination of policy matters pertaining to the health of the public. The Institute acts under the responsibility given to the National Academy of Sciences by its congressional charter to be an adviser to the federal government and, upon its own initiative, to identify issues of medical care, research, and education. Dr. Harvey V. Fineberg is president of the Institute of Medicine.

The **National Research Council** was organized by the National Academy of Sciences in 1916 to associate the broad community of science and technology with the Academy's purposes of furthering knowledge and advising the federal government. Functioning in accordance with general policies determined by the Academy, the Council has become the principal operating agency of both the National Academy of Sciences and the National Academy of Engineering in providing services to the government, the public, and the scientific and engineering communities. The Council is administered jointly by both Academies and the Institute of Medicine. Dr. Bruce M. Alberts and Dr. Wm. A. Wulf are chair and vice chair, respectively, of the National Research Council.

www.national-academies.org

COMMITTEE ON THE CONSEQUENCES OF UNINSURANCE

MARY SUE COLEMAN (*Co-chair*), President, University of Michigan, Ann Arbor

ARTHUR L. KELLERMANN (*Co-chair*), Professor and Chairman, Department of Emergency Medicine, Director, Center for Injury Control, Emory University School of Medicine, Atlanta, Georgia

RONALD M. ANDERSEN, Wasserman Professor in Health Services, Chair, Department of Health Services, Professor of Sociology, University of California, Los Angeles, School of Public Health

JOHN Z. AYANIAN, Associate Professor of Medicine and Health Care Policy, Harvard Medical School, Brigham and Women's Hospital, Boston, Massachusetts

ROBERT J. BLENDON, Professor, Health Policy and Political Analysis, Department of Health Policy and Management, Harvard School of Public Health and Kennedy School of Government, Boston, Massachusetts

SHEILA P. DAVIS, Associate Professor, The University of Mississippi Medical Center, School of Nursing, Jackson

GEORGE C. EADS, Charles River Associates, Washington, D.C.

SANDRA R. HERNÁNDEZ, Chief Executive Officer, San Francisco Foundation, California

WILLARD G. MANNING, Professor, Department of Health Studies, The University of Chicago, Illinois

JAMES J. MONGAN, President, Massachusetts General Hospital, Boston

CHRISTOPHER QUERAM, Chief Executive Officer, Employer Health Care Alliance Cooperative, Madison, Wisconsin

SHOSHANNA SOFAER, Robert P. Luciano Professor of Health Care Policy, School of Public Affairs, Baruch College, New York

STEPHEN J. TREJO, Associate Professor of Economics, Department of Economics, University of Texas at Austin

REED V. TUCKSON, Senior Vice President, Consumer Health and Medical Care Advancement, UnitedHealth Group, Minnetonka, Minnesota

EDWARD H. WAGNER, Director, McColl Institute for Healthcare Innovation, Center for Health Studies (CHS), Group Health Cooperative, Seattle, Washington

LAWRENCE WALLACK, Director, School of Community Health, College of Urban and Public Affairs, Portland State University, Oregon

IOM Staff

Wilhelmine Miller, Project Co-director
Dianne Miller Wolman, Project Co-director
Lynne Page Snyder, Program Officer
Tracy McKay, Research Associate
Ryan Palugod, Senior Project Assistant

Consultants

Gerry Fairbrother, Research Director, Child Health Forum, New York
Academy of Medicine
Hanns Kuttner, Senior Research Associate, Economic Research Initiative on
the Uninsured, University of Michigan

Foreword

Health Insurance Is a Family Matter is the third in a series of six reports planned by the Institute of Medicine (IOM) and its Committee on the Consequences of Uninsurance. This series of studies represents a major and sustained commitment by the IOM to contribute to the public debate about the problems associated with having more than 38 million uninsured people in the United States. This very broad research effort also represents a significant contribution from The Robert Wood Johnson Foundation for which we are grateful.

Health Insurance Is a Family Matter adds to the IOM's history of related contributions. Most relevant for this report on families is a consensus report issued by the Committee on Children, Health Insurance, and Access to Care in 1998, *America's Children: Health Insurance and Access to Care*. That committee concluded that all children should have health insurance. Because this has not yet become a reality, the Committee on the Consequences of Uninsurance provides further evidence and confirmation of the effects on children of being uninsured, as well as the impact of uninsurance on the whole family.

As we prepared to issue the Committee's first report last fall, *Coverage Matters: Insurance and Health Care*, two hijacked airliners destroyed the World Trade Center and another severely damaged the Pentagon. After the initial shock and recovery began, attention turned to the families of the victims. Around the country people began asking what could be done for families who had lost their health insurance and their family's income along with their loved ones. As the economy slowed and more people lost their jobs, the fear of becoming uninsured grew and Congress began debating what to do about the problem of health coverage interrupted by a job loss. These circumstances make this report on the family effects of being uninsured all the more important and relevant to current efforts to understand the problem and find solutions.

The members of the Committee on the Consequences of Uninsurance are experts in a wide range of disciplines, including clinical medicine, epidemiology, health services research and delivery of services, economics, strategic planning, small business management, and health communications. They carefully considered the pertinent evidence, and here present a coherent picture of the various effects that being uninsured has upon family well-being.

This report shows that a family's chance of having an uninsured member at some point is significant and that a lack of coverage can have negative effects on the uninsured child or pregnant woman. In addition, some of the ill effects of uninsurance spill over to other family members, even if they have coverage, and can jeopardize the family's well-being and put the family unit at risk of financial disruption. Children are our nation's future, and families are the place for raising and protecting them; it is crucial to the strength of the country that we consider the contribution health insurance makes to family well-being. This report will provide much material for reflection by policy experts, decision-makers, and the general public as they consider the various ways that being uninsured can erode the strength of America's families—and what can be done about it.

Harvey V. Fineberg, M.D., Ph.D.
President, Institute of Medicine
September 2002

Preface

Health Insurance Is a Family Matter is the third report that the Institute of Medicine (IOM) Committee on the Consequences of Uninsurance is issuing since it began its research efforts in autumn 2000. Three more reports will be issued before the completion of the project in 2003. These reports represent the Committee's efforts to review and assess the evidence concerning a wide range of causes and effects of being uninsured. The Committee is concerned with both the effects of lacking health insurance for individuals and the broader effects of having more than 38 million uninsured people in our nation.

The Committee is following a carefully designed research plan so that each report builds on previous ones and provides a foundation for future reports. The first report, *Coverage Matters: Insurance and Health Care,* provides essential background information for understanding the dynamics of health insurance, who is uninsured and why, and provides evidence to dispel many public misperceptions. Coverage does indeed matter. The second report, *Care Without Coverage: Too Little, Too Late,* presents an overwhelming body of evidence documenting the fact that adults without insurance suffer worse health. Now the third report widens the focus from the individual to the family.

Health Insurance is a Family Matter analyzes the effects being uninsured can have on the health, finances and general well-being of the family. It also examines the health of uninsured children and pregnant women to see whether they also receive less care and suffer worse health outcomes than do those who are insured. The next report will expand the focus of attention even more to examine how having part of a community's population uninsured can affect the community as a whole, including those with insurance. Then the Committee looks at the economic costs to society of sustaining an uninsured population of more than

38 million people. The final report will consider aspects of various programs, strategies, and policy options designed to expand coverage and reduce the problems of uninsurance.

This report comes at a time when personal concerns about being uninsured and about having such a large uninsured population in the country have fueled public debate yet again. The report echoes the messages of the first two reports that coverage matters and that being uninsured is bad for one's health. Being uninsured similarly affects the health and well-being of the family. We hope that *Health Insurance Is a Family Matter* will provide a fresh perspective on the issues and the solid analysis needed to move the discussion further along toward solutions.

Mary Sue Coleman, Ph.D.
Co-chair
Arthur Kellermann, M.D., M.P.H.
Co-chair
September 2002

Acknowledgments

Many individuals contributed to *Health Insurance Is a Family Matter.* The Committee acknowledges the assistance of those who helped with the analyses on which the report is based.

The Committee especially recognizes the members of the Subcommittee on Family Impacts of Uninsurance, which developed this report: George Eads, who served as its chair, Sheila Davis, Cathy Schoen, Shoshanna Sofaer, Peter Szilagyi, and Barbara Wolfe. They provided a wide range of expertise, devoted significant amounts of time, and assisted in guiding the development of the critical literature review and analyses of data that form the basis of this report's findings and conclusions.

Gerry Fairbrother, of the New York Academy of Medicine, served as principal consultant to the Subcommittee and prepared background papers on insurance coverage patterns within families and on the interactions within families that are related to insurance coverage and family health. She also conducted a major literature review of the evidence concerning health outcomes for pregnant women, infants, and children. Gerry was always available for advice during preparation of this report, generous with her assistance to staff and the Committee, and her expertise improves the whole report. The Committee is grateful to the New York Academy of Medicine for its generosity with her time and that of her assistants.

Hanns Kuttner, of the Economic Research Initiative on the Uninsured at the University of Michigan, assisted the Committee by drafting background papers analyzing and synthesizing the research on the financial effects of health insurance on the family and effects over the life cycle of the family. He also generously provided ongoing economic advice and assistance. Matthew Broaddus provided new tabulations of the latest census data on insurance status, which formed the basis for much of the analysis in the report. The Committee is grateful to the Center on Budget and Policy Priorities and to the David and Lucile Packard Foundation for making Matt's time and expertise available to us. Consulting editor Cheryl Ulmer assisted in preparation of the literature review on health outcomes for pregnant women, infants, and children and the short summary of the report.

The Committee recognizes the hard work of staff at the Institute of Medicine. This work is conducted under the guidance of Janet Corrigan, director, Board on Health Care Services. All members of the project team, directed by Dianne Wolman and Wilhelmine Miller, contributed to this report. Dianne was lead staff in working with the Subcommittee and the Committee in developing and managing the research and drafting of *Health Insurance Is a Family Matter.* Wilhelmine and Program Officer Lynne Snyder reviewed and edited multiple drafts and background documents and contributed in many ways to the final report. Research Associate Tracy McKay researched and drafted a summary of public insurance programs, conducted systematic literature searches for the Committee's review, and prepared the whole manuscript for publication. In addition to collecting the large number of articles and references used for this report and maintaining the reference database, Senior Project Assistant Ryan Palugod efficiently supported communications with Committee members and meetings logistics.

Funding for the project comes from The Robert Wood Johnson Foundation (RWJF). The Committee extends special thanks to Risa Lavisso-Mourey, senior vice president, and Anne Weiss, senior program officer, RWJF, for their continuing support and interest in this project.

Finally, the Committee would like to thank Co-chairs, Mary Sue Coleman and Arthur Kellermann, and Subcommittee Chair George Eads for their guidance in the development of *Health Insurance Is a Family Matter.*

Reviewers

This report has been reviewed in draft form by individuals chosen for their diverse perspectives and technical expertise, in accordance with procedures approved by the NRC's Report Review Committee. The purpose of this independent review is to provide candid and critical comments that will assist the institution in making its published report as sound as possible and to ensure that the report meets institutional standards for objectivity, evidence, and responsiveness to the study charge. The review comments and draft manuscript remain confidential to protect the integrity of the deliberative process. We wish to thank the following individuals for their review of this report:

RON J. ANDERSON, President and Chief Executive Officer, Parkland Memorial Hospital, Dallas, TX

JANET CURRIE, Professor, Department of Economics, University of California, Los Angeles

GARY L. FREED, Professor, Department of Pediatrics, University of Michigan, Ann Arbor

JOHN HOLAHAN, Director, Health Policy Center, Urban Institute, Washington, DC

EMBRY HOWELL, Principal Research Associate, Health Policy Center, Urban Institute, Washington, DC

SARA ROSENBAUM, Director, Center for Health Services Research and Policy, The George Washington University, Washington, DC

AMY K. TAYLOR, Senior Economist, Department of Health and Human Services, Rockville, MD

Although the reviewers listed above have provided many constructive comments and suggestions, they were not asked to endorse the conclusions or recommendations nor did they see the final draft of the report before its release. The review of this report was overseen by **Hugh H. Tilson, Clinical Professor, School of Public Health, University of North Carolina, Chapel Hill,** appointed by the Institute of Medicine and **Joseph P. Newhouse, John D. MacArthur Professor of Health Policy and Management, Harvard University**, appointed by the NRC's Report Review Committee, who were responsible for making certain that an independent examination of this report was carried out in accordance with institutional procedures and that all review comments were carefully considered. Responsibility for the final content of this report rests entirely with the authoring committee and the institution.

Contents

Health Insurance Is a Family Matter

BOX ES.1
Preview of Selected Committee Findings

Here is a preview of the Committee's most important findings concerning the impact on the family of not having health insurance and the health effects on children, pregnant women and infants of being uninsured. Chapters 1 through 7 include background and discussion of these and other Committee findings. The following Executive Summary provides an overview of the full report.

Insurance Coverage of Families

- If parents have health insurance, children are likely to be covered as well.
- In one-fifth of the more than 38 million families that include children, there are one or more family members uninsured.[1]
- Many uninsured children are eligible for, but not enrolled in, public programs. More than half of the 8 million children who remain uninsured are eligible for Medicaid or State Children's Health Insurance Program (SCHIP) coverage.
- Family insurance coverage is strongly and positively related to income. Just 59 percent of families with children and with income less than 50 percent of the federal poverty level (FPL) have all members covered, compared with 90 percent of families whose income is above 200 percent of FPL.

Insurance Transitions over the Family Life Cycle

- The structure of public health insurance programs and the cutoff age for dependents' eligibility in private insurance plans make it more likely that dependent children will become uninsured as they grow up.
- The link between health insurance and employment for most families creates many opportunities for loss of coverage. In order to obtain or maintain coverage, family work choices may be constrained. Work choices for families enrolled in public insurance programs may also be constrained because of the income ceilings for eligibility.
- Marriage increases the chances of having employment-based health insurance for the whole family. Getting separated, divorced, or being widowed may increase the risk that family members lose their employment-based coverage.

Financial Characteristics and Behavior of Uninsured Families

- Families with at least one uninsured member are predominantly lower-income families.
- Most uninsured families would not have sufficient funds in their budget to purchase health insurance without a substantial premium subsidy.
- On average, families with some or all members uninsured spend less on health care in absolute dollars and they use fewer services than do families with all members covered by private insurance. Paradoxically, families with uninsured members are more likely to have high health expenditures as a proportion of family income than are insured families.

---

[1] The CPS data used in this report considers a person to be uninsured if they are without coverage for a full year or more.

- Among families with no health insurance the entire year and incomes below the poverty level, more than one in four have out-of-pocket expenses that exceed 5 percent of income; 4 percent of *all* uninsured families have expenses that exceed 20 percent of annual income.

Family Well-Being and Health Insurance

- Extension of publicly supported health insurance to low-income uninsured parents is associated with increased enrollment among children.
- Uninsured parents have poorer health, have poorer access to the health care system, are less satisfied with the care they receive when they gain access, and are more likely to have negative experiences around bill collection compared with insured parents.
- The health of one family member can affect the health and well-being of other family members. In particular, the health of parents can play an important role in the well-being of their children.

Health-Related Outcomes for Children, Pregnant Women, and Newborns

- Uninsured children have less access to health care, are less likely to have a regular source of primary care, and use medical and dental care less often compared with children who have insurance. Children with gaps in health insurance coverage have worse access than do those with continuous coverage.
- Previously uninsured children experience significant increases in both access to and more appropriate use of health care services following their enrollment in state-sponsored health insurance expansions.
- Lower-income, minority, non-citizen, or uninsured children consistently have worse access and utilization than do children with none of these characteristics. These factors overlap to a large extent. However, each exerts its own independent effect on access and utilization.
- Uninsured children often receive care late in the development of a health problem or do not receive any care. As a result, they are at higher risk for hospitalization for conditions amenable to timely outpatient care and for missed diagnoses of serious and even life-threatening conditions.
- Undiagnosed and untreated conditions that are amenable to control, cure, or prevention can affect children's functioning and opportunities over the course of their lives. Such conditions include iron deficiency anemia, otitis media, asthma, and attention deficit–hyperactivity disorder.
- Uninsured women receive fewer prenatal care services than their insured counterparts and report greater difficulty in obtaining the care that they believe they need. Studies find large differences in use between privately insured and uninsured women and smaller differences between uninsured and publicly insured women.
- Uninsured women and their newborns receive, on average, less prenatal care and fewer expensive perinatal services. Uninsured newborns are more likely to have low birthweight and to die than are insured newborns. Uninsured women are more likely to have poor outcomes during pregnancy and delivery than are women with insurance. Studies have not demonstrated an improvement in maternal outcomes related to health insurance alone.

Executive Summary

A FAMILY PERSPECTIVE

In America the family is the basic social unit. Strong families are essential to America's future. We all share an interest in the collective well-being of our national community and in providing the conditions for families to succeed in raising the next generation. This report views the consequences of having more than 38 million people in the country lacking health insurance from the perspective of families, in contrast to most research, which examines the impact on individuals. The vast majority of uninsured individuals live in families. Having one or more uninsured individuals in a family can have an impact, even if some or all of the remaining members of the family have health insurance.

In its previous report, *Care Without Coverage: Too Little, Too Late*, the Institute of Medicine's (IOM) Committee on the Consequences of Uninsurance concluded that being uninsured can adversely affect an individual adult's health. In this report the Committee examines two sets of literature, one concerning the relationship between health insurance status and the health of pregnant women, infants, and children and the other on whether having an uninsured member in the family can have a deleterious effect on the family as a whole.[1] The Committee acknowledges that it may take more than simply providing insurance coverage to have a positive health impact. Health insurance is, however, an important factor in reducing barriers to care. The Committee addresses these questions:

---

[1]The Committee's rigorous evaluation of the literature encompassed a wide range of research; its findings are based on the most methodologically sound studies; and results reported are generally significant at the $p = 0.05$ or better, unless otherwise specified.

- How does the presence of an uninsured family member affect the health of the rest of the family? Even if only one member of the family is uninsured, could that affect the family's finances and economic stability?
- Because parents act as the health care seekers and decision makers for their children, does being uninsured affect their functioning in that capacity? What if their children have no health coverage?
- Because a family's health and insurance needs tend to change as its members reach maturity and grow older, how well do the current insurance mechanisms and programs match those needs?

Our nation encompasses a rich variety of family structures that reflect how individuals view themselves, the people they live with, and their emotional, social and economic interrelationships. The Committee purposely chooses to view families as self-defined responsibility units whose members' lives are emotionally and economically entwined. It recognizes that the concept is broadly encompassing, not neat and uniform, but it reflects reality. A person's own definition of family does not necessarily correspond to the definition of family used by employment-based insurance plans for coverage eligibility. As a result, some self-defined family members may not qualify for coverage. In addition, most of the publicly financed health insurance programs provide coverage for individuals rather than for families as a whole, although people generally function economically and socially as part of a family unit. This mismatch between insurers' eligibility criteria and a family's definition of itself affects the coverage patterns of families and, ultimately, the family's well-being. The mismatch and resulting uninsurance within the family also have important implications for the public debate about expanding coverage.

The source of health insurance available to families directly affects whether all members are covered. Employment-based plans are more likely to offer coverage for the entire family than are other types of insurance. The Committee concludes that if all family members are covered, the chances increase that they will get the health care they need in a timely fashion and that the costs of those services would likely have a less destabilizing impact on the family's finances than if some or all members are uninsured. The Committee also concludes that the health of children and their long-term development would likely be enhanced if the children are covered by insurance. Box ES.1 presents the Committee's specific findings regarding the nature of the consequences of uninsurance on families.

COVERAGE PATTERNS OF FAMILIES AND THEIR SIGNIFICANCE

There are 85 million families in the United States, and 17 million of them—about one in five—have one or more members who are uninsured. The more than 38 million *uninsured people* nationally live with roughly 20 million *insured family members*, which means that 58 million lives may be affected by the consequences of uninsurance. There are more than 38 million *families* with minor children; 20 percent do not have all their members insured.[2]

Employment-based insurance is the most common type of coverage. Usually workers purchase coverage when it is offered on the job and buy additional coverage for their dependent family members if they consider it affordable and alternative coverage does not exist. Thus, when parents are insured, whether they are in single- or two-parent families, more than 95 percent of the time all their children are also covered.

Among the almost 20 percent of families with some or all members lacking coverage, specific social and demographic characteristics are more common, including lower income, single parenthood, racial and ethnic minority status, and immigrant status.

• Family insurance coverage is strongly related to family income; families with lower incomes are less likely to be fully insured. Similarly, single-parent families are less likely to have all members covered than are two-parent families (71 percent compared with 85 percent).

• Lower-income *parents* are more likely to lack coverage than are their *children*, because public programs provide coverage for children up to higher family income levels than they do for adults. Nonetheless, many children remain uninsured although they are eligible for public programs. Of the estimated 8 million uninsured children in 2000, most are eligible for Medicaid and SCHIP, but not enrolled (Urban Institute, 2002a). The proportion of uninsured children who are eligible for public programs will likely continue to decrease, if enrollments continue increasing.

There are 9.1 million uninsured parents (Lambrew, 2001b). One-third of these uninsured parents have incomes below the federal poverty level (FPL) and another third have incomes between 100 percent and 200 percent FPL.[3] The fact that many of the parents are uninsured is significant because parents obtain health care for their children. Even if their children may be eligible for coverage or are actually enrolled, children are dependent upon their parents' enrolling them in public programs and taking them for treatment. The parents' decisions on whether, when, and from whom to seek care for their children may be influenced by their own experiences with and knowledge of the health system. When states have expanded Medicaid coverage broadly to include low-income parents as well as their children, the enrollment of eligible children has increased more than it has in

---

[2]Committee analyses are based on tabulations of the Census Bureau's 2001 Current Population Survey public use file designed to aggregate data by family units prepared by Matthew Broaddus, Center on Budget and Policy Priorities. Families with heads under age 65 are included as well as children under age 18.

[3]For 2000, the FPL is $11,250 for a family of two and $14,150 for a family of three. See Appendix D, Table D.1.

states without broader parental coverage (Ku and Broaddus, 2000; Dubay and Kenney, 2002). Parents' lack of knowledge about the programs and their confusion about eligibility, which traditionally are barriers to the enrollment of eligible children, are lower when parents themselves enroll.

A parent's own use of health services is a strong predictor of their children's use. Uninsured parents are more likely to have negative experiences with the health system than are those with insurance, and this may affect their perception of the value of health care and their willingness to take their children for needed care. Parents without coverage are more likely to report that they are in poorer health than are privately insured parents; they have more trouble gaining access to care when they need it, and more often lack a regular source of care. In addition, as the Committee concluded in *Care Without Coverage: Too Little, Too Late*, uninsured adults are more likely to delay seeking care for themselves and to suffer poorer health and even premature death than are their insured counterparts.

INSURANCE TRANSITIONS OVER THE FAMILY LIFE CYCLE

The current patchwork of insurance programs in the United States makes it common for family members to experience periods of uninsurance. Americans take health insurance into account when making decisions about jobs and work and report that their choices are constrained by coverage considerations. As children grow up they are increasingly likely to be uninsured because public programs tend to have more generous family income limits for younger children than for older children and both public and employment-based coverage for children usually ends around their nineteenth birthday. While teenagers or those graduating from college may be ready to go to work, they are less likely than their older coworkers to find jobs that include health benefits or to earn enough to purchase insurance independently (IOM, 2001; Quinn et al., 2000). At an age when serious injuries are most common, some young adults may assume their health needs will not be large or may find health insurance unaffordable, although independently-purchased plans are generally less expensive for them than for older persons.

The predominance of employment-based coverage in this country means that families may lose their health insurance when working parents change jobs, are laid off or die. When an older worker carrying employment-based coverage for a younger spouse and dependents reaches age 65, retires, and qualifies for Medicare, the other family members may be left without any health coverage. Alternatively, the parents' choices about work may be constrained by the need to obtain and maintain health benefits with the job (sometimes referred to as job lock). While having two parents in the family increases the chances of having employment-based coverage for the whole family, it does not preclude dependents' losing coverage upon separation, divorce, or death of the parent carrying the insurance. Many life transitions, whether resulting from age, employment or a change in marital status, are unavoidable or unpredictable and result in loss of coverage.

FINANCIAL CHARACTERISTICS AND BEHAVIOR OF UNINSURED FAMILIES

Even in the healthiest of families, if one member has an accident the resulting medical bills can affect the economic stability of the whole family. The impact depends, in part, on whether the injured person was insured, the size of the bills, and the family's income and other resources. Families with at least one member lacking insurance predominantly have lower incomes (below 200 percent FPL). Not surprisingly, families with uninsured members also have few if any assets and are unlikely to be able to borrow to pay their medical bills. Often they do not have the budgetary resources to purchase health insurance without a premium subsidy, given the relatively high cost of family coverage outside of group plans.

The annual out-of-pocket expenses for health care for an uninsured family on average are less in actual dollars and less relative to their income than those expenses for families with coverage. Uninsured families do not have the expense of insurance premiums and are less likely to use *any* health care services; but those who do generally use fewer services. Paradoxically, uninsured families are also more likely than insured ones to face health costs that are high relative to their income. At the low end of the spectrum, families without health insurance are more likely to have no health care expenses than are families with health insurance because they are fortunate enough to be healthy or they forgo needed care. In the middle of the spectrum, the average annual out-of-pocket expense for families without health insurance is less than that of families with coverage. However, at the high end of the spectrum, families without health insurance are more likely to have health expenses that exceed 5 or 10 percent of their income than are families with health insurance. For all family types and for single adults, the burden of out-of-pocket expenditures rises as incomes fall. The burden is also greater for uninsured families with members in poorer health compared to those with better health status. More than half of all working-age adults uninsured now or in the recent past report difficulties paying medical bills, compared with less than a quarter of insured adults (Duchon et al., 2001).

How do families cope with the burden of medical bills? Some families delay payment and may be dunned by collections agents. Among all working-age adults with medical bill problems, almost 60 percent are currently or were recently uninsured. Of those with severe bill problems and in those uninsured groups, two-thirds report borrowing from family or a friend and a quarter got a loan or mortgage on their home in order to pay (Duchon et al., 2001). Some families resort to declaring bankruptcy and put their future credit rating in jeopardy. Medical bills are a factor in nearly half of all bankruptcy filings. However, it is not known whether bankruptcy is more likely for uninsured families than for those with coverage.

When a family is uninsured, has very limited income, and cannot pay all its medical bills, the financial burden falls on the providers of services and on the broader community, which offer various supports. These supports include charity care, the use of sliding fee schedules based on family income, and the availability of safety-net providers. While uninsured families absorb more than 40 percent of the costs for their medical services on average, the proportion varies widely, depending on the type of service used. For example, prescription costs are unlikely to have subsidies or external support, and families pay 88 percent of that expense. Because of the availability of various subsidies for the care that hospitals provide uninsured people, families ultimately bear only about 7 percent of these expenses. It is difficult to determine the sources of the various supports available to those who cannot afford to pay for their care, who bears the burden financially, and whether free or reduced-cost care is fairly and equitably distributed to needy families and individuals. Some of these issues will be examined in more detail in the Committee's following reports on community-wide effects and societal costs of uninsured populations.

HEALTH INTERACTIONS WITHIN THE FAMILY

The health of one member of the family can affect the health of the other members and of the unit as a whole. Particularly for children, their early development is dependent on the health and well-being of their parents. Children's early development can have lifelong consequences for them (Shonkoff and Phillips, 2000). Public health insurance programs have expanded coverage to children, but insuring children *alone* may not be enough. This is because parents are a key part of the process of obtaining health care for their children.

The Committee's analyses show that in families with some members uninsured, parents are more likely than the children to lack coverage. The Committee's previous report shows that uninsured adults are more likely to have poorer health, to receive delayed diagnoses and treatments and to die prematurely. Lower-income parents not only are more likely to be uninsured, but also are more likely to suffer from poorer health compared with wealthier parents. This report presents evidence that parents in poorer physical or mental health have greater difficulty fulfilling their parental roles and responsibilities than do healthy parents. Studies that relate these family circumstances to insurance status do not yet exist.

Family stress, found more frequently in lower-income families than in those with higher incomes, is associated with higher levels of behavioral, emotional, and physical health problems for the children. While there are many contributing factors to the level of stress within the family, uncertainty about health care may be one of them. Research to further clarify the relationships between health insurance, family health, and emotional well-being is needed.

HEALTH-RELATED OUTCOMES FOR CHILDREN, PREGNANT WOMEN, AND NEWBORNS

It is important to examine the relationship between the insurance status of children and pregnant women, their use of health care, and ultimately their health outcomes. Uninsured families are parsimonious in their use of health services. *Uninsured* adults are more likely to report going without care that they feel is needed than are *insured* adults. Not surprisingly, delaying treatment and not using services can adversely affect health, even though they avoid costs in the short term.

The Committee has reviewed the extensive body of research on the relationship between health insurance and access, use, and outcomes for children, pregnant women, and newborns and concludes that having health insurance coverage improves these health-related outcomes. This conclusion is based on both individual and population-level studies. However, insurance does not guarantee appropriate use of health services and is only one of many factors affecting health, along with poverty, diet, exercise, smoking, and other behavioral factors.

Health insurance promotes children's use of routine and appropriate care and facilitates a regular source of care, or "medical home." Well-child care and a regular care provider are very important for monitoring childrens' development and detecting potential problems early before they can cause long-term health consequences. Uninsured children use medical and dental services less frequently than do insured children, even after taking into account differences in family income, race and ethnicity, and health status. Children with gaps in health insurance coverage are less likely to have a regular source of care and are less likely to see a health care provider when their parents believe they need one than are children with continuous coverage.

Children who are both uninsured and poor or uninsured and a member of a racial or ethnic minority or immigrant group have added difficulties in gaining access to and using primary care services. Although these factors frequently overlap, each independently adds to a child's likelihood of reduced access and use. Uninsured children with special health needs are particularly disadvantaged since they need considerably more than routine care. Uninsured children with special health needs are less likely to have a usual source of care, less likely to have seen a doctor in the previous year, and less likely to get needed medical, mental health, dental, prescriptions, or vision care than are their insured counterparts.

Adolescents as a group are particularly at risk of not having a regular source of care or any physician visits in the past year. They have the highest uninsured rate of all children even though their need for some kinds of health care services, such as mental health screening and treatment for drinking and other risky behaviors, increases in their late teenage years.

Because uninsured children are more likely to receive no or delayed care, they are at greater risk of hospitalization for conditions that could have been treated on an outpatient basis. Health conditions that are readily treatable and that could affect a child's long-term development and life chances if untreated, may be more likely to go undetected when children are not insured. Conditions such as asthma, iron deficiency anemia, and middle-ear infections, if left untreated or improperly controlled, can affect mental development and school performance, language development, and hearing. Although long-term studies linking insurance status to these conditions and later life outcomes have not been conducted, the lack of routine care that would detect these conditions in uninsured children remains a concern.

Being uninsured may affect the health of pregnant women, the care that they receive, and birth outcomes. Uninsured women have greater difficulty in getting the care that they believe they need than do insured women. The differences in the use of medical care between uninsured women and those who are privately insured are larger than those between uninsured and publicly insured women.

Uninsured women and their newborns receive, on average, less prenatal care and fewer expensive perinatal services, such as cesarean sections. Sick newborns who are uninsured average shorter hospital stays.

Uninsured newborns are more likely to have poorer health outcomes than are insured newborns, such as low birth-weight, which is a risk factor for developmental problems. Uninsured babies are also more likely to die prematurely. However, evidence of improvements in low birth-weight for newborns based on population studies of Medicaid expansions is not definitive. While uninsured women more frequently have poor outcomes during pregnancy and delivery than do insured women, insurance coverage alone may not be enough to improve maternal outcomes.

CONCLUSIONS

The Committee demonstrated in *Coverage Matters* (IOM, 2001) that the uninsured population includes people from all social and economic groups. The uninsured are, however, predominantly in working families, and two-thirds are from families that have incomes below 200 percent of the federal poverty level. *Care Without Coverage* (IOM, 2002a) concluded that adults without coverage do not get the care they need and are more likely to suffer poor health and premature death than are insured adults. The consequences of being uninsured are certainly significant for the *individual.* Now *Health Insurance Is a Family Matter* documents that having one or more uninsured members within the family can have adverse consequences for the whole family.

The Committee concludes that the financial, physical, and emotional well-being of all members of the family may be in jeopardy if any individual within the family lacks coverage. In the United States there are more than 38 million *uninsured* individuals and an additional 20 million *insured* individuals who live in a family with one or more persons who lack health insurance. This means that approximately 58 million people, fully one-fifth of the U.S. population, is affected by lack of health insurance.

NOTES

BOX 1.1
A Family Perspective

This report, the third of the Committee on the Consequences of Uninsurance, examines the impacts on America's families of not having health insurance for all their members. On the basis of a literature review this report provides new analyses of the consequences of a lack of insurance within families and the effects on the health of children and pregnant women. The Committee looks at the phenomenon of uninsurance from the perspective of the family, which is important for several reasons:

• The health of one family member can affect the health and well-being of the family as a whole. For example, an uninsured parent may delay seeking care and suffer sufficiently debilitating ill health that it is difficult to continue working or caring for children. Even if there is only one uninsured member, if that person has a serious illness or accident, it could generate medical bills that threaten the economic stability of the whole family.

• Publicly financed health insurance usually covers individuals. Examining the complicating effects on families broadens the perspective of public policy debate.

• Within the family, parents make decisions for their children about seeking care. Whether and how they use the health system for themselves may affect whether their children receive needed, timely care.

• A family's health care and insurance needs change over time as its members grow up and mature. Many common aging and family transitions, such as retiring after a lifetime of work, can affect coverage of individual members and the whole family.

1

A Family Matter

When a member of a family is sick, the whole family can be affected. This report examines whether having an uninsured member of the family might affect the entire family, also. More than 38 million Americans are uninsured.[1] In addition to the personal consequences for those people without coverage, another nearly 20 million immediate family members who *are* insured may also be affected by the lack of coverage of others in the family.[2,3] This report will assess the literature on the physical and psychological health consequences as well as financial effects on the entire family unit of having one or more members uninsured.

This report of the Institute of Medicine (IOM) Committee on the Consequences of Uninsurance provides new analyses of the effects of not having health insurance within families (see Box 1.2). The Committee builds on the first report, *Coverage Matters*, which examines the dynamic, fragmented structure of health insurance in the United States, the causes of uninsurance, and which individuals

---

[1]The Committee's earlier reports refer to roughly 40 million uninsured individuals, based on the 1999 and 2000 Current Population Surveys (CPS). The 2001 CPS was available for this report and shows a dip to 38.7 million uninsured persons (Mills, 2001).

[2]Analyses in this report are based on tabulations of the March 2001 Current Population Survey (CPS) public use file designed to aggregate data by family units conducted by Matthew Broaddus, Center on Budget and Policy Priorities.

[3]The CPS estimates those who have been uninsured for the complete year. It has been criticized for probably over-estimating that number and underestimating the number covered by Medicaid. For example, in 1996 the CPS estimate of the number of nonelderly uninsured persons was 41 million and Medical Expenditure Panel Survey estimated 32 million for that year (Lewis et al., 1998; Fronstin, 2000). For a discussion of the main national surveys including insurance status see *Coverage Matters*, Appendix B.

BOX 1.2
Committee Terminology

The Committee specifies particular meanings for terms used in this report as follows:

- A *family* is any combination of more than one person living together whose lives are emotionally and/or financially intertwined. The report notes when the term refers to a family with minor children, a two-parent family, a one-parent family, a family joined by marriage, or a self-defined family not related by blood or marriage. At times restrictive definitions of family are dictated by the definitions used in surveys or other data sources.
- The term ***uninsured family*** is used as shorthand to refer to families in which one or more members have been uninsured for at least one year. When the report uses data that relate to particular members of the family being uninsured it will specify, for example, families with *all* members uninsured or *some* members uninsured, families with *parents* uninsured or families with *children* uninsured.
- ***Family well-being*** means more than the absence of medical problems or the physical health of individual family members. Family well-being encompasses the psychological, social, and financial soundness of the individual members and the family unit as a whole, including their physical health.
- ***Family stress*** is used in its broad, conventional sense, as any kind of mental, emotional or physical tension or strain, particularly changes in the body and brain in reaction to overwhelming threats to physical or psychological well being.

are likely to be uninsured. It also extends the second report, *Care Without Coverage*, which concludes that health insurance is a vital factor in promoting good health for adults. This report provides analyses of two distinct sets of evidence: 1) studies of insurance effects on the health of children and pregnant women and 2) studies of the interactions within families that may be affected by the lack coverage of individual members.

The Committee recognizes that insurance coverage alone is not enough to ensure improved health outcomes. There are nonfinancial barriers to care as well, such as insufficient education to realize when health care is needed, inability to take time off from work to go to the doctor, lack of needed specialists in the immediate area, lack of culturally and linguistically appropriate services, and psychological inhibitions or fears about seeking care. In addition, there are lifestyle choices, such as smoking, diet, exercise, and alcohol use, that can affect health status and outcomes, even when appropriate care is sought. Nevertheless, insurance remains a very important factor in individual health.

This chapter first presents the purpose of the report and the rationale for using a family perspective to examine the impact of not having insurance. These sections are followed by a brief discussion of how families get health coverage—whom the family may consider to be its responsibility, whom insurers consider family for coverage purposes, and how families evolve and change in relation to these definitions. Finally, the conceptual framework that guides the Committee's work is briefly presented, as well as an overview of the report.

PURPOSE OF THE REPORT

The first of two main purposes of this report is to examine the patterns and consequences of having uninsured members within the family.[4] The report looks at the health and financial impacts on families with and without children. As such it represents a departure from most research on the uninsured, which focuses on the effects of health insurance on individuals. Much of the current debate does not capture the impact on the family of having some or all members uninsured.

The family constitutes a useful vantage point because most people do not live alone but rather in family units. The Committee examines whether the poor health or impaired functioning of one member can affect the physical, psychological, social, and economic well-being of the unit as a whole. In fact, in this country, more than 85 percent of individuals live in families.[5] Not all members of a family have the same opportunities for health coverage or can be insured by the same plan or program. The patterns of coverage within a family result in part from the sources and structure of health insurance plans and programs. This report documents the effects that a lack of coverage may have not only on the uninsured members and their health status but also the care that insured members, particularly children, receive.

The second purpose of this report is to update and reassess analyses of the impact of insurance status on the health of children and pregnant women. The Committee reviewed the literature to determine whether there are documented clinical differences associated with the insurance status of pregnant women, infants, and children. Health insurance or lack of coverage affects and is affected by family interactions, so the Committee has given particular attention to research on health outcomes in the context of the family.

Whether family members have coverage or not was the critical variable of interest in the studies reviewed. However, some studies also considered the differing impacts of public and private coverage. Distinctions based on variations in benefit levels and aspects of underinsurance are generally not addressed by this report.[6] In its previous report, *Care Without Coverage*, the Committee shows that

---

[4]Generally the Committee focuses on families with uninsured individuals, defined as those having no coverage for any health benefits and no assistance in paying for health care other than what is available through charity and safety-net institutions. Since the federal Medicare program provides almost universal coverage for individuals at least 65 years old, the Committee concentrates analyses on the population under age 65. (See Appendix B for a description of Medicare.)

[5]The data used in this report generally exclude families with all members over age 64 because Medicare covers almost all of them.

[6]The Committee recognizes the importance of underinsurance but in this project focuses primarily on family members with no insurance.

uninsured adults suffer diminished health and experience reduced life expectancy. This report determines whether pregnant women, newborns, and children without insurance experience similar negative effects.

NEED FOR A FAMILY PERSPECTIVE

Social and economic life in America is organized around families. The health and well-being of families is especially important in determining children's opportunities later in life (Shonkoff and Phillips, 2000). The health of any member can affect the whole family. Yet our most important means to obtain health services—health insurance—is frequently offered on an individual basis or with only partial regard to an individual's family circumstances. The mismatch between families' functioning as a social and economic whole and the qualification for insurance coverage as individuals is at the root of many of these negative consequences for family members and the family unit.

Four aspects of family experience distinguish the consequences of uninsurance for families from the consequences of uninsured persons considered strictly as individuals: (1) the health of one member can affect other family members; (2) public programs designed to provide coverage for individuals frequently do not consider the implications for family units; (3) parents make decisions about their children's care that may be influenced by their own experiences with and attitudes toward the health system; and (4) as individuals within the family mature and age, transitions of age, work, and marital status can trigger loss of coverage for the family.

First and foremost, the health of one family member can influence the health and well being of other individuals within the family and the family as a whole. *Care Without Coverage: Too Little, Too Late* documented how being uninsured compromises the health of individual adults. This report examines how individuals' lack of insurance affects the health of pregnant women, children, and families as a whole. When parents' health is impaired, their ability to care physically and emotionally for their children may be adversely affected as well. A focus on the consequences within a family of having no insurance draws our attention to the relationship between parental health and its impact on children.

Second, examining uninsurance in a family context highlights the fact that most publicly financed health insurance programs have been designed to provide coverage to individuals. If *all* individuals were entitled to the insurance, there would be no issue of a mismatch of family definitions or a gap in coverage. Without universal coverage, however, the issue of who qualifies for coverage and who does not is real. Families may find that different members are eligible for different programs, while some members are not eligible at all. When family members have different sources or types of coverage, each family member may be required to use a different doctor, hospital, or clinic. Considering the family as the unit of analysis leads to an examination of the effects that a patchwork of programs may have on access to health services and health outcomes for family members.

Third, parents or other adults in the family unit often make decisions about health care for younger members. Parents' experiences with the health care system, their beliefs about health care, and their ability to negotiate that system on their children's behalf may influence whether and how even children with coverage actually use appropriate services. The fact that family members may be eligible for coverage does not guarantee that they will enroll. Furthermore, being enrolled does not assure use of services. This report examines some of the financial and nonfinancial barriers to use of services that can affect health outcomes.

Fourth, looking at the family as a whole highlights how individuals' insurance needs and opportunities change over the life cycle of the family. This broad view of families across age categories encompasses the interplay in young families between parents' and children's health coverage status and use, changes in health care coverage as children approach adulthood, and evolving relationships to work as couples approach retirement. For example, late-middle-age couples are likely to have increasing health needs and one or both may feel ready to retire, but neither may be eligible for Medicare (IOM, 2002a,b).

HOW FAMILIES GET HEALTH INSURANCE COVERAGE

The rate of uninsurance for families stems, in large part, from differences between how families manage their finances, make decisions about health care, and define themselves as a functional economic unit on the one hand, and how employers, insurers, and public programs set the rules for individual and family coverage on the other. There are many, often inconsistent, definitions of family. This definitional mismatch has implications beyond limiting the data available for research. Definitions of family used by insurance companies often do not fit actual dependency relationships. Public programs may ignore family links altogether. Because both family composition and opportunities for health insurance change over time, gaining and keeping health insurance for all of its members pose a challenge for families. These factors contribute to a mixture of coverage patterns within families.

Individuals' perceptions of what makes up a family and who is a member reflect a richness and variety of human experiences. This richness is often lost when researchers attempt to count and measure what happens to and within families because demographic analysis relies on uniform definitions and historical conventions in order to count people and families consistently. The definition of family used for statistical purposes and the constraints it imposes are discussed further in Chapter 2.

The Insurance Unit

Most health insurance coverage in the United States is provided by employers and governments. Insured family members receive coverage through their job or that of a family member or through a government program such as Medicaid or Medicare. Public programs and employers may limit who gets insurance, under what conditions, and for how long.

Employers offer health insurance to their employees as a pre-tax workplace benefit. Generally they also offer coverage to the immediate family members of their workers but often contribute a lower proportion of the premium compared to their worker-only contribution. Virtually all larger firms (200 or more workers) and 65 percent of small firms (3–199 workers) offer at least some of their employees health insurance benefits, usually with the employer paying part of the premium, and generally make health insurance coverage available to family members as well (Kaiser-HRET, 2001).[7] In this way, employers facilitate insurance of *families*. Employers and the health insurance plans that they sponsor decide which family members are eligible. Family coverage includes the spouse and children of the employee, but policies vary in how long a dependent child can stay on as part of the family policy.

Insurance companies, employers, and the public sponsors of coverage define a family-based "insurance unit," which may be different from a *family-defined* "responsibility unit." A grandmother taking care of her grandchildren, a brother and sister living together and, in some cases, long-term companions might consider themselves family and feel responsibility toward each other. If one member of the unit became ill, the other would see to it that care was provided and paid for, to the best of his or her ability. Yet individuals in these family responsibility units might not be able to provide insurance for all the members through traditional employment-based insurance and they may not be eligible for public insurance coverage. The family responsibility unit might also extend to members living outside the immediate household. For example, parents of a 22-year-old recent graduate living independently with an entry-level job and no insurance might assume responsibility for some of the adult child's health care costs in the event of an illness or injury. In fact, one-third of the public has someone outside their household—an elderly parent (13 percent), a grown child (8 percent), another family member, or a friend (14 percent)—for whom they feel responsible for seeing that they get proper medical care (NPR-Kaiser-Kennedy School of Government, 2002). One-third of those with this responsibility said that the person had problems getting medical care.

Government programs, in contrast to employment-based coverage, often insure *individuals*. For publicly funded coverage in programs such as Medicaid, Medicare, and the State Children's Health Insurance Program (SCHIP), the public at large through its legislatures decides what groups of individuals are eligible. (All

---

[7]In 2001 employment-based premiums, including both the employer's share and the worker's share averaged $2,650 for the worker's coverage and $7,053 for a family plan. On average, employers contribute 85 percent of employee-only health insurance premiums and 73 percent of family health insurance premiums (Kaiser-HRET, 2001).

three programs are described in Appendix B.) Currently, these groups include lower-income persons, sick people with high medical expenses, the disabled, and those over 65 years of age.[8] Within the lower-income group (i.e., persons in families with incomes below 200 percent of the federal poverty level [FPL]), children, the disabled, and pregnant women have priority and to a lesser extent, so do parents. In addition to the federal and federal–state programs, several states have independently designed health insurance programs and subsidies using state revenues. Because the rules for these government programs are written to make it easier for people in priority age groups and in particular circumstances to get insurance, within a given family some members may be eligible for government insurance programs and others not. For example, a pregnant woman and later her infant might be covered through Medicaid because the income eligibility standard is relatively generous for these categories, but older siblings of the infant and the woman's husband might not be eligible for coverage because the income eligibility standard is more restrictive for older children and most restrictive for adults (other than pregnant women). Often adults who are neither pregnant, disabled, nor over 65 are ineligible regardless of how little income they have.

Dynamic Nature of Families and Society

Changes in a family's circumstances may lead to the gain or loss of eligibility for insurance coverage by one or more family members. Even when public policy or private insurance practices include family members initially, a change in a family's circumstances can create new exclusions, some of which may be surprising. Many of the family transitions related to age, employment and marriage that can trigger a withdrawal of coverage are normal life occurrences that most of us experience. For example, a 62-year-old woman insured through her 65-year-old husband's employer might find herself uninsured when he retires at 65. The husband would be covered through Medicare, but the wife might be without insurance for the three years before she turns 65 and becomes eligible for Medicare.

Broader social, political, and economic developments may also lead employers and the government to change the terms for offering coverage, which may in turn result in family members gaining or losing eligibility for coverage. Insurance

---

[8]Family income levels are defined as follows:

- *Low income*: an annual income of less than 100 percent of the federal poverty level (FPL), which is established on a yearly basis for different types of family groups that comprise a given household, for example, one adult, or one adult and two children;
- *Lower income*: an annual income less than 200 percent of FPL; and
- *Moderate income*: an annual income between 200 and 400 percent of FPL for a given family group.

See Appendix D, Table D.1, for federal poverty levels.

rules are not static but change with fluctuating public policy, business practices, and economic conditions. Insurance rules also reflect a changing social consensus about who should be covered or considered "family." Since the mid-1980s, beginning with Medicaid eligibility expansions for pregnant women and young children, and extending through the enactment and implementation of SCHIP in the late 1990s, public programs have reflected a growing commitment to ensuring health coverage for lower-income children. Another example of social values changing toward a broader definition of family and influencing insurance rules is that in the private sector, almost 20 percent of workers are employed in firms that have extended their definitions of family to include nontraditional partners— same-sex partners and unmarried heterosexual couples (Kaiser-HRET, 2001).

Changes in economic conditions can also affect how employers and the public sector define who is eligible for family coverage and on what terms. In the past, a rapid rise in health care costs and a downturn in the economy have led employers to reduce coverage to dependents and increase premiums and copayments for their employees. This has begun to happen again (Gabel et al., 2001; Kaiser-HRET, 2001; Freudenheim, 2002). Likewise, public programs may decrease efforts to expand coverage to uninsured individuals, cut back on existing coverage, or be less aggressive in encouraging enrollment. Reductions in public coverage can result from explicit policy changes to limit enrollment or tighten eligibility requirements or through administrative actions to make enrollment and re-enrollment more difficult. Forty-seven states report having instituted in fiscal year 2002, or planning to introduce in fiscal year 2003, policies to reduce Medicaid expenditures, including increased copayments, reduced provider payment rates, and reduced optional benefits and eligibility groups (NASBO, 2002). In the past, during some periods of decline in employment-based insurance coverage, Medicaid expansions served to mitigate the impact of the decline on the number of uninsured people, but that cushion may be reduced (IOM, 2001).

In an attempt to capture some of these dynamics of the economic and social factors affecting family units that may not be clear from the statistics and to add a human dimension, some of the following chapters begin with a vignette or example of family circumstances based on the research in the chapter. These vignettes are composites of circumstances documented in the research literature that illustrate family experiences related to not having health insurance. The vignettes integrate that information to enrich understanding of the issue and broaden the perspectives on family.

CONCEPTUAL FRAMEWORK

To guide its assessment of the literature on the health, social, and economic consequences for families of having one or more uninsured members, the Committee uses a conceptual framework based on a widely accepted behavioral model of access to health services (Andersen, 1995; Andersen and Davidson, 2001). This framework provides a common grounding to the Committee's six reports.

The conceptual framework as adapted for the family-level analysis in this report extends the framework or model introduced in the Committee's first report, *Coverage Matters*, to highlight the findings regarding family effects; see Figure 1.1. It makes explicit the interdependence and shared decision making within families and suggests how such interdependence may influence the relationship between the health insurance status of family members and the receipt of health care. Appendix A provides a further description of the framework.

Characteristics such as income, race, and family structure, which are discussed in the next chapter, are included in the parent and child boxes in the middle panel of Figure 1.1. These characteristics may affect the individual and family-level determinants of coverage in the panel on the left. For example, the family's income level can determine whether the children in the family will be eligible for public health insurance and may affect whether and how frequently parents will seek care for their children. The relationship between the availability of insurance plans and family members' eligibility for them is examined in relation to family characteristics and needs in Chapters 2 and 3.

The use of health services by children, influenced both by the insurance status of the child and the parent and by other family and individual characteristics and needs, can affect the child's health and long-term development as well as the family's economic health. These relationships are depicted as one moves from left to right across Figure 1.1. The financial and health consequences of uninsurance on the individual pregnant woman, child, and the whole family are the main focus of this report (Chapters 4–6). The health effects of uninsurance on working-age adults was the subject of the Committee's previous report and is not discussed here. The health outcomes of pregnant women were not discussed in the previous report, however, and are covered in Chapter 6. In Figure 1.1 feedback loops operate among most of the boxes but not all are indicated, in the interest of clarity. For example, the poor health outcome for one child in the family (in the panel on the right) could cause health problems for another family member, possibly affecting the health needs and insurance status of a parent (boxes in the middle panel).

The mix of health services providers and institutions, their numbers, and their costs and revenues are factors at the community level that influence a family's process of obtaining care—where it chooses to go for treatment as well as how frequently its members might seek care. The factors in the boxes labeled community level and effects on communities also are affected by the health care obtained in aggregate by all families. The economic and health outcomes of all families in aggregate can influence where doctors may choose to locate and what level of service quality hospitals can afford to provide. The quality of care that patients receive, as well as the costs of that care at the community level, reflect the care-seeking behavior of parents and children. The various community effects will be discussed in more detail in the Committee's next report on community effects of uninsured populations.

22

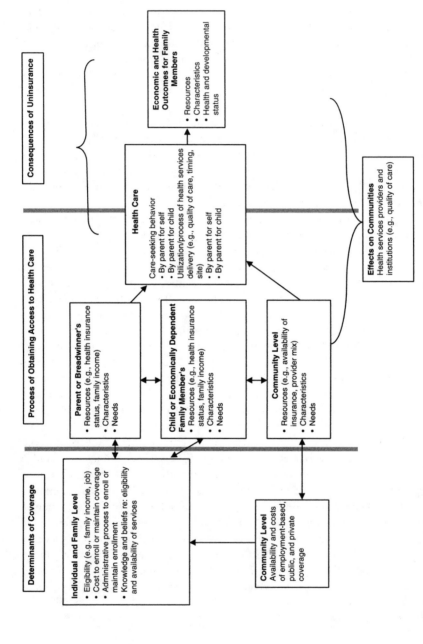

FIGURE 1.1 Conceptual framework for evaluating the consequences of uninsurance on the family.

REPORT OVERVIEW

This report provides new analyses of the consequences of a lack of insurance within families and the effects on the health of children and pregnant women. In the second chapter, the Committee examines insurance coverage patterns within families, including sources of coverage. The chapter describes the types of families that are most likely to have uninsured members and the characteristics associated with having some or all members uninsured. Chapter 3 considers the key transitions over a family's life cycle that may affect insurance coverage, including aging and changes in employment and marital status. Chapter 4 discusses how family income, assets, and spending patterns affect and are affected by family choices about health insurance and purchases of health care and how being uninsured affects family economic stability. Chapter 5 describes the factors that may influence the health care decisions that parents make for their children, including their own experiences with the health care system. In addition, that chapter discusses the effect of parents' health on the family environment and their children's health. Chapter 6 assesses evidence on health and developmental outcomes associated with health insurance status for children, infants, and pregnant women. The Committee's conclusions are presented in the seventh and final chapter.

BOX 2.1

The Rodriguez family of four in Oakland, California, fell through the cracks.[1] Both Mr. and Mrs. Rodriguez work at low-paying jobs without health insurance coverage; they make ends meet only by picking up as much overtime as possible. Because of their extra efforts, the family's income is too high for them to be eligible for Medicaid but too low to cover the cost of independently purchased health coverage. When they checked, they found that reasonable coverage in a health maintenance organization (HMO) could cost more than $4,000 just for the annual premium for Mr. Rodriguez, and he is basically a healthy 50-year-old.[2] Mrs. Rodriguez had developed lupus a couple of years ago, which is currently under control. She requires periodic medical attention and drugs, however, and cannot get affordable independent insurance to help cover the costs. They have never thought of themselves as needing or wanting charity.

Mrs. Rodriguez had been covered by a state program Access for Infants and Mothers (AIM) when her last child was born five years ago, but the coverage only lasted for two months after delivery. Maria, the baby, is covered by the state Medicaid program, called Medi-Cal, and she belongs to an HMO not far from their home. The older daughter, Joanna, is now 10 and is covered by Healthy Families, the State Children's Health Insurance Program (SCHIP). She had to register in a different HMO from her sister. Now Mrs. Rodriguez goes to a county health department clinic when she has to, but has difficulty getting referred to the specialty care she needs, particularly when the disease flares up. Fortunately, the Rodriguez family's problem will soon be addressed by a public–private partnership created by the Alameda Alliance, the Family Care program, which provides seamless family coverage, including comprehensive health and dental coverage for those family members not eligible for Medi-Cal and Healthy Families. The Alliance Family Care Program includes all families in Alameda County with incomes up to 300 percent of the federal poverty level (FPL).

---

[1]This vignette is a composite of circumstances documented in the research literature and statistics.

[2]Based on a quote from https://www.quotesmith.com/cgi/indmed/emd3. Accessed May 16, 2002.

2

Insurance Coverage of Families

The health and economic stability of families may be affected by the variety of health insurance arrangements within families. There is much variation in uninsured rates and in patterns of insurance coverage among different types of families. Sometimes not all members of a family are covered, or if they are, each may have coverage from different sponsors and different terms of insurance. This variation is influenced by the rules, policies, and requirements of public coverage programs as well as those of employment-based insurance plans. In addition, the socioeconomic and demographic characteristics of families influence these patterns of coverage. In *Coverage Matters* the Committee described the characteristics of uninsured individuals. This chapter aggregates the data on individuals into family groups and describes various family configurations as a unit.

This chapter describes coverage variations, the reasons for them, and some of the implications for families. The first section gives an overview of the sources of health insurance coverage, including employment-based, individually purchased, and public coverage. Because each source or type of insurance has distinctive rules for eligibility and they do not necessarily match a family's perception of its members, many families have some members who are uninsured. The second section examines the resulting coverage patterns of various types of families in the United States and describes how coverage varies within different families and for different family members. It also takes a closer look at specific characteristics, such as income level, racial and ethnic identity, and immigrant status of families with children that may affect a family's likelihood of having one or more uninsured members. Many of the social and economic characteristics associated with individual uninsurance are, not surprisingly, also related to family uninsurance. There is a summary section at the end of the chapter.

OVERVIEW OF SOURCES OF COVERAGE

There are differing eligibility rules and benefit packages for each source of health insurance that result in some family members having coverage and others not. Insurance plans operate in the context of state and local economies and politics as well as local health services markets, leading to geographic variation in family insurance patterns as well as different patterns within families. The size and other characteristics of a state's employers and the types of industries making up a state's economy all influence the level of employment-based coverage, the proportion of the population who may need other sources of coverage, and family coverage patterns. These economic factors, and the nature of a state's fiscal and political circumstances, can affect the proportion of its population covered by employment-based or public insurance and the proportion that remains uninsured.

Employment-Based Insurance

Most of America's families and their members obtain health insurance through their job or that of a family member. Provision of health benefits is routine for many jobs, particularly those at relatively high wages. Nonetheless, more than 80 percent of uninsured adults and children live in working families, but insurance either is not offered with the job or is not affordable for them (IOM, 2001).

For those with employment-based coverage, the employer typically pays some portion of the cost and the employee is responsible for the remainder. Employment-based plans generally are more expensive when they include coverage for dependents in addition to the employee. Children are less likely than working parents to be covered by this type of insurance. The total premium cost of employment-based plans for family coverage is on average two and a half times greater than that for employee-only coverage, $588 compared to $221 per month. Employers tend to pay a smaller portion of the insurance cost for coverage for the entire family (73 percent) than for the employee only (85 percent) (Kaiser-HRET, 2001). Employees cite the cost of coverage as the most common reason for not taking an employer's offer and for not covering their family members (Cooper and Schone, 1997). Most workers, even those from lower-income families, take this workplace coverage when it is offered (IOM, 2001).

Individually Purchased Insurance

When family members are not offered or do not take health benefits on the job, they can sometimes, if they are healthy, purchase health insurance in the individual, nongroup market. Such insurance, however, would likely cost the purchaser considerably more than employment-based insurance for comparable coverage, both because there is no employer contribution to premiums and because premiums are higher than those employers obtain. (If the person is not completely healthy, private insurers may refuse to offer a policy or may increase the premium, limit the benefits, or exclude coverage of the particular condition.) The lower premiums for employment-based coverage mainly reflect lower underwriting costs because the risks are pooled and administrative and marketing costs are lower. As a result, individually purchased insurance is relatively rare. According to the most recent Current Population Survey (CPS), only 7 percent of the population under age 65 had individually purchased coverage (Fronstin, 2001).[1] A national telephone survey of adults from ages 19 to 64 finds, however, that 27 percent of working-age adults had considered the purchase or had bought it in the previous three years (Duchon and Schoen, 2001). The financial aspects of a family's decision to purchase health insurance independently are discussed further in Chapter 4.

Public Programs

Individual family members who are not covered through employment-based plans may qualify for Medicaid, the State Children's Health Insurance Program (SCHIP), Medicare, or state-regulated high-risk pools if they meet certain eligibility criteria. In general, different eligibility requirements in Medicaid and SCHIP make it more likely for children to be covered than their parents; see Appendix B. Medicaid and SCHIP cover more than 40 million poor and disabled Americans, half of whom are children. They include over half of the children living in families with incomes below the federal poverty level (FPL) (8.5 million) and 30 percent of children living between 100 and 199 percent FPL (4.5 million) (Hoffman and Pohl, 2002).[2]

Income eligibility thresholds for public programs differ by state. Within each state, these income thresholds vary by age group, family type, and health status and include different limits on family income, assets, and methods for deducting and disregarding certain costs and income (see Appendix B and Appendix D, Table D.2). Although Medicaid has the advantage of limited or no cost sharing for participants and may have more generous benefits than either employment-based or individually purchased coverage, small increases in family income can disqualify the family, or particular family members such as older children or adults, from the program. Discontinuities in coverage also may result from the administrative requirements for periodic recertification of eligibility.

INSURANCE PATTERNS BY FAMILY CHARACTERISTICS

This section details the different types of families in the United States and their social and economic characteristics that can affect their insurance coverage. It looks particularly at distinctive coverage patterns for families with children.

---

[1]See Committee's report *Coverage Matters*, Appendix B, (IOM, 2001) for a discussion of the main national population surveys on insurance.

[2]The federal poverty guideline in 2000 was $13,738 for a family of three, and 200 percent FPL is $27,476. (See Appendix D, Table D.1, for the federal poverty guidelines.)

Demographic Overview

Because in this report the Committee is concerned mainly with the consequences of uninsurance on *families* and particularly on dependent children, it examines patterns of health insurance coverage within families and across families with different social and economic characteristics. This is a challenge because much of the readily available data are based on the *individual* rather than the *family unit.* Another challenge in drawing parameters around the family unit stems from definitional inconsistencies among various surveys and program statistics. The Committee's analyses in the following chapters demonstrate that the presence of an uninsured family member has the potential to affect the health and well-being of all the members of that family. For this reason, it is important to consider not only the number of families but also the total number of people living within the families with uninsured members.

In addition to the more than 38 million *uninsured* individuals, almost 20 million *insured* family members live with them. Thus, a total of approximately 58 million, or one-in-five, people in the United States potentially may be affected by the lack of insurance within their family.[3] Most of the Committee's population analyses in this report are based on data collected in the March 2001 CPS and reflect insurance coverage during calendar year 2000. These data are available in public use files of the Census Bureau and the tables presented in Appendix D. Box 2.2 explains how the CPS elicits information on familial relationships and Box 2.3 provides a demographic overview.

The experiences that *families with children* have in gaining, maintaining, and losing coverage are distinctive because of the role that parents play in obtaining coverage, as well as care, for their dependent children and because of the broad public policy commitment to insuring all of the nation's children. The Committee focuses on a subset of families and excludes people living alone and families with all members over age 65.

Almost 85 million *families* comprised of 232.6 million *individuals* are the main focus of this report. Families with minor children account for more than 38 million of these families and include roughly 146 million individuals; see Figure 2.1 and Appendix D. Within these families with children, 26.3 million individuals either are uninsured or live with someone who is uninsured. Table 2.1 shows these families with children, along with married couples with no children at home, at the top of the table because they are the family types most likely to be eligible for coverage as dependents of a working family member.

---

[3]This calculation is based on the total U.S. population, excluding those living in group quarters (0.2 million). Unlike most other calculations in this report, it includes both uninsured individuals over age 65 (less than half a million) and insured family members living with them regardless of their age. It does not include family members who live in different households but who, nonetheless, might be affected by the uninsured member's circumstances.

BOX 2.2
Who Counts as "Family"?

Each person has his or her own sense of who counts as family. Surveys that ask about health insurance use a uniform definition of who counts as family to facilitate the survey process. Likewise, private insurance plans and policies use certain conventional definitions of who is eligible for coverage within a family unit. Public programs also use family relationships as a criterion for determining individual eligibility for coverage.

This report relies largely on data from the Current Population Survey carried out by the Bureau of the Census to describe the nature of families and the extent of health insurance coverage. The CPS is a *household survey*. The sampling process selects dwelling places, not people. A household consists of all the persons who occupy a housing unit (most often a house or apartment). CPS interviews begin by establishing a list of all persons who live in the unit. The list, called a *household roster*, includes individuals who are temporarily absent and who have no other usual address. College students account for most absent household members; those in institutions such as nursing homes or the military are not included. The interviewer asks the respondent to start with the name of a person who owns or rents the housing unit. This person is termed the *reference person*.

The interviewer presents a card to the household respondent that lists relationship categories (e.g., spouse, child, grandchild, parent, brother or sister, unmarried partner, non-relative). The interviewer asks the respondent to report each household member's relationship to the reference person.

The responses about relationships are used to group *families*. A family is defined as a group of two or more individuals residing together who are married or related by birth or adoption. A *housing unit* might contain *subfamilies*, defined as families that live in housing units where either none of the members of the family are related to the reference person or the related person has his or her own spouse or child living with them. In this report, subfamilies are considered separate family units in the data analysis. For example, an apartment with a man and a woman, their grown daughter, and her infant would appear in the tabulations in this report as two families. The grandparents would be a "married couple no children at home" and the daughter and her baby would be a single-parent family. Family income is calculated separately for each subfamily unit, including income from all the members of the subfamily.

Note: In this report the Committee recognizes that self-defined families may include members unrelated by birth, marriage, or adoption. By including households with persons other than legal family members in some of the data analyses, the Committee recognizes that it likely also includes some individuals who do not consider themselves family and are not closely related financially or emotionally. (See Table D.4 for a list of the various population groupings.)

SOURCE: Census Bureau. 2000a.

BOX 2.3
Demographic Overview

The Committee has chosen to focus on families and how they experience being uninsured. However, few of the data related to health insurance coverage are available based on family units so special tabulations of the March 2001 Current Population Survey public use tapes were prepared for Committee analyses.[1] To put these data in context, consider the following:

- The total population in the United States in 2000 was 276.5 million.
- The Committee has focused on the population under age 65 by excluding families comprised *entirely* of adults over age 65, 24.6 million people.

The Committee has also excluded from consideration in this report the following:

- People living in group quarters, 0.2 million;
- Unmarried childless persons living alone, 17.9 million people; and
- Families with a child under age 18 as householder or reference person, 1.1 million people.

The remaining families total 84.9 million and include 232.6 million individuals.

_____

[1] By Matthew Broaddus, Center on Budget and Policy Priorities.

The other family configurations, listed in the bottom half of Table 2.1, are less likely to have the opportunity for dependent coverage, although they may function much like the families listed in the top half of the table. This remaining one-quarter of American families include people living with relatives other than their own children under age 18 and those living with people other than legally recognized kin. While members of these families are not generally able to obtain coverage as dependents on another member's employment-based insurance policy, they may nonetheless bear financial responsibility for the health care needs of others in their unit. Examples of these types of families include adult siblings living together, grandparents caring for grandchildren, and unmarried mixed-sex or same-sex couples.[4]

_____

[4]This analysis includes roommates and renters among the households with unrelated members as "families." Thus, the financial and emotional ties that exist in self-defined family units may not be present in all such configurations included here.

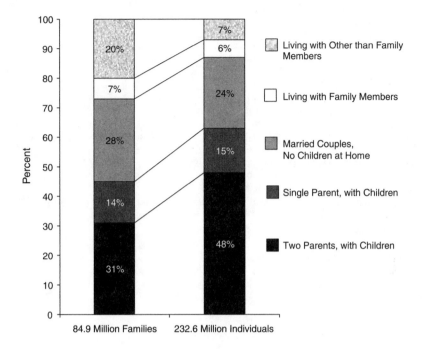

FIGURE 2.1 Percent of families and individuals in various types of families.
NOTES: Percentages are subject to rounding error. Includes all two-or-more person households with at least one person under age 65. Excludes single adults under 65 living alone, 17.9 million adults.
SOURCE: See Appendix D.

Families of Married Adults with No Children at Home

One-quarter of people included in this analysis of families are married and have no children under age 18 at home: 85 percent of these 23.7 million couples are fully insured, 9 percent have only one member covered, and 6 percent have neither member insured (see Figure 2.1 and Table 2.1). The proportion of those insured increases as family income increases. Many married couples in late middle age fit this family category and are of particular interest because their health status tends to worsen as they age and the need for health care and insurance is greater. In the next chapter, "Insurance Transitions over the Family Life Cycle," the insurance status of pre-retirement families is examined.

TABLE 2.1 Extent of Insurance Coverage By Family Type And Income Group, 2000

Living Arrangement or Family Type	Number (in thousands)		Percentage of overall total	Within family configuration
Family Configurations Where Dependent Coverage Is Likely				
Two-parent family	26,442		31.2	
All insured		22,427		84.8
Some insured		2,393		9.0
None insured		1,622		6.1
Married, no children at home	23,681		27.9	
All insured		20,010		84.5
Some insured		2,196		9.3
None insured		1,475		6.2
Single-parent family	12,118		14.3	
All insured		8,637		71.3
Some insured		1,929		15.9
None insured		1,552		12.8
Configurations Where Dependent Coverage Is Less Likely				
Living with others than family members	16,798		19.8	
All insured		11,963		71.2
Some insured		—		—
None insured		4,835		28.8
Living with family members	5,837		6.9	
All insured		4,647		79.6
Some insured		—		—
None insured		1,191		20.4
Total		84,876		
Families of this income class as percentage of all families				

NOTE: Among families whose head is age 65. Not included in this table are persons living alone and families with children as householder/reference person.

SOURCE: March supplement to the 2001 Current Population Survey; see Appendix D.

By Income Group

Under 100% FPL		100–200% FPL		>200% FPL	
Number	Percentage (share of row)	Number	Percentage (share of row)	Number	Percentage (share of row)
1,679		4,006		20,757	
812	3.6	2,669	11.9	18,946	84.5
475	19.8	831	34.7	1,087	45.4
392	24.2	506	31.2	724	44.6
902		1,856		20,923	
491	2.5	1,211	6.1	18,308	91.5
168	7.7	319	14.5	1,709	77.8
243	16.5	326	22.1	906	61.4
4,252		3,468		4,398	
2,650	30.7	2,335	27.0	3,652	42.3
865	44.8	661	34.3	403	20.9
737	47.5	472	30.4	343	22.1
3,531		3,343		9,924	
1,761	14.7	2,024	16.9	8,178	68.4
—	—	—	—	—	—
1,770	36.6	1,319	27.3	1,746	36.1
506		1,127		4,204	
309	7.6	815	17.4	3,522	75.0
—	—	—	—	—	—
197	16.5	312	26.2	682	57.3
10,870		13,800		60,206	
	12.8		16.3		70.9

Families with Children

Finding: If parents have health insurance, children are likely to be covered as well.

Almost 12 percent of children nationally are uninsured (Fronstin, 2001). Figure 2.2 illustrates that in almost all families, if the parents are covered, the children are too. In two-parent families, if both adults are covered, virtually all the children are as well, but if *neither* of the parents is covered, children are covered in only a third of the families. The patterns are similar for single-parent families; children are more than twice as likely to be covered if the custodial parent is covered than if he or she is not.

Finding: In one-fifth of the more than 38 million families that include children, there are one or more family members uninsured.

There are 7.5 million families (19 percent) with at least one family member *lacking insurance* and 31.1 million families (81 percent) with *all members insured*. More than 6 million children live in families where *everyone is uninsured*. An

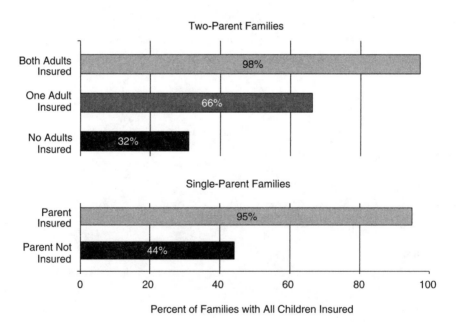

FIGURE 2.2 Percent of families with children, where all children are insured, by parental coverage.
NOTE: Percentages are subject to rounding error.
SOURCE: See Appendix D.

additional 9.4 million children live in families where *at least one member is lacking insurance.* Chapters 4 and 5 discuss related financial, economic, and psychosocial consequences of uninsurance that can affect the whole family.

Finding: Single-parent families with children are less likely to have all members covered than are two-parent families. Single-parent families are twice as likely as two-parent families to have no insured members.

Family composition influences insurance status directly and indirectly as well, through income. Patterns of coverage differ for single-parent and two-parent families, in part because having two parents may increase the family's income and improve its chances of being offered affordable employment-based coverage that includes dependents (see Figures 2.3 and 2.4). Of all *two-parent families with children,* 85 percent have all members insured, compared with 71 percent of *single-parent families.* In addition, single-parent families are more than twice as likely to have *no members insured* than are two-parent families, and a greater proportion of single-parent families *have at least one uninsured member,* compared with two-parent families.

Single-parent families with at least one uninsured member are more likely than two-parent families with at least one uninsured member to have coverage either for the children but not the parent(s) or for only the parent(s). This distinctive pattern reflects the availability of public coverage (Medicaid, SCHIP) for lower-income children, who are disproportionately in single-parent families. It also reflects the relative difficulty of securing affordable employment-based dependent coverage for single mothers, who are likely to be lower-income workers. Families in which some but not all children have coverage often include an ill or disabled child who may qualify for federal or state programs designed to insure disabled persons.

There are 9.1 million *uninsured parents* in the United States, representing about one-third of all *uninsured adults* (Lambrew, 2001b). Parents are more likely to be uninsured than their children and have less access to public programs because of more restrictive income eligibility requirements (see Appendix D). *Half* of the uninsured parents with incomes below 200 percent FPL had *all* their children insured. That is a better record than might be expected from Figure 2.2, which shows that only 32–44 percent of families at all income levels with both or one parents uninsured had all their children covered. In part, the better coverage of children in *lower-income* families compared with wealthier families reflects the eligibility limits of public coverage for children. In 1997, more than two out of five low-income uninsured parents—1.5 million people—had at least one child covered by Medicaid (Dubay et al., 2000). Since then, states have implemented SCHIP programs and have launched major education and outreach efforts aimed at uninsured children who may be eligible for Medicaid as well as SCHIP. States also have taken steps to make the enrollment process easier for both programs (Edmunds et al., 2000).

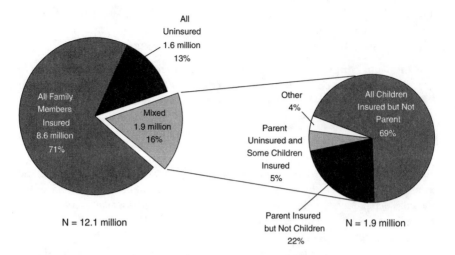

FIGURE 2.3 Patterns of insurance coverage in single-parent families with children.
NOTES: Other: parent covered, some but not all children covered. Percentages are subject to rounding error.
SOURCE: See Appendix D.

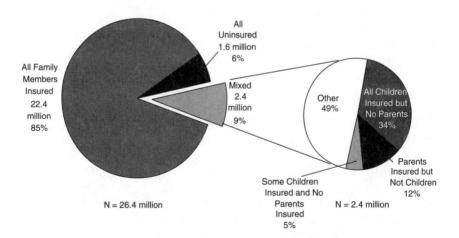

FIGURE 2.4 Patterns of insurance coverage in two-parent families with children.
NOTES: Other: one parent covered; all, some, or no children covered. Percentages are subject to rounding error.
SOURCE: See Appendix D.

Finding: Many children who are eligible for publicly sponsored coverage do not participate and remain uninsured.

A long-standing policy concern is that many children who are eligible for publicly sponsored coverage are not enrolled and remain uninsured. Nearly 5 million uninsured children, more than half of all uninsured children, are eligible for Medicaid and SCHIP but not enrolled, according to an eligibility simulation model designed by the Urban Institute (Urban Institute, 2002a).[5] The uninsured rate for the under-age-18 population overall is almost 12 percent (Mills, 2001). Some of this gap between eligibility and enrollment has been attributed to sharp declines in Medicaid enrollment following federal welfare reform in 1996 (Kronebusch, 2001). Other contributing factors include the administrative complexities of signing up for and maintaining public coverage and limited general knowledge about the programs.

Many more children on Medicaid and SCHIP have uninsured parents rather than parents covered privately. Only about 2 percent of these children have a different type of insurance from that of their primary parent (e.g., the parent with employment-based coverage and the child with Medicaid or SCHIP) (Davidoff et al., 2001b).[6]

Children in lower-income households (less than 200 percent FPL), minorities, immigrants, and those with parents who work in less than full-time, full-year positions are more likely than average to be uninsured (Ku and Blaney, 2000; IOM 2001; Hoffman and Pohl, 2002). In *Coverage Matters* the Committee examined the effects of many of these characteristics on the *individual's* likelihood of being uninsured; here the perspective of the *family* is examined. Social, economic, and demographic characteristics are strongly related to a family's chances to gain and keep health insurance coverage. These characteristics may be influenced by coverage as well as influencing whether the family is covered. The existence and strength of causal relationships among family characteristics may thus be hard to distinguish. The discussion that follows addresses the characteristics of income level, residence with one or two parents, racial and ethnic identity, and immigrant and citizenship status (see Figure 2.5). From a policy perspective, the key characteristic for families is income, since it determines both the eligibility of individual family members for public insurance and the ability to purchase health insurance independently or health care out of pocket, without insurance. Chapter 4 examines these financial concerns.

---

[5]The model combines data from the 2000 and 2001 CPS in order to calculate state estimates. The model uses state-specific eligibility criteria and runs the CPS data through the Urban Institute's Transfer Income Model Version 3 (TRIM 3).

[6]Survey respondents identified the parent most knowledgeable about the child's health care.

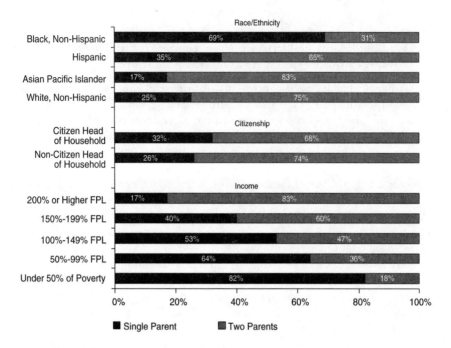

FIGURE 2.5 Structure of families with children by race/ethnicity and citizenship, and income.
NOTE: Percentages are subject to rounding error.
SOURCE: See Appendix D.

Income Levels

> **Finding: Family insurance coverage is strongly and positively related to income. Just 59 percent of families with children and with income less than 50 percent of FPL have all members covered, compared with 90 percent of families whose income is above 200 percent of FPL.**

Higher-income families are more likely to have employment-based coverage (because it is more likely to be offered in businesses with higher-wage employees) and lower-income families are more likely to have public insurance.[7] Of the 38.6 million American *families that include children*, two-thirds (25.1 million families)

---

[7]Data on family income are self-reported and does not include non-cash assistance from government programs.

earn more than 200 percent FPL, about 19 percent (7.5 million families) earn between 100 and 200 percent FPL, and the remaining 16 percent (5.9 million families) live below the official poverty line (100 percent FPL) (Table 2.1).

As family income increases, the likelihood that *all* members will be uninsured decreases (see Figure 2.6). For families with children and with incomes less than 50 percent of FPL, 59 percent have *all members covered* (1.5 million families), 20 percent (0.5 million families) have *some insured members*, and another 20 percent have *no insurance at all*. Families with children and with earnings above 100 percent FPL fare better, with the proportion of insured members increasing as family income increases. Not until families' incomes rise above the poverty level are parents likely to gain access to employment-based insurance, counteracting a slight decline in coverage as they lose their income-linked eligibility, while children may

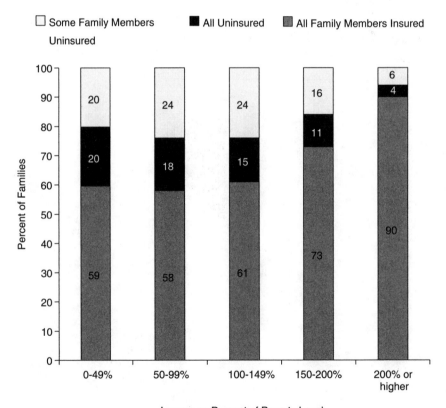

FIGURE 2.6 Insurance status of members of families with children, by income.
NOTE: Percentages are subject to rounding error.
SOURCE: See Appendix D.

still maintain their eligibility for public coverage. This can be seen in the increase in the proportion of families with *some members uninsured* in the 50-149 percent FPL level.

Approximately one-third of uninsured parents have incomes below 100 percent FPL. Another third of uninsured parents have incomes between 100 and 199 percent FPL (see Figure 2.7). Of all lower-income parents (<200 percent FPL), about one-third are uninsured and another 16 percent are covered by public programs (Lambrew, 2001b). Lower-income parents are more likely to be uninsured than are their children, and the parents' uninsured rate is growing. In 33 states, adults lose their eligibility for public insurance when they earn more than 50 percent FPL. Nevertheless, having family income below half the poverty level does not ensure public coverage; 40 percent of families below that income level have uninsured parents and/or uninsured children (Lambrew, 2001b; Appendix D). There is a gap between eligibility and enrollment for lower-income parents as well as their children.

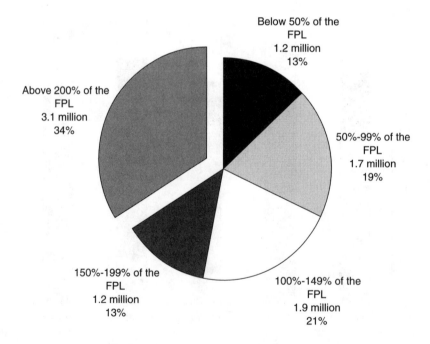

Total number of uninsured parents = 9.1 million

FIGURE 2.7 Income distribution of uninsured parents in families with children.
NOTE: Percentages are subject to rounding error.
SOURCE: See Appendix D.

Race or Ethnicity

Finding: Among families with children, Hispanic families are most likely to have at least one uninsured member (41 percent), followed by non-Hispanic African-American families (23 percent), and non-Hispanic white families (13 percent).

Ethnic and racial minority group members are more likely than non-Hispanic whites to be uninsured and to be members of families with at least one uninsured member (see Figure 2.8). For all adults, with and without children, uninsurance rates are higher for minority populations, with Hispanics having the highest uninsurance rate of all (Holahan and Brennan, 2000; IOM, 2001). All members *are insured* in only 60 percent of Hispanic families (3.4 million families), compared with 77 percent (4.4 million) of African-American, non-Hispanic families and 80 percent (1.3 million) of Asian or Pacific Islander families. In contrast, all members

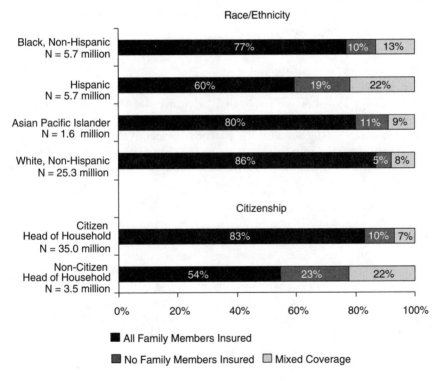

FIGURE 2.8 Insurance coverage within families with children, by race or ethnicity and citizenship.
NOTE: Percentages are subject to rounding error.
SOURCE: See Appendix D.

are insured in 86 percent (21.8 million) of white, non-Hispanic families. The coverage pattern for families generally follows that among all adults.

The greater likelihood that minority families have *at least one uninsured* member may contribute to the decreased access to care and lower quality of care that minority group members experience, relative to non-Hispanic whites. However, the relative importance of insurance coverage, compared with such factors as income, health status, and the cultural competency of health service institutions and practitioners, has yet to be fully explained. Even after taking health insurance status into account, racial and ethnic minorities tend to receive lower-quality and less health care than do non-minorities (IOM, 2002b). Health insurance coverage, however, plays a part in reducing disparities. Population groups that most often lack stable health insurance coverage and have relatively worse health status, including racial and ethnic minorities and lower-income adults, would stand to benefit most from increased levels of health insurance coverage (IOM, 2002a). The Committee concluded in its previous report *Care Without Coverage* that increased coverage would likely reduce some of the racial and ethnic disparities in the utilization of appropriate health care services and may also reduce disparities in morbidity and mortality among racial and ethnic groups. (See chapters 5 and 6 of this report for further discussion.)

Citizenship and Immigrant Status

Finding: Families whose head is a non-citizen are more likely to have some or all members uninsured than are families headed by citizens, 45 percent and 17 percent, respectively. However, most families with children that have at least one uninsured member are headed by U.S. citizens. Families headed by a non-citizen comprise only one-tenth the total number of families in the United States.

The length of time of residence in the United States, together with income level, public insurance eligibility criteria, and race and ethnicity, influences the likelihood that one or more members of immigrant families are uninsured. The uninsured rate for individuals who are *immigrants*, including naturalized citizens, is significantly higher than it is for *U.S.-born* citizens, with the uninsured rate for immigrants declining with increasing length of residency in the United States (IOM, 2001).[8] Proportionally fewer families headed by non-citizens have *all members insured*, compared with families headed by U.S. citizens. All members are covered in 54 percent of immigrant families (1.9 million families) compared with 83 percent of families headed by citizens (29.1 million families) (see Figure 2.8).

Higher uninsured rates among immigrant families reflect lower rates of

---

[8]The CPS includes immigrants who have been naturalized and native-born people in the category of citizen. Non-citizens are immigrants who have not been naturalized.

employment-based coverage, the impact of legislative changes in 1996, and more restricted access to public insurance, compared to families headed by a U.S. citizen (Rosenbaum, 2000; Ku and Freilach, 2001; Ku and Matani, 2001). First- and second-generation immigrant children are at significantly higher risk of being uninsured than are third- and later-generation children. This pattern holds true for all ethnic groups, although the uninsured rate varies substantially by country of origin (Brown et al., 1999). The cost of health insurance is given by immigrant parents as the main reason for lack of coverage of their children (Brown et al., 1999).

SUMMARY

One-fifth of the total U.S. population, 58 million people, may be directly affected by being uninsured or indirectly affected by living with an uninsured family member. Nearly one in five families with children has at least one member uninsured. For these families, public programs are more likely to provide coverage for the children than for their parents, and employment-based insurance is more likely to cover the parents than the children. Most uninsured children are SCHIP- and Medicaid-eligible but not enrolled. Among the families with some lack of coverage, there are more families with *some members covered* than there are families with *no one covered* (see Box 2.4).

Insurance coverage of families follows patterns similar to those of coverage for individuals. Families with at least one uninsured member tend to have low incomes, have a single parent, and/or be of a racial or ethnic minority. The risk is relatively high that Hispanic families and those headed by an immigrant lack coverage for all their members compared with non-Hispanic whites and citizen-headed families. Also, children are at greater risk of being uninsured if their parents do not have coverage.

The financial risks to families of having an uninsured member are studied in Chapter 4. The risks to family well-being and access to care for children, particularly if a parent is uninsured, are explored in Chapter 5.

Often the gain or loss of coverage is linked to common family transitions related to aging, employment, or marital status. These issues are considered in Chapter 3 which contains an analysis of key transition points in the family life cycle that have a particular impact on whether the family maintains insurance coverage or not. The focus is on understanding the gaps in coverage just discussed. These gaps are endemic to the current system of health insurance in the United States. The next chapter examines how and why so many people slip through them.

BOX 2.4
Summary of Findings

- If parents have health insurance, children are likely to be covered as well.
- In one-fifth of the more than 38 million families that include children, there are one or more family members uninsured.
- Single-parent families with children are less likely to have all members covered than are two-parent families (71 percent compared with 85 percent). Single-parent families are twice as likely as two-parent families (13 percent compared with 6 percent) to have no insured members.
- Many children who are eligible for publicly sponsored coverage do not participate and remain uninsured.
- Family insurance coverage is strongly and positively related to income. Just 59 percent of families with children and with incomes less than 50 percent of FPL have all members covered, compared with 90 percent of families with children and with incomes above 200 percent of FPL.
- Among families with children, Hispanic families are most likely to have at least one uninsured member (41 percent), followed by non-Hispanic African-American families (23 percent) and non-Hispanic white families (13 percent).
- Families whose head is a non-citizen are more likely to have some or all members uninsured than are families headed by citizens, 45 percent and 17 percent, respectively. However, most families with children that have at least one uninsured member are headed by U.S. citizens. Families headed by a non-citizen comprise only one-tenth the total number of families in the United States.

NOTES

BOX 3.1

Amelia and her family live in a suburb of Chicago.[1] She is 60 and has been married for 35 years. Amelia has worked at part-time jobs in retail stores most of her life while caring for her children and now her grandchildren. Her husband Bob worked in a tire company all of his life, where he made foreman before retiring at 65. His company had provided health insurance coverage for him and the family throughout his life, and Bob had always expected they would still be providing coverage for him when he retired. Unfortunately, however, about 10 years ago the company realized that it could no longer afford to provide health insurance to retirees and their families. The business had just gotten too competitive and costs had to be cut somewhere.

It was a real shock when Bob and Amelia realized that, while Bob would automatically go on Medicare, Amelia would be without any kind of coverage until she turned 65. In addition, when they found out the gaps in Medicare coverage, they realized they would have to get an insurance supplement for Bob, who has a history of heart problems. Amelia, too, has a health problem—she has suffered from situational depression for more than a year, since their eldest son was killed in a car crash. Otherwise she has been healthy. While they were not worried much about the depression, which was under control with treatment, they also knew that anything could happen at Amelia's age. When Amelia applied independently for insurance, several companies rejected her, offered limited benefits that would exclude the mental health treatments and drugs she needs, or increased the premium.

Amelia was able to get an offer of private insurance. However her health history meant that the price was high relative to their limited income, especially in combination with the $180 a month Bob was paying for a Medicare supplement with prescription coverage. Bob and Amelia spend a lot of time at the kitchen table with the calculator, trying to figure out whether they should spend some of their retirement savings to purchase coverage for Amelia at $400 a month or whether that would jeopardize their future income too seriously. On top of the premium, insurance for Amelia would require her to pay an annual deductible of up to $500 and a $20 copayment for each office visit. It is not an easy choice to make.[2] An opportunity for Amelia to "buy-in" to Medicare would probably be a better deal, but it remains an idea whose time has not yet come.

---

[1]This vignette is a composite of circumstances documented in the research literature and statistics.

[2]Premium and Amelia's age and health condition taken from Pollitz et al. (2001).

3

Insurance Transitions over the Family Life Cycle

The Committee noted in its first report, *Coverage Matters,* that U.S. insurance arrangements function like a sieve, with many holes through which individuals and whole families may slip. This chapter focuses on the transitions in a family's life cycle where this slippage is most likely to occur (see Box 3.2).

Many of these transitions and their insurance consequences could affect anyone and some are essentially unavoidable. These transition points, which sometimes threaten continuous insurance coverage, represent targets of opportunity for policy action. Some of the transitions indicate where families bump up against the rules of coverage set by private insurers and public programs.

In this chapter, three kinds of transitions are particularly relevant:

1. *Age*: As individuals within families age, their health insurance status may change because of rules in public programs and private plans.

2. *Employment status*: How and where family members are employed may affect the family's insurance status.

3. *Marital status*: Family issues relating to marriage, divorce, widowhood, single parenting, cohabiting, and separating may affect coverage.

There is considerable overlap among these three types of changes in status when one considers how each may influence coverage. For example, a child may reach age 19, get a job, and get married all around the same time. Decisions for each change may be interrelated and each can have insurance implications. In the following pages, each kind of transition is described and their interactions are discussed.

BOX 3.2
How Family Members Gain, Maintain, and Lose Coverage

Transitions related to the age, employment, and marital status of family members may influence the chances to gain or maintain health insurance coverage for themselves and for their whole family. Some of the transitions expand opportunities for coverage, while others narrow the options or even lead to the loss of coverage. Below is an overview of the transitions discussed in this chapter.

How Family Members Gain or Maintain Coverage

Age

- Sixty-fifth birthday brings individual coverage under Medicare.

Employment

- A new job is obtained where affordable insurance is offered for the worker and coverage for dependent family members is both offered and affordable.
- Change from part-time to full-time work within the same company may bring an offer of employment-based coverage.
- Change from one job to another at different companies may permit maintaining coverage without excluded conditions when the worker is eligible for protections through the Health Insurance Portability and Accountability Act (HIPAA).
- Change or loss of job may allow maintaining coverage for a limited time period, often at significantly higher cost, if the worker is eligible for protections through the Consolidated Omnibus Budget Reconciliation Act (COBRA).
- Loss of a job and drop in income (if low enough) may qualify for Medicaid or other state program.

Marital Status

- Marriage may offer family coverage tied to spouse's employment.
- Divorce or separation may allow children to maintain coverage on at least one parent's plan.

How Family Members Lose Coverage

Age

- Birthdays of infants and young children receiving coverage under either Medicaid or the State Children's Health Insurance Program (SCHIP), may put them into a category with more stringent income eligibility standards.
- Young adults age out of employment-based insurance of the parent.

Employment

- Increase in family income because of a pay raise or new employment exceeds the eligibility limit for public coverage, with no offer of (affordable) employment-based coverage.
- Loss of job or lay-off of the worker carrying the coverage for the family occurs.

- There is an unaffordable increase in the cost of employment-based insurance premiums.
- The worker carrying the policy retires, but no retirement benefit is available for either the worker or dependents' coverage. The younger spouse of a Medicare-eligible retiree may lose employment-based coverage.

Marital Status

- Divorce or separation may result in loss of coverage under a spouse's or parent's plan.
- Death of the spouse carrying the family coverage may result in loss of coverage for surviving spouse or children.

The dynamic processes that create transitions mean that some individuals move back and forth between having and not having health insurance. Table 3.1 shows how these transitions relate to the social characteristics of individuals and to who has health insurance for all of the year, who has no health insurance for the entire year, and who has health insurance for at least one month during the calendar year. For example, widowed or divorced individuals are almost twice as likely to have been uninsured for the previous year (18.2 percent) as are people who were married all year (9.8 percent). Similarly, those with a family income below 100 percent of the federal poverty level (FPL) are twice as likely to be uninsured during part of the year (20.3 percent) as are those with incomes above 200 percent FPL (9.9 percent). When these individuals are grouped into families and considered as a unit, the number of people affected by the experience of uninsurance within the family is enlarged and the points of transition can come more frequently.

Comparing "uninsured" with "insured" at a given point in time overlooks the fact that many families may have members uninsured for short or long periods that cannot be detected simply by knowing their current insurance status.[1] A lack of continuity in health insurance coverage can adversely affect access and health outcomes (IOM, 2001; 2002a).

Gaps in health care coverage are more common for lower-income families than for wealthier families. On average, those under age 65 with coverage through public programs are more likely to be uninsured at some time during the year than

---

[1]Using the Current Population Survey (CPS), only individuals who report no coverage at all during the previous calendar year are classified as uninsured. A person gaining coverage in the last month of the year might suffer the effects of uninsurance but be counted as insured by the CPS. Other surveys may count persons as insured or uninsured according to their status at the time of inquiry. A person who lost coverage the previous week would be counted as uninsured but may be more likely to resemble those in the insured category.

TABLE 3.1 Transitional Points and Health Insurance Status of the Population Under Age 65, 1996

Characteristic	Population (thousands)	Insured All Year	Insured Part of Year	Uninsured All Year
		Percentage		
Total	229,325	73.0	13.3	13.8
Employment status				
Employed all year	114,545	76.5	11.1	12.4
Employed part year	25,437	53.2	22.9	23.9
Not employed all year	26,286	70.8	11.6	17.5
Marital status				
Married all year	86,758	80.9	9.3	9.8
Widowed all year	2,293	73.4	8.4	18.2
Divorced all year	11,459	68.4	13.4	18.2
Separated all year	3,574	55.9	19.6	24.6
Never married all year	49,925	60.8	17.6	21.7
Changed marital status	13,007	60.2	19.3	20.4
Age				
Under age 7	24,229	76.9	14.7	8.4
7–17	43,340	75.5	13.1	11.4
18–24	24,798	54.5	22.8	22.7
25–34	39,587	65.2	17.8	17.0
35–54	76,769	77.8	9.1	13.0
55–64	20,602	82.1	7.2	10.8
Race or ethnicity				
White	162,084	77.9	11.6	10.5
Black	29,924	64.1	18.5	17.4
Hispanic	27,202	53.5	17.8	28.7
Other	10,114	71.8	11.6	16.6
Income				
Up to 100% FPL	30,489	55.2	20.3	24.5
100–200% FPL	40,029	53.4	21.1	25.6
Above 200% FPL	158,256	81.4	9.9	8.8

NOTES: Total includes persons with unknown marital or employment status or income. Marital status is for persons age 16 and over.

SOURCE: Monheit et al., 2001b.

are those with private health coverage (19 percent and 7 percent, respectively) (Monheit et al., 2001b). Only 75 percent of those with public coverage maintain it for the full year compared to 92 percent of those with private coverage (Monheit et al., 2001b). African-American males are somewhat more likely to retain public coverage for the full year than are Hispanic males, and the uninsured rate for the whole year is higher for Hispanics than for other ethnic groups. For some families, the annual or more frequent recertification process for Medicaid and the State Children's Health Insurance Program (SCHIP) may pose a barrier to maintaining coverage. For some immigrant families, public coverage is not an option.

The remainder of this chapter focuses on the age, employment, and marital transitions that affect the insurance status of individuals and the gaps in coverage they experience.

AGE ISSUES AFFECTING INSURANCE PATTERNS WITHIN FAMILIES

Finding: The structure of public health insurance programs and the cutoff age for dependents' eligibility in private insurance plans make it more likely that children will become uninsured as they grow up.

The probability that a person will be without health insurance varies with age and the type of family in which he or she lives. From the consumer's perspective, the most important age for insurance purposes is 65, the point at which almost everyone qualifies for and is enrolled in Medicare. Through this federal program, basic coverage is ensured for the rest of the person's life and is not directly influenced by any of the age, employment, marital status, or health-related transitions that can affect coverage for younger individuals. However, for families with at least one member younger than age 65, aging may cause the loss of coverage. A family member's transitions can precipitate not only his or her own but also other family members' loss of coverage

Children and Public Programs

Families with Medicaid or SCHIP coverage for their children may face tightened income eligibility limits as their children get older (see Appendix B). Thus, within a family, only younger children may be covered. Depending on how close a family's income is to the limit, an infant could lose Medicaid coverage when he or she reaches a first birthday. For example, in Florida the infant would be covered with a family income up to 185 percent FPL, children between the ages of 1 and 6 are covered if family income is less than 133 percent FPL, and children between ages 6 and 18 are covered if family income is not over 100 percent FPL. Figure 3.1 shows that the likelihood of having public insurance gradually decreases for children through age 17 (see Appendix C, Table C.2). There is a drop of almost 6 percentage points in public coverage of young adults aged 18–20, but the almost

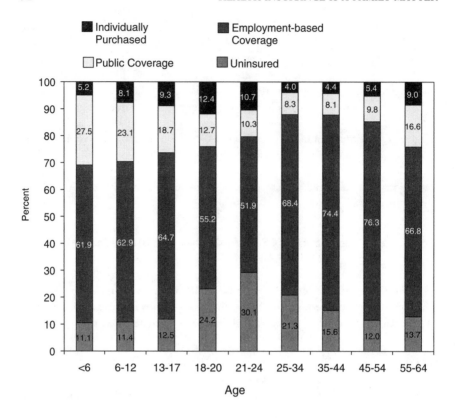

FIGURE 3.1 Health insurance status, by age
NOTE: Percentages may not total 100 percent because individuals may receive coverage from more than one source.
SOURCE: Fronstin, 2001.

12 percentage-point increase in their uninsured rate results from a larger drop-off (more than 9 percentage points) in private coverage, too.

For Medicaid, eligibility based solely on family income usually ends at age 19, although states have the option to cover youth through age 21. Within their SCHIPs, most states also cover youth through their nineteenth birthdays. Generally, for people beyond their nineteenth birthday, Medicaid requires more than just a low income to qualify. Most commonly, low-income people above age 18 who are disabled or who are pregnant are able to maintain or gain Medicaid eligibility.

Dependency Coverage Ends

The age at which young people often leave home (18–24) coincides with the age at which the risk of traumatic injury is the highest and the risk of being without health insurance is the greatest (see Figure 3.1). Among those aged 13 to 17, most of whom are still part of their parents' households, 12.5 percent are without health insurance. In the next older group, those ages 18 to 20, the risk of being without health insurance almost doubles, to 24.2 percent. The uninsured rate jumps to more than 30 percent for people aged 21–24, the highest rate observed for any age group.

The large increase in young people losing coverage beginning at age 19 is a result of how both private insurers and public programs define eligible family members. The rules for private insurance vary somewhat. Workers who elect family coverage from their employer usually find that children above some age can no longer be included as part of the family's health insurance unit except under specific circumstances. Many employment-based plans set that limit at age 19 but may make exceptions for full-time students. The Federal Employees Health Benefits Program (FEHBP), the single largest employment-based health plan in the United States covering 9 million federal workers, their dependents, and retirees, takes another approach. The FEHBP has a cutoff age of 22 and permits children with a disability that prevents them from living independently to continue coverage as part of their parent's family plan (Office of Personnel Management, 2001). While children age 18 and older may continue to live with their parents or return to their parents' home (there are more than 21 million people who have reached their majority living with their parents), they are more likely to be without health insurance than they had been previously. Twenty-five percent of children who live with their parents and are age 18 and older are without health insurance, nearly twice the share who are under age 18 (Census Bureau, 2000b).

A majority of those who graduate from high school continue in some form of training or higher education. This increases their chances of maintaining private insurance coverage. One-third of the 18 million young adults ages 19 to 23 are full-time students (Quinn et al., 2000). More than half of the 6 million full-time students have health insurance as dependents through their parents' family coverage. Another fifth have coverage through plans organized by their educational institution and an additional eighth have coverage through other means. The remaining one-fifth are uninsured.

As young people obtain more education, form new families, and become more attached to the labor market, the share without health insurance drops, to 21.3 percent among 25–34-year-olds. Young people follow various paths in leaving their parents' homes, including marriage, childbearing and rearing, education, and joining the labor force. Leaving home may mean living as a household of one or with roommates. While these young people may have a separate residence from their parents, they continue to look to their parents for many needs, often including health insurance.[2] Depending on the rules defining when a child can no longer be a dependent, the parents may or may not be able to provide that coverage through the family's insurance plan. In any case, should the independent young adult be in need of health care, the family may feel some responsibility to help financially if it can.

EMPLOYMENT ISSUES AFFECTING FAMILIES

Finding: The link between health insurance and employment for most families creates many opportunities for loss of coverage. In order to obtain or maintain coverage, family work choices may be constrained. Work choices for families enrolled in public insurance may also be constrained because of the income ceilings for eligibility.

Employment can have a positive effect on coverage by making an insurance plan available to family members in addition to the employee as a benefit of the job. Alternatively, a job that increases family income but that does not offer affordable or any health insurance coverage can have a negative effect on coverage by precluding a family's eligibility for public coverage. It is important to remember that most of those without insurance are in working families, but many jobs do not offer coverage. Transitions into and out of the work force, as well as the terms of participation, affect coverage. Decisions whether to work full-time, part-time or not at all, to change jobs, or to retire from a job each have implications for a family's eligibility for private or public health insurance. A critical literature review of more than 50 studies provides evidence of the impact that insurance has on work-related choices (Gruber and Madrian, 2002). These transitions highlight many of the gaps in the current insurance system through which individuals and families may lose coverage or remain uninsured.

Transitions into the Work Force

Young adults who do not pursue full-time education move into the work force at a younger age than those who choose postsecondary education, and they are much less likely to obtain the kind of job that brings health insurance with it. Compared to the 19 percent of young people age 19 to 23 who are in school full-time and are without health insurance, a much larger share of those not pursuing full-time schooling is without health insurance, 43 percent of men and 35 percent of women (Quinn et al., 2000). Racial minorities are less likely to be full-time students than are whites, and those not in school full-time are even more likely to

---

[2]The dimension of family that goes beyond living together is not recognized in most government surveys. For example, the usual unit in Bureau of the Census surveys is the "household." Part of the definition of household used in Census Bureau surveys is "living together."

be uninsured: 47 percent of African-American men ages 19 to 23 who are not in school full-time are without health insurance, as are 62 percent of men of Hispanic descent. Much of this may be due to higher unemployment and part-time or part-year employment among minority men.

The transition from school to work for young adults may be direct and full-time or may combine work with part-time schooling. Either route is likely to mean that the new worker holds a job for a shorter period than those who have been in the work force longer, that the work is more likely to be part-time rather than full-time, that it is more likely to be with a small employer, and that it is more likely to have lower pay. For older workers, all of these factors—longer job tenure, employment by larger employers, and higher wages—increase the likelihood that they will be able to maintain employment-based health insurance over time.

To Work (Full-Time) or Not

Families with two wage-earners may have two chances to obtain employment-based health insurance. Coverage of one spouse through an employer may influence the other spouse's decisions about whether to work, for what firm, and how much to work. When husbands are not insured through their jobs, their wives are much more likely to work, to work more hours, and to work in jobs that offer health insurance (Gruber, 2000). In families where one spouse has employment-based coverage, the probability that the other spouse works full-time is 6 to 12 percent lower than if the spouse did not have employment-based coverage. The effect is specific to the likelihood of working full-time; part-time work, which is less likely to bring health benefits than full-time work, is unaffected (Buchmueller and Valletta, 1999).

To Change Jobs or Not

Another labor market decision that may be shaped by the availability of health insurance is the decision to change jobs. An extensive literature review documents a phenomenon known as "job lock," or reduced mobility between jobs, that stems from fear that a new job will bring a disruption in health insurance (Gruber and Madrian, 2002). Families with spouses who both work may avoid job lock if both have access to employment-based coverage with similarly generous benefits and affordable premiums. One study found that the job mobility of husbands is 25 to 32 percent lower when their wives do not have employment-based health insurance and the mobility of wives is 49 percent lower when their husbands do not have health insurance compared to their counterparts with insured spouses (Buchmueller and Valletta, 1996). The federal Health Insurance Portability and Accountability Act (HIPAA), designed to minimize the occurrence of job lock, is discussed below. The studies noted by the Committee are based mainly on data from the period before HIPAA became law.

HIPAA

The Health Insurance Portability and Accountability Act, which became law in 1996, protects health insurance coverage for workers and their families when they change or lose their jobs. It limits the use of preexisting condition exclusions from coverage by health insurance and guarantees, in most cases, that health insurance can be renewed regardless of health condition. It does not limit pre-existing condition exclusions for those who have not had health insurance, nor does it limit the premium charged for the insurance (Health Care Financing Administration, 2002).

Work and Public Insurance Programs

Single-parent families have only one opportunity to obtain employment-based coverage through the employment of an adult family member. Some working parents who do not have employment-based insurance are covered by public programs and may lose their own and their children's coverage if their earnings exceed the state-set level. For some, the possible loss of coverage may be a factor in deciding whether to work or to change employment and may be a deterrent to increasing earnings above the eligibility level because comparable coverage may not be available or affordable even with the increase in income.

With the decoupling of Medicaid and public assistance eligibility in 1996, however, and increases in upper income limits for children to participate in Medicaid and SCHIP, parents who no longer qualify for Medicaid themselves may still retain Medicaid eligibility for their children. The variation among states in the extent to which Medicaid eligibility has been expanded has created a natural experiment: how much more would single parents work if their children could still participate in Medicaid? An evaluation of these expansions over the 1980s, prior to the decoupling mentioned above, found that for each increase of 25 percent of the poverty threshold in the Medicaid eligibility standard for children, labor force participation by single parents rose by 3.3 percent (Yelowitz, 1995). Single parents were more willing to work if their children could retain Medicaid coverage.

One factor that may constrain the work behavior of a family receiving public assistance is the presence of a disabled child. There are two limited but suggestive studies of this effect. Families with a disabled child that receive public assistance face a double challenge in moving from welfare to work. First, the child's disabilities may make it more difficult to both care for the child and work; helping a disabled child with activities of daily living, medical treatments, and frequent visits to the doctor can require full-time attention by the parent. Second, earnings beyond some level threaten Medicaid eligibility for both the parents and children. (One might term this the "welfare lock," a counterpart to job lock, rooted in concern that going to work would endanger a child's Medicaid eligibility.) Families caring for disabled children are substantially less likely to exit welfare than are families with children who are not disabled (Brady et al., 1998).

A random, stratified sample phone survey of welfare recipients and their families (Aid to Families with Dependent Children [AFDC]) in selected California counties in 1995 found 12 percent of the children had some disability or chronic illness, including 7 percent with a severe disability or chronic illness (Meyers et al., 1998).[3] About 20 percent of AFDC families were caring for such children, defined in the survey as children with a disabling or chronic condition that required the child to need a lot more help than other children. Roughly half the children classified in the survey as having severe illness received Supplemental Security Income (SSI), which automatically brings with it Medicaid eligibility. Since SSI provides the child with Medicaid eligibility on his or her own, the parents could move to work, potentially working enough hours at a high enough wage that they would lose their own Medicaid benefits, but the child would remain eligible for Medicaid. Parents whose children did not receive SSI faced loss of both their and their children's Medicaid when moving to work. Parents in families that received AFDC were more likely to work and leave welfare when their disabled children received SSI than AFDC families whose disabled children were not SSI recipients.

Risk of Job Loss and Layoffs

The loss of a job can result in the loss of employment-based insurance not only for the worker but also for all family members. At a time when family income is significantly if not drastically reduced, families may face difficult choices about purchasing health insurance or taking the risk of being uninsured. A recent survey shows that working-age adults going without insurance for even brief periods have problems getting to see a doctor, filling a prescription, or paying their medical bills, problems similar in magnitude to those of adults who have been uninsured over the long term (Duchon et al., 2001).

Even in stable economic periods, the normal turnover in jobs can put families at risk of being uninsured. Based on statistical modeling, economists have estimated that for every percentage point rise in the unemployment rate, about 1.2 million people become uninsured. This implies that 85 people become uninsured when 100 people lose their jobs (Gruber and Levitt, 2001). During the economic downturn with mass layoffs in the last half of 2001, Congress turned its attention to the plight of workers losing their insurance coverage because of job loss. It attempted to expand an existing program, the Consolidated Omnibus Budget Reconciliation Act of 1986 (COBRA) and proposed alternative approaches to protect former workers and their families, but did not reach political agreement on the best approach.[4]

---

[3]Welfare reform legislation, the Personal Responsibility and Work Opportunity Reconciliation Act of 1996 (PRWORA), has changed the link of welfare benefits to Medicaid coverage.

[4]Title II of the Trade Act of 2002 (P.L. 107-210, signed into law August 6, 2002) provides for a federal income tax credit of 65 percent of the premium cost of health insurance coverage for unemployed workers (and their dependents) who qualify for trade adjustment assistance, i.e., whose job loss is recognized as a result of international trade.

COBRA

Part of the Consolidated Omnibus Budget Reconciliation Act facilitates coverage for certain workers who lose employment-based health insurance because of a job change or loss or a related family transition. Generally, persons who lose coverage for work-related reasons are guaranteed access to their former coverage for 18 months. An estimated two-thirds of all workers would qualify for COBRA assistance. However, for workers with incomes below $20,000 this falls to only 40 percent, and for Hispanic workers to 50 percent because they are more likely to work at jobs that are not covered by the law (Doty and Schoen, 2001). Those workers who are eligible under COBRA must pay both the employer and the employee share of their insurance premium (and up to 2 percent more for administrative costs) if they wish to continue coverage. Under COBRA, workers who leave their jobs, or experience a reduction in hours worked below the level that would qualify them for health benefits, may continue in their employer's plan. Those who lose coverage for family-related reasons are guaranteed access for 36 months, for example, if a spouse becomes entitled to Medicare or following divorce.

Federal COBRA exempts employers with fewer than 20 employees, and it does not apply to the federal government and some church-related employers. These exemptions, along with the fact that many workers do not have access to employment-based insurance, explain why many workers and their dependents are not protected during job and family transitions. Of those workers unemployed in 1999, only 7 percent actually took advantage of COBRA coverage (Zuckerman et al., 2001). For many workers, particularly those with low wages, the cost of the full premium (more than $2,700 for an individual plan or $7,000 for a family plan, on average) would be prohibitive (Kaiser-HRET, 2001). Although the majority of lower-income workers would not be eligible for COBRA, if the premiums were affordable, millions of other workers and their families could continue group health coverage.

Retirement

Retirement is the employment-related decision that most strongly affects insurance status for older persons. The economics literature also shows that retirement decisions are strongly influenced by the availability of insurance after retirement (Gruber and Madrian, 2002). Nearly all Americans become eligible for Medicare, although a majority retire before reaching age 65. Between ages 55 and 65, labor force participation by men declines from 81 percent to 33 percent (Burkhauser et al., 1996). Employment-based insurance is particularly important for adults in late middle age because they are at greater risk of having health problems and opportunities to purchase insurance individually can be limited and too costly (IOM, 2002a). This expense may deter workers from retiring before they become eligible for Medicare. On the other hand, some workers may suffer from debilitating health conditions that make it difficult for them to continue work even though they are not yet eligible for full retirement benefits or Medicare. The uninsured rates for men and women are about even—more than 13 percent—for those workers aged 60–64 (Monheit et al., 2001a).

Some firms offer retiree health insurance, but the percentage of firms doing so has been declining since the 1980s and varies substantially by the size of the firm. Two-thirds of all large firms (more than 200 workers) offered retirees coverage in 1988, but that is down to one-third now and only 3 percent of small businesses still offer it (Kaiser-HRET, 2001). Among firms still offering such coverage, the cost sharing for the employee has been increasing, and these increases are expected to continue (Freudenheim, 2002; Kaiser-HRET-Commonwealth, 2002).

Retirement at or after age 65 can result in a married couple with an older, retired spouse insured through Medicare and an uninsured younger spouse. Women tend to be the younger spouse and are more likely dependent upon their husband's coverage than the reverse (Lambrew, 2001a; Monheit et al., 2001a). Working women aged 55–59 are more likely to be uninsured than are working men, reversing the pattern seen in younger adults, when men are more likely to be uninsured. Among women who are younger than their husbands, 10 percent become uninsured when their husbands begin Medicare eligibility (Lambrew, 2001a). Because women are more likely to have chronic conditions than are men in this age group, their opportunities for purchasing independent insurance may be more limited by higher premiums and restrictions on benefits, if they are offered coverage at all (National Center on Women and Aging, 2001).

MARITAL ISSUES AFFECTING FAMILIES

Finding: Marriage increases the chances of having employment-based health insurance for the whole family. Getting separated or divorced or being widowed may increase the risk that family members lose their employment-based coverage.

Decisions about marriage, cohabitation, having children, and divorce are intimate family choices that may include consideration of health insurance issues, and the decisions may affect the family's coverage. In addition, the death of a spouse or parent may also change the insurance status of surviving family members.

Marriage

Marriage brings the opportunity to obtain health insurance coverage through one's spouse's employer, if it is offered. If both spouses work, they might obtain health insurance coverage from either employer. These factors contribute both to persons in married households being more likely to have health insurance and to health insurance being more common in families with two workers compared to those with one. Married adults are more likely to have health insurance than those who are not married, and children who live in families headed by a married couple are more likely to have health insurance than are children who live in single-parent families. Among children in married-couple families, 10 percent were uninsured in 2000, compared to 15 percent of children in single-parent families (Census Bureau, 2001a).

The share of young people who are married has been shrinking. The rate at which people marry has declined during much of the period since World War II. Among women ages 20 to 24 who are white or African American, the percentage who had ever married dropped by 32 points from 1975 to 1998 (Teachman et al., 2000). Approximately one in four 20–24-year-olds, of either sex and all races, was married in 1998.

The relatively high uninsured rate for young adults reflects both the declining marriage rate and the increasing age at first marriage. As young people age they tend to marry and increasingly they gain coverage through their spouse. Of those aged 19 to 23, 15 percent are married and 3 percent have coverage through a spouse's employer. Those rates increase to 68 percent married and 18 percent obtaining coverage through a spouse among those from age 30 to age 64 (Quinn et al., 2000).

Cohabitation

Lower rates of marriage and later ages of first marriage might be related to cohabitation, which may affect health insurance because members of cohabiting couples are not as likely as are married ones to obtain health insurance as a dependent of their partner. Only one in five workers in the private sector works for an employer that offers coverage to nontraditional partners such as same-sex and unmarried heterosexual couples (Kaiser-HRET, 2001).

Young adults are more likely to cohabit than are members of older age groups, although cohabitation is increasing among all age groups (Bumpass and Sweet, 1989; Chevan, 1996). A total of 4.1 million couples were regarded as cohabiting as of 1997, which represents an increase of 46 percent since 1990 (Casper and Cohen, 2000). Among families headed by cohabiting couples, about half include children. Cohabiting couples make up one-fourth of all stepfamilies (Bumpass et al., 1995). Children in these stepfamilies are unlikely to have health insurance coverage through their parent's partner's employer, although they may retain coverage through their absent parent.

Most employment-based insurance plans technically exclude an unmarried couple from dependent coverage, although insurance may be offered to the worker alone (Kaiser-HRET, 2001). It is unclear where cohabiting people fit in Figure 2.1, which depicts different family types, because of the variety of ways that people respond to the census survey. Some couples may consider themselves married and respond as such, so they would be noted in either the two-parent or the married-without-children categories. Other cohabiting couples might be in the "living with non-relatives" category.

Separation, Divorce, and Children

Decisions of parents to divorce or to separate affect the likelihood that their children will have health insurance. Children in one-parent families, including those where parents are divorced, separated, or never marry, are less likely to have health insurance than are children in two-parent families. The lower rate of health insurance coverage in single-parent families reflects, in part, lower incomes on average in single-parent households.

As adults increasingly spend fewer years in marriage, more children live in families without two married parents. Nearly half of white children and two-thirds of African-American children are likely to spend part of their lives before age 18 in a single-parent household (Bumpass and Sweet, 1989).

Marriage confers some insurance advantage on children, even after separation or divorce. Almost half of children in ever-married single-parent families had private health insurance, often provided through the employment of either the parent in the household or the absent parent, compared to one-fifth among children in never-married single-parent families (Weinick and Monheit, 1999).

Children living apart from a parent may obtain coverage through the absent parent as a consequence of a legal or informal child support agreement or award. Overall, 24 percent of noncustodial parents provide health insurance for their children (Grall, 2000). This share reflects both the proportion of noncustodial parents who have jobs that allow for dependent coverage and the share of child support awards that include health insurance. Health insurance for children through a noncustodial parent was most common where a child support award or agreement was in place and the award or agreement included health insurance. In these 4.6 million cases with agreements to provide health insurance, custodial parents reported that the absent parent provided health insurance 44 percent of the time. Having health insurance from noncustodial parents was about equally likely where there was an agreement or award that was silent on health coverage (13.5 percent) and where there was no agreement (15 percent). Among the 21 million children eligible for child support, the federal government reports that approximately 15 percent are uninsured (Medical Child Support Working Group, 2000).

The federal government first took steps in 1984 to increase the share of absent parents who included their children in employment-based coverage both to increase coverage for children and to minimize Medicaid enrollment by children who could be privately covered. (This is an early example of federal efforts to prevent the substitution of public insurance programs for private coverage, a phenomenon described as "crowd out"). Legislation required states to include provisions for health coverage in their child support guidelines and to pursue private coverage where the noncustodial parent could obtain it at a reasonable cost. By 1998, 93 percent of support orders had provisions requiring medical support. Compliance went up 18 percentage points from 1989 to 1998 (Medical Child Support Working Group, 2000).

Evidence of increased compliance might be seen in the reported increased share of private coverage for children in single-parent families that came from someone outside the household, presumably the absent parent, between the 1987 and 1996 rounds of the Medical Expenditure Panel Survey (MEPS) (Weinick and Monheit, 1999). Coverage from outside the household for children with never-married parents increased from 4 percent to 12 percent and to 21 percent for children of ever-married parents. However, the absolute level of private coverage remained the same, which suggests some combination of custodial parents being less likely to have jobs that bring coverage for dependent children, and custodial parents moving children to the absent parent's coverage.

Divorce and Women

Divorce diminishes the probability that an individual will have health insurance through his or her spouse's employer. Because more women than men are covered through their spouses' job (26 percent of women and 11 percent of men), women are more likely to suffer an insurance loss through divorce (Lambrew, 2001a). The rate of divorce showed a pronounced increase from 1968 to 1980 with less change since then (Teachman et al., 2000).

When spouses divorce, loss of health insurance is part of a broader decline in economic status among women (Hoffman and Duncan, 1988; Weir and Willis, 2000; National Center on Women and Aging, 2001). Among women between 35 and 64 years of age, divorced women are about twice as likely to lack health insurance as married women, and divorced women are more likely to be uninsured than widows or women who have never been married (Berk and Taylor, 1983).

Widowhood

Although both men and women can be widowed, widowhood is more common among women than among men and is more likely to mean a loss of health insurance for women than it is for men. Eighty-three percent of those widowed by age 65 are women. The probability of widowhood increases with age. Widows and widowers comprise 4 percent of people aged 50–55 and 16 percent of those aged 62–64, an increase of 400 percent (Weir and Willis, 2000).

Widows are more likely to be without health insurance than married persons of the same age. With one-quarter of widows aged 51–61 not having health insurance, they are almost twice as likely to be uninsured as married women in the same age group (Weir and Willis, forthcoming). For women, widowhood carries adverse economic effects (Weir and Willis, 2000). Widowhood does not provide any exception to the general rule that initial eligibility for Medicare begins at age 65.

SUMMARY

Given the many transitional events that affect the life of a family and its chances to gain or lose health insurance, it is not surprising that so many families lack full coverage. When the choice of a spouse or job or the date of retirement can affect health coverage for oneself and others within the family, family decisions become more complex. Even families with the best of intentions and making the most rational choices cannot ensure that all of their members will be able to get and maintain coverage. Many of the factors affecting coverage are beyond the immediate control of the family, are unpredictable, and have no apparent rationale. Not all workers have a choice of a job with affordable employee and dependent coverage. Not all lower-income families are fortunate enough to live in a state with expansive public programs.

A common thread runs through most of the family transitions that result in the loss of coverage. Often, uninsurance results from a combined loss of income and loss of access to employment-based coverage.

The nature of these family transitions make it easier to understand the patterns discussed in the preceding chapter—why single-parent families are at greater risk of uninsurance and why, within the same family, children may be covered and parents not. The following chapters look at the impacts on families of not having all members insured. Nevertheless, it is also important to keep in mind that 81 percent of all families with children *do* have coverage for all their members. If they are lucky, they will be able to maintain that coverage until they all reach Medicare age.

BOX 4.1

David doesn't know where to turn.[1] He's facing mounting medical bills and can't pay them off. He and 900 of his colleagues were laid off when the bank he worked for merged with another. They were told their health benefits were protected by the Consolidated Ominibus Budget Reconciliation Act (COBRA) and they could maintain coverage if they wanted to, but they would have to pay the full amount of the premium plus 2 percent extra. That's $600 per month for family coverage, four times more than they had been paying on the job. Without a salary, David as well as many of his colleagues decided they could not afford to maintain the coverage. David's wife had given up her job with an accounting firm 10 months ago to be an independent contractor because it looked as if she would eventually make more money, could work from home, and would have more time to spend with the kids. Unfortunately, her business has been growing very slowly and she has no access to group health benefits.

Then John, the oldest boy, broke his ankle at a neighborhood soccer game. He had a multiple fracture that was treated quickly at the emergency room. John needed follow-up surgery, had complications from the anesthesia, and stayed in the hospital for four nights, and the bills are starting to pile up from the doctor, surgeon, lab, and radiology. Soon John will need physical therapy to regain full functioning of the joint, and they will have to pay cash up front for each visit. The medical bills already have eaten into the savings they need until David finds another job. David is afraid to let their 8-year-old play sports now because they cannot risk another injury. David has been having stomach pains but refuses to go to the doctor since he cannot pay the bill now. He hopes it is just stress and not too serious. He fears the growing debt might force them into bankruptcy if he doesn't find a job soon.

---

[1]This vignette is a composite of circumstances documented in the research literature and statistics.

4

Financial Characteristics and Behavior of Uninsured Families

Though it is much more than this, a family can be thought of as a collection of individuals that is grouped into a single financial unit sharing both resources and risks. In this sense, health insurance coverage can be viewed as a shared family resource. It is often obtained through the employment of a single member of the family, but it reflects a shared resource in other ways as well. When individuals in a family obtain coverage through means-tested government programs, their eligibility often depends on the combined income of the family unit. Conversely, the risk that out-of-pocket health care expenditures will severely strain a family's finances can be seen as a shared family risk. So can a family's decision about how many of its members to cover if employment-related family health care coverage is available to a member of the family.

This chapter examines the impact of health care expenses on the finances of families where one or more of the members are *not* covered by employer-provided or publicly provided health insurance. It first offers a picture of the typical financial position of such families—their income, assets, and borrowing capacity. Then it examines their health care expenditures. Next, the ways in which they meet these expenditures and the burden this imposes on family finances are explored. The chapter ends with a brief summary.

INCOME, ASSETS, AND BORROWING POWER OF UNINSURED FAMILIES

Finding: Families with at least one uninsured member are predominantly lower income.

As discussed in Chapter 2, uninsured families have lower family incomes on average than do families with health coverage. More than half of all families with at least one uninsured member have incomes that are at or below 200 percent of the federal poverty level (FPL). Two out of every five lower-income[1] families have at least one uninsured member, whereas just 9 percent of families with moderate and high incomes have at least one uninsured member.[2] Poverty, lack of insurance, and poor health are factors that are often present in families concurrently, and are interrelated so that it is difficult to identify the causal directions and impacts.

This relationship between lack of insurance coverage and low family income is underscored by the insurance and income characteristics of families with children. The median income for two-parent families in which both parents are covered by insurance is $67,000 compared to $30,000 for two-parent families in which neither parent is covered. The median income of one-parent families in which the single parent does not have health insurance is only $14,280 (Figure 4.1). As noted in Chapter 2, virtually all (98 percent) families with *both parents insured* have all of their children covered by insurance and are associated with the higher median income, while only 44 percent of one-parent families in which the *parent is uninsured* have all children covered.[3] Given the lower median income of uninsured single-parent families, many of their uninsured children would be eligible for public coverage.

Finding: Families with uninsured members tend to have fewer assets than do fully insured families and are unlikely to have the capacity to borrow to cover major unexpected health care costs.

Not only do families with uninsured members have lower incomes than fully insured families, they also have extremely limited financial resources such as savings and lines of credit with which to pay medical expenses. Public insurance programs have both income and asset requirements for eligibility that leave many low-income families with uninsured members. Among families in which no one had health insurance in 1989, 45 percent had *no* financial assets. (Starr-McCluer, 1996).[4] In 1989, the median amount of financial assets for families with no members insured was $50.

---

[1]"Low-income family" is defined as a family reporting its income to be at or below 100 percent of FPL and, "lower-income family" is a family reporting its income to be at or below 200 percent of FPL.

[2]Calculated from data in Table 2.1.

[3]Analyses conducted for this report are based on tabulations of the 2001 Current Population Survey (CPS) public use tapes by Matthew Broaddus of the Center on Budget and Policy Priorities.

[4]This survey includes singles and childless couples as families. Assets include balances in checking and savings accounts, stocks, bonds, mutual funds, and individual retirement accounts (IRAs) and other retirement savings. The statements about asset levels are based on the Survey of Consumer Finances (SCF). The SCF is a national survey carried out every three years by the Board of Governors of the Federal Reserve Board. In the SCF, a family is a subset of the household unit referred to as the

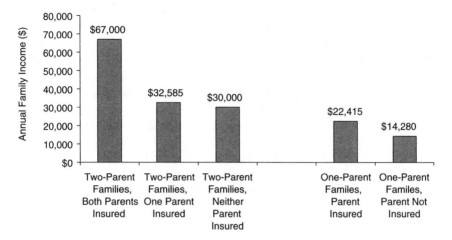

FIGURE 4.1 Families with children, median family income, 2000, by extent of parental health insurance coverage.
SOURCE: See Appendix D.

People of late middle age who are uninsured are at a higher risk of needing to use their assets for health services because they have an increased risk of chronic disease (IOM, 2002a). They also have fewer years before retirement to replenish savings depleted by health care costs. Families with older members in which no one has health insurance have only marginally greater financial assets than younger uninsured families (Starr-McCluer, 1996). Among uninsured families headed by 55 to 64-year-olds in 1989, median financial assets were $200.

Other assets beyond financial ones could help a family cope with medical expenses, but a majority of families in which no one has health insurance have limited assets of any kind. Net worth is the broadest measure of accumulated wealth. It is the sum of financial wealth and other assets, including homes, other real estate, business equity, and vehicles, minus liabilities. Liabilities include mortgages, home equity loans, automobile loans, other loans, and credit card debt. Across families of all ages, median net worth for families with all members uninsured was $1,000 in 1989, compared to $60,175 for families with all members insured (Starr-McCluer, 1996).

"primary economic unit" (PEU). In brief, the PEU consists of an economically dominant single individual or couple (married or living as partners) in a household and all other individuals in the household who are financially dependent on that individual or couple. The same survey has been carried out since 1989, most recently in 2001, but 1989 is the only round for which tabulations of wealth by health insurance status are currently available.

A third way in which uninsured families might cover health care costs, especially non–routine health care costs such as hospitalization, is through borrowing, but this avenue is also likely to be of limited help to many uninsured families. The large share of families with lower incomes have a limited ability to pay off loans from future income. Because they do not have significant assets, they cannot offer such assets as security to a lender. Families who own their own homes have their home equity as a resource for meeting health care expenses, but uninsured families are less likely to be homeowners. In 1987, half of the families in which some or all members did not have health insurance were homeowners, compared to two-thirds of families of all types and ages in which everyone had health insurance (Miller, 1990). Low income and very limited assets and borrowing capacity are all indicators of poverty among uninsured families (see Box 4.2).

BOX 4.2
Poverty Standards

• The poverty threshold is one of the most commonly used measures to define family income so low as to be unable to support a minimal standard of living.[1] Thirty-one percent of families (including single people and childless couples) in which all members lack health insurance have incomes below the poverty threshold, compared to 5 percent of families in which at least one member is covered by private insurance and no one has public coverage and 41 percent of families in which at least one member has public insurance (Banthin et al., 2000).
• However, not all of a family's income may be available to purchase goods and services that contribute to its standard of living. For example, if a family member works, the share of income used to pay taxes, obtain transportation to and from work, and pay for child care cannot be used for food, shelter, or clothing or health care (Citro and Michael, 1995).
• By subtracting out-of-pocket expenditures for health services from income, the poverty rate among households in which no members have health insurance would have been 33.1 rather than 31 percent in 1999 (Banthin et al., 2000).
• In addition, if health care expenditures were excluded from income, some uninsured families currently above the poverty line would slip below that line if they purchased insurance. After meeting the expense of health care, both out-of-pocket costs for services and premium costs, an additional 10 percent of previously uninsured families would fall below the poverty line if their expenses for health care and insurance were deducted from resources. Thus the poverty rate among families with all members previously uninsured would rise from the nearly one-third (31 percent) observed to an estimated two in five (42 percent) (Banthin et al., 2000).

---

[1]The poverty threshold and poverty guidelines are slightly different versions of the federal poverty measure. Poverty thresholds are used mainly for statistical purposes. The federal poverty guidelines, commonly called the federal poverty level, are a simplification of the poverty thresholds for administrative purposes such as determining program eligibility. The 2001 poverty guidelines are roughly equivalent to the poverty thresholds for 2000 (Institute for Research on Poverty, 2000).

HEALTH SERVICES COSTS FOR UNINSURED FAMILIES

Finding: On average, families with some or all members uninsured spend less on health care in absolute dollars than do families with all members covered by private insurance and they use fewer services. Paradoxically, families with uninsured members are more likely to have higher health expenditures as a proportion of family income than are insured families.

One reason that uninsured families have lower health spending than insured families is because they use fewer health services on average. An examination of family spending patterns of those with and without health insurance provides an indication of how the uninsured family might accommodate health bills and the costs of purchasing insurance.

Across households, regardless of insurance status, housing is the largest expenditure, transportation (primarily automobile ownership and operation) the second largest, and food eaten at home the third.[5] These three basic necessities accounted for 59 percent of consumption for fully insured families and 64 percent for uninsured families. In terms of absolute dollars spent for these three purposes, fully insured families spend more than families with no insurance (Paulin and Weber, 1995). After spending for housing, transportation, and food, uninsured families spend both a smaller percentage of income and fewer dollars on other items compared to insured families. Among all uninsured families, those in the lowest quartile based on total spending use their "extra" money (not spent on insurance premiums) for more or better food at home and housing, while those in the top quartile spend their "extra" money across all expenditure categories, not just necessities (Levy and DeLiere, 2002). Figure 4.2 shows the average annual expenditures of families with no members insured and the share they spent on different consumption categories in 1993. Their health spending was 3 percent of total spending. In 2000, the median income for a two-parent family with neither parent insured was $30,000. If such a family spent 3 percent of income on health, it would have health expenditures of roughly $900.

Forty-three (43) percent of working-age adults without health insurance and 31 percent of those currently insured but recently uninsured report that in the past year they did not seek a physician's care when they had had a medical problem, compared to 10 percent of those who were insured all year. In families with incomes below $35,000, 40 percent of those without insurance went without a doctor's visit when sick, compared to less than 10 percent of those with coverage

---

[5]Expenditure data come from the Consumer Expenditure Survey (CES.) A family in the CES is a unit that shares resources. The survey includes single persons and units without children. The Bureau of Labor Statistics uses CES data to benchmark consumer purchases for calculating the Consumer Price Index (CPI).

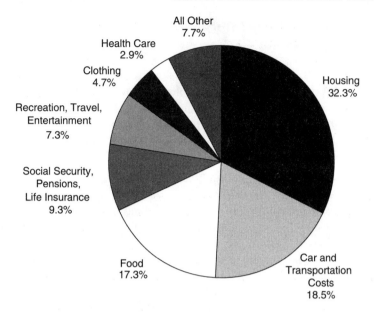

FIGURE 4.2 Spending in families with no members insured.
NOTE: Expenditure units include single people.
SOURCE: Data from 1993 Consumer Expenditure Survey in Paulin and Weber, 1995.

(Duchon et al., 2001). Fifteen (15) percent of uninsured adults reported being unable to pay for basic necessities because of medical bills (Duchon et al., 2001).

Utilization differs between insured and uninsured children. Children who were uninsured for all of 1996 were less likely to use any health care services than were those with insurance, particularly office visits, dental visits and prescription medicines (see Table 4.1 and Box 4.3). Utilization by insured adults also tends to be higher than that by uninsured persons (IOM, 2002a). While the greater use by insured people may be for needed and appropriate services and the uninsured may be lacking needed care, it is also possible that some of the increased care for those with insurance may be unnecessary and contribute to excessive costs.

Average health care expenditures of uninsured families are lower than those of insured families because there are disproportionately more uninsured families with no or very limited use of services. However, uninsured families with health problems requiring care are more likely to find themselves at the other end of the spending spectrum with out-of-pocket costs that can be very large. One example comes from a study of uninsured people between ages 51 and 61 who experienced the onset of cancer, heart conditions, stroke, or lung disease.[6] In that group, half

---

[6]The Health and Retirement Survey, which began in 1992 with a sample of 7,600 households with at least one member between ages 51 and 61, includes more than 22,000 Americans over age 50.

TABLE 4.1 Children Age ≤ 17 Using No Health Care Services, 1996

	Percentages					
	Hospital Inpatient	Hospital Outpatient	Hospital Emergency Department	Office Visits	Dental Visits	Prescription Medicines
Any private	97.6	92.2	87.5	23.8	49.9	38.6
Public only	94.6	92.7	84.5	33.2	71.4	44.0
Uninsured	98.1	96.3	89.2	49.3	79.3	57.2

SOURCE: MEPS 1996 data in McCormick et al., 2001.

BOX 4.3
What Counts as an Expense for Health Care Services?

The most comprehensive data on who uses what health care services and how much is paid for those services comes from the Medical Expenditure Panel Survey (MEPS). MEPS began in 1996 and is ongoing. Similar surveys in earlier years were the National Medical Care Expenditure Survey (NMCES) in 1977 and the National Medical Expenditure Survey (NMES) in 1987. The data presented in this chapter on who pays how much for health care are derived from MEPS.

In the MEPS, an *expenditure* is what is paid for health care services. Total expenditures are the sum of amounts that patients and their families pay out-of-pocket and payments by private insurance, Medicaid, Medicare, and other sources. Payments for over-the-counter drugs such as aspirin or cold remedies and for alternative care services such as massage or homeopathy are not included.

This definition of expenditure requires someone to make a payment in order for a medical service to generate an expenditure. Amounts that are not collected from patients, including both bad debt and charitable care, are not counted as expenditures because no payment has been made, even though a provider may have incurred some cost to provide those services. An exception is made for public clinics and hospitals. For those settings, amounts are counted toward expenditures even in the cases where no one makes a payment for a service.

The payment-based definition of expenditure is a change from the 1977 and 1987 surveys, in which the definition of an expenditure was tied to a provider's cost rather than the payment the provider received. The 1996 definition is more useful for this report, which examines health expenditures from the perspective of the family, but it does not give a complete picture of the value of services rendered from the health care provider's perspective.

had out-of-pocket costs below $1,060 over a two-year period; 1 in 10 had out-of-pocket payments that exceeded $16,500, 1 in 20 had payments that exceeded $30,500, and at the very top, 1 in 50 paid more than $64,700 out-of-pocket over the two years (Smith, 1999).

Unless a new health condition is disabling, even persons with large health expenses are unlikely to qualify for Medicaid unless they have a very low income and meet other eligibility criteria. Among families with uninsured members who *are* eligible to enroll in Medicaid but who are not enrolled (primarily families with children), out-of-pocket costs could be reduced if eligible family members enrolled. As noted in Chapter 2, most uninsured children are eligible for Medicaid and SCHIP but are not enrolled. Almost 85 percent of Medicaid-eligible uninsured children live in families that have some health care costs; in 1993 and 1994, 29 percent had out-of-pocket expenses greater than $500 (Davidoff et al., 2000a). An analysis of the 1997 National Health Interview Survey shows that only about half of Medicaid-eligible working-age adults are enrolled and more than a quarter remain uninsured. Those families with an uninsured adult are twice as likely to report out-of-pocket spending of between $500 and $2,000 as are families of Medicaid-enrolled adults, 21 percent and 10 percent, respectively (Davidoff et al., 2001a).

Among all individuals under age 65, the average out-of-pocket cost in 1996 was lower for persons who did not have health insurance ($253) than for those who had private insurance ($326), including costs of the latter that some would view as examples of underinsurance.[7] Among those who actually used any health care service and paid for it out-of-pocket, however, the difference in mean levels of expense paid out of pocket is roughly the same for insured and uninsured patients (around $400) (Taylor et al., 2001a). Although those with health insurance had some expenses covered by their plan, their out-of-pocket expenses were about the same as those of uninsured persons because, on average, insured people use more services.

Lack of insurance affects the health care costs of uninsured families in another way. Insurance plans serve a less obvious purpose of negotiating competitive prices with providers of services. Uninsured families do not enjoy the agency of a large insurer or managed care company when they pay for their own care. Thus uninsured persons may be charged and pay a higher price for the same service than the price paid by an insurer on behalf of an enrollee. Anecdotal evidence suggests that the prices providers charge the uninsured can be two to three times the payment amount negotiated by insurers on behalf of the privately insured (Wielawski, 2000; Kolata, 2001). This pricing practice can affect both the out-of-pocket expenses a family pays for services used by an uninsured member and the amount of debt resulting if the uninsured family cannot pay the full amount

---

[7]Calculations by Hanns Kuttner based on data in Cohen et al. (2000).

charged. This practice also affects the amounts paid by other sources on behalf of uninsured medically indigent patients.

Finding: Most uninsured families would not have sufficient funds in their budget to purchase health insurance without a substantial premium subsidy.

The primary reason that uninsured families spend a smaller share of their family budget on health is that they do not pay for health insurance (Acs and Sabelhaus, 1995). Surveys show that the most common reason given for not being insured is the perceived unaffordability of the premium (Thorpe and Florence, 1999; Orne et al., 2000). This section shows how purchasing health insurance would affect the budget of the typical uninsured family.

Determining the cost of purchasing private health insurance other than an employment-based group plan is not easy. A wide range of plans and premiums are available, with substantial variation in benefits covered and cost sharing required, including copayments and deductibles. In addition, an individual's age and medical condition will affect whether the person can get coverage at all and, if so, at what price and whether certain conditions are excluded from coverage. Given all these variables affecting the cost of independently purchased insurance and a lack of comprehensive data, it is impossible to put a specific price tag on an average policy. However, a 1999 study of web-marketed policies available in 15 major cities reports a median premium for a plan with a $250 deductible of $1,700 for a 25-year-old and $5,700 for a 60-year-old (Simantov et al., 2001). With a deductible of $1,000, the median premiums for a 25-year-old and 60-year-old were $1,100 and $4,000, respectively. A related survey of 1,500 people aged 50–64 reports that half of those with individually purchased coverage for a single person paid more than $3,500 in premiums and out-of-pocket expenses, compared with 17 percent of those in employment-based plans who had that level of expenses. A policy with terms similar to those in a group plan would likely cost more if purchased independently, however, because of the higher administrative costs and greater risks faced by the insurer.

Figure 4.3 shows the relationship between the cost of employment-based health insurance and income for a four-person family. For the cost of insurance, the figure uses the cost for the average employment-based health plan. At the 2001 FPL of $17,650 for a four-person family, the full premium represents 40 percent of income, a larger share than either food or shelter typically consumes. Individuals who sought to purchase that average plan on their own would likely pay even more; they might also seek to reduce their costs by purchasing a plan with less generous benefits and greater out-of-pocket costs than provided in the average employment-based plan. In any case, the family that purchases coverage outside employment would lose the tax advantage that comes from not paying income tax on the employer contribution, which averages 73 percent of the total premium for family coverage (Kaiser-HRET, 2001). If a middle-income family received the employer's share of the insurance premium as income instead of a health benefit,

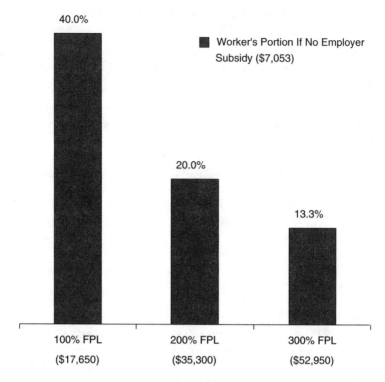

FIGURE 4.3 Share of a four-person family's income compared to premium costs to purchase family coverage in 2001.
SOURCE: Kaiser-HRET, 2001.

it would owe taxes of about 15 percent on the Federal Insurance Contributions Act (FICA) for Social Security and Medicare and 28 percent on federal income tax.

At the median income of families in which neither parent has health insurance ($30,000 in 2000, Figure 4.1) the annual cost of a typical plan would have required that more than one-fifth of family income be devoted to health insurance. Among single-parent families where the parent did not have health insurance, the median income in 2000 was $14,280, and the typical plan would have required almost half of the family's income. If a family were to spend that amount on health insurance, its remaining income would place the family below the poverty threshold (Kaiser-HRET, 2001).

Affordability of health insurance can also be evaluated in terms of a "minimally adequate" family budget. In contrast to the "privation" standard of the poverty threshold, assessments based on family budgets have tried to estimate the amount of income that provides for a modest standard of living, one that is more generous than that provided by the poverty threshold and that reflects the variety of goods and services a family typically buys.[8] Such a "basic needs" budget that included costs for housing, transportation, food, health care, telephone service, and taxes, using prices in Baltimore as a reference amount, was estimated to be $34,732 for a family of four in 1998. This amount is twice the poverty threshold for the same size family. Still, a family with an income below the basic needs level must do without or with fewer of the things than most families have. This budget includes $3,200 for employment-based health insurance and out-of-pocket expenses, based on typical costs for a family of this size. In this basic needs budget, health care amounts to 9.2 percent of a family's spending (Bernstein et al., 2000). This contrasts sharply with the 21 percent of family income cited above as being required just to purchase private health insurance for a non-insured family having a median income of $30,000 per year. Uncovered out-of-pocket health expenses for such a family would be an additional expense.

FINANCIAL BURDEN OF HEALTH CARE COSTS FOR UNINSURED FAMILIES AND HOW THESE FAMILIES COPE

The average levels of health care expenditures faced by uninsured families cited above mask a high variation in such costs. Lack of insurance exposes the uninsured to the financial risks represented by this high variation. Most vulnerable, clearly, are uninsured families in which one or more members have significant needs for health care.

Finding: Among families with no health insurance the entire year and incomes at or below the poverty level, more than one in four have out-of-pocket expenses that exceed 5 percent of income. Among *all* uninsured families, 4 percent have expenses that exceed 20 percent of annual income.

Low-income families with no members insured for the full year are at greater risk of incurring high medical expenses (greater than 5 percent of income) than are totally uninsured families with higher incomes (Taylor et al., 2001b). Regardless of income, 4 percent of uninsured families experience exceedingly high medical expenses (greater than 20 percent of income) (Taylor et al., 2001a). Having some insurance in the family for at least part of the year tends to reduce the risk of high expenditures relative to income. Families with some members insured and others uninsured are somewhat more likely to have out-of-pocket costs for medical services that exceed 5 percent of income in a year than are families with all

---

[8]For example, rather than referencing the Department of Agriculture's *thrifty* food plan originally used in defining the poverty threshold, the *low-cost* food plan might be used, and consumption areas that are likely not affordable in the poverty threshold budget, such as a telephone and health care, would be included. The latter plan also recognizes the variation in housing costs from city to city.

members insured (Table 4.2). Families with *no* members insured at any time in the year are almost twice as likely as those with *all* members insured for the full year to exceed the 5 percent threshold. Insurance offers protection against large, unpredictable expenses. The higher the threshold, the higher must a family's expenses relative to income be to exceed the threshold. Families without health insurance will be at greater risk than insured families of exceeding each higher threshold. Families with some insurance, either for some members or for some part of the year, are 1.5 times as likely to exceed the 10 percent threshold as fully insured families, and families in which no one has health insurance are 2.7 times as likely to have out-of-pocket costs exceeding 10 percent of family income. Table 4.3 provides a finer breakdown of out-of-pocket expenses among uninsured families of different types and shows that those who are uninsured for the full year are more likely to have no expenses during the year than are those families insured for part of the year. That is true whether the uninsured families are single- or two-parent or a single person or couple with no children at home. However, families uninsured for the full year are also more likely to have expenditures that exceed 5 percent of income than are those that are uninsured for part of the year.

Health care expenses in a year equal a small proportion of income for many families but a large proportion for a small share of families (Table 4.3). A majority of families, whether their members were with or without health insurance, have medical expenses that are less than 2 percent of income.

Lower incomes, poorer health, and lack of health insurance interact to create financial hardship. For example, a person with serious health problems may have difficulty holding a job, particularly one that would offer health benefits. Such an individual would also be more likely to have trouble obtaining coverage independently because of underwriting practices. The health problem could result in both a limited income and many health bills. Being uninsured is associated with poor health and financial problems paying bills, but the causal relationships are unclear.

TABLE 4.2 Out-of-Pocket Expenses as Percent of Family Income, by Insurance Coverage and Duration, Non-Medicare Families, 1996[a]

	Families Exceeding Threshold (percent)	
	5% or More of Income	10% or More of Income
All members insured for entire year	8.8	3.0
Some members uninsured and/or some period without health insurance	10.7	4.6
All members uninsured for entire year	15.4	8.0
All families	10.0	4.0

[a]These out-of-pocket expenses cover medical services; they do not include insurance premiums.
SOURCE: Medical Expenditure Panel Survey 1996 data across families of all sizes in Merlis, 2001.

TABLE 4.3 Out-of-Pocket Health Care Expense as a Share of Income, by Family Type and Insurance Status, 1996[a]

| | Percent of Families | | | | |
| | Out-of-Pocket Expenses as a Share Of Income | | | | |
	No Expenses	Less Than 2% of Income	2%–5% of Income	5%–10% of Income	More Than 10%
Single person					
Full year privately insured	12.6	60.3	15.5	5.1	4.6
Part year uninsured	20.3	48.1	15.2	6.0	7.2
Full year uninsured	32.1	28.8	11.7	6.1	10.9
Couple, no children at home					
Full year privately insured	1.6	70.0	18.6	7.4	2.2
Part year uninsured	7.3	66.0	14.6	4.4	4.3
Full year uninsured	12.3	48.5	21.4	11.7	5.1
Singe-parent families					
Full year privately insured	5.7	63.6	19.0	6.6	4.9
Part year uninsured	13.4	57.1	20.0	2.2	6.0
Full year uninsured	19.8	42.6	19.1	4.7	4.5
Two-parent families					
Full year privately insured	0.7	69.9	20.4	5.8	2.6
Part year uninsured	2.2	69.8	15.3	7.4	5.0
Full year uninsured	6.3	53.9	23.7	8.7	6.6

[a]These out-of-pocket expenses cover medical services; they do not include insurance premiums.
SOURCE: Tabulations from the 1996 Medical Expenditure Panel Survey, Center for Cost and Financing Studies, Agency for Healthcare Research and Quality.

A recent national survey of working-age Americans reports that 55 percent of those who were currently or recently *uninsured* had problems paying medical bills and about three in ten of those *uninsured* report needing to change their way of life in order to pay medical bills (see Box 4.4 for a description of procedures used for collecting medical bills). Only one-quarter of *insured* adults had problems paying medical bills and one-tenth of *insured* adults had to change their life-style (Duchon et al., 2001).[9]

---

[9]The sample of 2,829 were asked if the following actions were attributable to health costs: (1) did not fill a prescription, (2) did not get needed specialist care, (3) skipped a recommended test or follow-up, (4) or had a medical problem, but did not visit a doctor or clinic. Among uninsured people, 55 percent cited at least one of these reasons compared to 21 percent of those insured all year.

BOX 4.4
Collections Procedures for Medical Bills

If a family experiences difficulty paying a bill for medical services promptly, it may also experience one or more common collection procedures. Standard references for hospital financial administrators suggest they use collection agencies to pursue debt (Herkimer, 1993). More than a third of uninsured adults in a national survey reported being contacted by a bill collector for payment of medical bills (Duchon et al., 2001). The process used to collect debt is regulated by the Fair Debt Collection Practices Act (15 U.S.C. § 1692) The act allows collection efforts by writing letters or making phone calls but forbids certain abusive practices such as using obscene language and threatening personal harm. Even if a health care provider does write off a bill as a bad debt a family could still face adverse effects if the provider reported the debt to a credit reporting agency. Credit agencies can continue to report the bad debt for seven years (Federal Trade Commission, 1999), thus affecting the family's credit rating for many years.

For families without health insurance the burden of out-of-pocket expenditures falls as income rises (Figure 4.4). Among all types of families and singles, those who live in families with low incomes are more likely to be burdened by health care expenses. The burden is also greater for families with poorer health (Taylor et al., 2001b). Among all families in which no members are insured, twice as many families report no out-of-pocket expenses when the household head reports his or her health as good or better, as when the family head reports fair or poor health (23 compared to 12 percent). Less than half as many are likely to have out-of-pocket expenses that exceed 5 percent of family income (13 percent where the household head has good or excellent health compared to 34 percent where the household head reports fair or poor health) (Taylor et al., 2001b).

The degree to which high out-of-pocket expenses persist year after year affects the strategies a family can use to meet high costs. Borrowing or using available savings might be feasible if high costs are a one-time event, but if high costs are ongoing they must be offset by reducing other spending. No currently available survey provides the data to determine what share of uninsured families face high out-of-pocket expenses year after year. The overlap in the sample between the 1996 and 1997 rounds of the Medical Expenditure Panel Survey (MEPS) does shed some light on the extent to which high costs persist over two years. Among all non-Medicare families, 17 percent (whether insured or not) experienced high out-of-pocket costs (more than 5 percent of income) in either of 1996 or 1997, and of these, one in five had high costs in both years (Merlis, 2001).

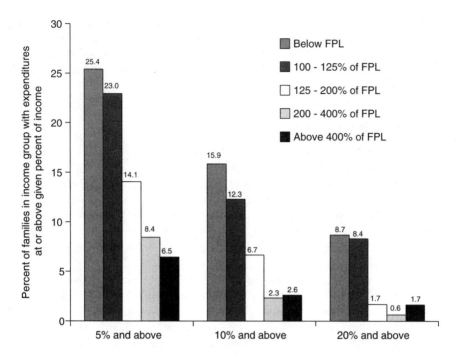

FIGURE 4.4 Uninsured families with high medical expenses, by poverty level, 1996.
NOTE: The dollar level of health expenditures required to reach 5 percent of income varies by family income. The 1996 FPL for a family of four was $15,600, 5 percent of expenditures at a family income of 100 percent FPL is $780; and at a family income of 400 percent FPL is $3,120.
SOURCE: Tabulations from the 1996 Medical Expenditure Panel Survey (MEPS), Center for Cost and Financing Studies, Agency for Healthcare Research and Quality, Taylor et al., 2001b.

How Uninsured Families Cope with the Financial Burden of Medical Expenses Borrowing

The Committee has noted earlier in this chapter that uninsured families typically have low borrowing power. Still, some do manage to borrow. A recent national phone survey of working-age adults reports that among uninsured people, almost 20 percent used all or most of their savings, 17 percent borrowed from family or friends, and 7 percent reported needing a loan or mortgage on their home in order to pay medical bills (Duchon et al., 2001).

The growing availability of credit cards provides another way for the uninsured to pay medical bills but at a very high cost in terms of interest. A family might use cash to pay health care bills and credit cards to purchase things that otherwise would have been purchased with cash. Alternatively, the family may make payment to a health care provider with a credit card. The debt arises as a result of health care expenses but would appear on a listing of family assets and liabilities as credit card debt. Thus, the extent to which medical expenses contribute to debt remains hidden, but some researchers consider it to be significant for middle-class families (Sullivan et al., 2000).

Declaring Bankruptcy

For some in financial stress, bankruptcy may be perceived as an option. The 1.5 million personal bankruptcy filings in 2001 were five times the level of a generation earlier (Administrative Office of the U.S. Courts, 2002). Bankruptcy is often described as a response by financially stressed families to some adverse event—losing a job, being sick, or becoming divorced (Stanley and Girth, 1971; Sullivan et al., 2000). Bankruptcy gives a "fresh start" to debtors, because many but not all unsecured debts can be discharged in bankruptcy. The largest class of unsecured debt for individuals is credit card debt.[10]

The most direct evidence on the relationship of bankruptcy and health insurance comes from a survey of almost 1,500 cases involving about 2,000 debtors in bankruptcy courts across eight judicial districts that asked if any family member did not have health insurance. Twenty-one (21) percent reported that no family members had health insurance (Jacoby et al., 2000). The survey did not ascertain whether an individual was without health insurance at the time of the survey or at the time the medical debt was incurred. The same survey of bankruptcy filers found medical problems associated with nearly half of all bankruptcies.[11] Those with no health insurance in their families do not disproportionately cite medical problems. Thus, it is difficult to determine from this survey what causal relationship may exist between being uninsured and bankruptcy.

The bankruptcy filings by some who are without health insurance may be attributed to high out-of-pocket medical expenses. While there is evidence that those who have medical debts that exceed 2 percent of income are far more likely to file for bankruptcy, it is not known what share of those who have high medical debts are currently uninsured or were uninsured at the time they incurred the debt (Domowitz and Sartain, 1999). None of the current surveys of nationally representative samples provide the detail about medical expenses, insurance status, and financial circumstances to illuminate how families with high out-of-pocket medical expenses deal with these costs. The relationship of high medical expenses and forms of financial stress such as bankruptcy is not clear.

---

[10]Much debt is secured—mortgages by homes, auto loans by autos—and thus cannot be discharged in bankruptcy.

[11]Medical reasons checked on the survey included substantial medical debt, medical bills not covered by insurance in excess of $1,000 in the past two years, birth of baby, or death in family, among 16 reasons listed.

Other Sources of Payments for Family Health Expenses

Not all health care expenses incurred by uninsured persons are borne by family budgets. Uninsured family budgets absorb 41 percent of total family health care expenses, but this varies by type of service; families pay for between 7 percent (hospital inpatient services) and 89 percent (glasses, other equipment, and services) of particular categories of service (see Figures 4.5 and 4.6). For example, while the average percentage paid out of pocket by uninsured families for a hospital stay is almost 7 percent (Figure 4.5), very few uninsured people under age 65 experience a hospitalization. Almost 3 percent of uninsured individuals have an inpatient expense (see Figure 4.7), and the average out-of-pocket amount paid by them is $567 (see Figure 4.8).

Apart from family spending, medical expenses for persons without health insurance are met by other forms of insurance such as automobile insurance and workers' compensation; public support for public hospitals, clinics, and community health centers; and philanthropy and provider sources.

Fifty-eight (58) percent of expenses for uninsured children are paid out of pocket (McCormick et al., 2001). In part, the larger share paid out of pocket for children reflects the fact that hospital services, where support from sources outside family budgets is greatest, are a smaller share of children's use of services than adults' use.

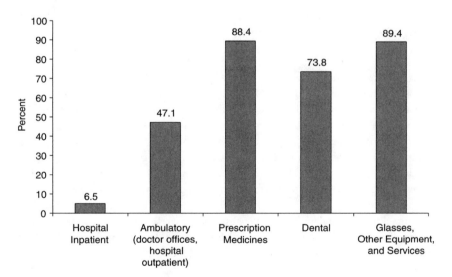

FIGURE 4.5 Share paid out-of-pocket by uninsured persons under age 65, within each type of service, 1997.
SOURCE: Data from Medical Expenditure Panel Survey in Agency for Healthcare Research and Quality, 2001a.

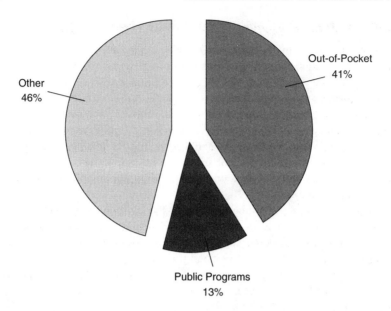

FIGURE 4.6 Sources of payment for expenses of the uninsured, 1997.
NOTE: Public programs exclude Medicare and Medicaid. They include state and local payments for clinics, health departments, and other programs and at the federal level some payments by the Department of Veteran Affairs, Indian Health Service, military treatment facilities, and other federally provided care. SOURCE: Data from Medical Expenditure Panel Survey in Agency for Healthcare Research and Quality, 2001b.

Prescription medicines and medical supplies receive the least external support, and the family's share of those expenses is greater than for other services. Almost as large a share of the uninsured had expenses for prescription medicines as had outpatient expenses in 1997 (40 percent compared with 47 percent) (Figure 4.7). Prescription expenditures were less than half those of outpatient costs among those who had any costs (mean of $517 for outpatient costs and $233 for prescription medicines; median of $164 for outpatient costs and $58 for prescription medicines). Despite the higher cost of outpatient services, average out-of-pocket payments for uninsured persons were nearly the same for these services, about $200 (Figure 4.8). The relative lack of subsidies for prescription drug costs, only 7 percent of expenses, largely accounted for an equal out-of-pocket burden from two categories so different in total expense (AHRQ, 2001a).

Hospital Care

A health event that requires an inpatient hospital stay leads to significant expense. Among those without health insurance who had a hospital stay in 1997, the average amount paid by all sources was $8,730 for the stay. However, just 6.5

percent ($567, on average) was paid by the uninsured or their families. About one-fifth (22 percent) came from government programs (other than Medicare and Medicaid) such as local programs to make payments for uncompensated care and services provided by the Department of Veterans Affairs. The largest share (72 percent) came from payments from other forms of insurance such as workers' compensation and automobile accident insurance and as hospital charity care. (MEPS counts uncompensated care as expenses when provided by public hospitals [AHRQ, 2001a]). The hospital sector differs from other providers of health care used by those without health insurance. Under the Emergency Medical Treatment and Active Labor Act (EMTALA), hospitals with emergency departments are required to provide treatment to patients needing emergency care whether they are insured or not.[12] Many hospitals, particularly those that are public or not for profit have as part of their mission serving uninsured patients. Regardless of ownership status, however, accounting standards require hospitals to have a standard set of procedures to decide who qualifies for charity care (Box 4.5).

Hospital inpatient stays and resulting out-of-pocket payments are comparatively infrequent; only 3 percent of those who were uninsured throughout the year had expenses for hospital inpatient stays in 1997 (Figure 4.7). Expenses for ambulatory services, including services provided in hospital outpatient departments, the area of a hospital that includes emergency departments and physician offices, are more common and account for a much larger share of the amount families with uninsured members pay from their own pockets. Almost half of uninsured people had expenses for ambulatory services in 1997. The average amount paid by families was $244 (see Figure 4.8).

Outside Supports, Trade-offs, Fairness, and Accountability

Because uninsured people do not bear all the costs of their care, the existence of outside financial support and the availability of services rendered at no or reduced charge enters the calculus for uninsured families when they weigh the value of insurance against competing demands on the family budget. Many of the largest financial risks families face from being without health insurance may be mitigated by a patchwork of arrangements involving trading off inconvenience or loss of dignity for avoidance of financial harm (Collins et al., 2002; Doty and Ives, 2002; Hughes, 2002). However, if families without health insurance have the resources and choose to buy insurance, they may lose access to these supports and face paying more in total (including premiums, copayments, and deductibles) for health care than they had previously. The greater financial cost of having health

---

[12]Under EMTALA hospitals are required to assess and stabilize all patients with a life- or limb-threatening or emergency medical condition or those who are about to give birth. Hospitals are not required to provide continuing care after stabilizing and releasing the patient. No federal funds directly support this mandate.

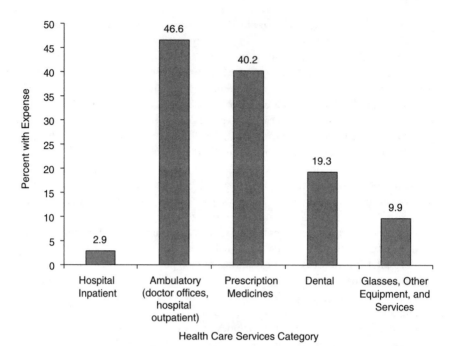

FIGURE 4.7 Share with expense in the service category, full-year uninsured individuals under age 65, 1997.
SOURCE: Data from Medical Expenditure Panel Survey in Agency for Healthcare Research and Quality, 2001a.

insurance creates a dilemma both for persons without health insurance and for a society that cares enough about those who do not have health insurance to not withhold all health care services from those who cannot pay for all services they receive (Coate, 1995). This conundrum will be examined further in the Committee's next report, which addresses community-wide impacts of uninsurance.

There are two issues related to the provision of financial support for families facing large medical expenses: (1) how to promote consistency and fairness across similar situations, and (2) how to ensure documentation of and accounting for what is spent. Laws and regulations ensure that the federal tax code treats families in similar circumstances the same way. Medicaid law and regulations at the federal level provide some consistency in establishing an eligibility floor while allowing considerable variability among states in the upper limits of eligibility and benefits. The financial support that uninsured families receive, most notably from hospitals, cannot be described by a set of rules and regulations to ensure that similarly situated persons are treated equally regardless of the institution where they are served. Likewise, physicians' provision of free or reduced-cost care to uninsured

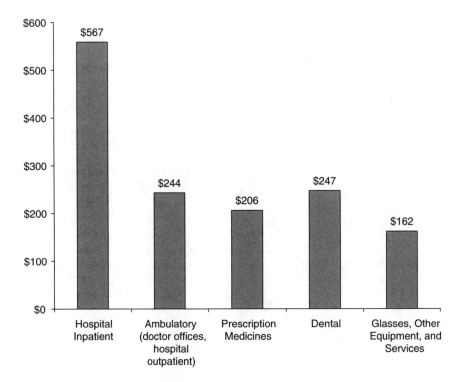

FIGURE 4.8 Mean out-of-pocket expense among uninsured persons with expense, in the service category, full-year uninsured individuals under age 65, 1997.
SOURCE: Data from Medical Expenditure Panel Survey in Agency for Healthcare Research and Quality, 2001a.

patients varies among practitioners and across communities (Cunningham et al., 1999). Data concerning bad debt and free care are very limited, particularly for health service providers other than hospitals.

Unlike assistance to families through Medicaid and the tax code, much of the financial support received by uninsured patients directly from providers of services and from charitable organizations is hard to document and quantify. The assistance is generally not allocated through a public or transparent process, and there are no consistent rules for reporting the costs. One year's data from seven hospitals in one state suggest that financial assistance from hospital decisions to offer charity care and write off bad debt flows to those with lowest income (Weissman et al., 1999). Eighty percent of the cost of free care went to individuals from families with incomes below the poverty threshold; another ten percent went to individuals with family incomes between the poverty threshold and twice the threshold.

BOX 4.5
How Do Hospitals and Community Health Centers
Handle Uninsured Families and Bill for Care?

Few generalizations are possible about what a person without health insurance can expect when seeking care. Some providers may be willing to offer services at a reduced price; others may not. Some hospitals may defer elective admissions until a financial plan for payment has been agreed upon. Some people without health insurance will find they are required to pay cash up front. Others without financial resources may be denied care.

The American Institute of Certified Public Accountants' audit and accounting guide requires hospitals to establish billing and collections policies to determine the circumstances under which uncompensated care is considered charity care. While data are limited on the nature of such policies, the Committee notes the following widely varying practices:

- Regardless of how hospitals arrive at the amount to charge, they appear to follow similar billing procedures, including an initial bill, mail and phone follow-ups, and if payment is not received, referral to a collection agency. These procedures would generally be followed after provision of care in the emergency department under EMTALA requirements also.
- In many hospitals, individuals who do not qualify for free care or payment set by a sliding scale receive bills for the full charge of each service.
- Hospitals often make decisions at the time a patient is admitted as to whether the patient meets the hospital's criteria for free care. Criteria for free care often includes a family income at or below the FPL. In one state, individuals with incomes below the FPL accounted for 80 percent of free care (Weissman et al., 1999). Hospitals that receive state or local government subsidies may exclude people from outside the jurisdiction from free care.
- Public hospitals, often in large cities, most frequently use a sliding scale based on income. They often expect payments from people below the poverty level. One such hospital charged those with incomes at or below 40 percent of FPL $15 for a stay, with expected payment rising with income, reaching $765 at 185 percent of FPL (Singer, 2000).
- A small community hospital considers charity care for people under 300 percent FPL, if asked, and decides cases individually by a committee established for that purpose.
- A survey of 20 community health centers (CHCs) found that half of these usually create a payment plan when the patient cannot pay. One-quarter continue to bill the patient. At least one CHC uses a sliding fee schedule based on a federal scale with no charges to patients below the poverty level (Fairbrother et al., 2002).

Families with incomes below the poverty threshold also accounted for two-thirds of the bad debt dollars written off. Even after the debt is written off by the hospital or other provider, a family may still lose its credit rating if the debt is reported to a credit bureau (see Box 4.4).

SUMMARY

Uninsured families are more likely to face high medical bills with less income, savings, and other assets than are insured families (see Box 4.6). Managing without health insurance is part of a broader experience for uninsured families of managing with fewer resources in general. Their choices are constrained and their limited resources may be a contributing factor to their lack of coverage. If workers are not offered heavily subsidized health insurance with their job (often the case for lower wage workers), it is unlikely that they would be able to afford to purchase a plan independently for themselves and their dependents. The Committee has shown that most uninsured families have little leeway in their budgets to accommodate payments for an insurance premium, given the relatively high costs of coverage. Such families could face difficulties with even routine medical bills; a major hospitalization or chronic condition requiring frequent medical services might easily destabilize them.

The evidence shows that uninsured families do not use the health system to the same extent that insured families do. This means that the children are less likely to see a doctor, receive hospital outpatient or emergency care, visit a dentist,

---

BOX 4.6
Summary of Findings

• Families with at least one uninsured member are predominantly lower income.

• Families with uninsured members tend to have fewer assets than do fully insured families and are unlikely to have the capacity to borrow to cover major unexpected health care costs.

• On average, families with some or all members uninsured spend less on health care in absolute dollars than do families with all members covered by private insurance and they use fewer services. Paradoxically, families with uninsured members are more likely to have higher health expenditures as a proportion of family income than are insured families.

• Most uninsured families would not have sufficient funds in their budget to purchase health insurance without a substantial premium subsidy.

• Among families with no health insurance the entire year and incomes at or below the poverty level, more than one in four have out-of-pocket expenses that exceed 5 percent of income. Among *all* uninsured families, 4 percent have expenses that exceed 20 percent of annual income.

or receive prescription medicines than are children who are privately insured or covered by public programs. Also, proportionally more uninsured families record no medical expenses during the year than do insured families. Limiting purchases is a common way for families to survive with reduced resources, but using health care is sometimes unavoidable and families may suffer ill effects when their members do not receive timely, appropriate care. Chapter 6 details the consequences for children and pregnant women of delaying care and not maintaining contact with a routine source of care.

Even though uninsured families are more likely than their insured counterparts to have *no* medical expenses, those at the other end of the spending spectrum who cannot avoid using services, are also more likely to have burdensome medical expenses of more than 5 percent of family income. The extent to which uninsured families resort to borrowing and filing for bankruptcy compared to insured families cannot be readily determined. It is clear, however, that high medical bills can cause problems for families with health insurance as well as for those without. It is unknown how many more uninsured families would face high levels of expenditures if it were not for the availability of subsidized care and the use of safety-net providers. These external supports exist to assist uninsured families; it is not clear how many families may benefit from them, or to what extent, and how many do not have these options or choose not to use them.

There is much that we do not fully understand about the interaction of economic and health pressures on families and what influences how they respond. It is an area ripe for further inquiry.

NOTES

BOX 5.1

Suzanne is a divorced mother, with three children under the age of 12.[1] She experiences severe pain from rheumatoid arthritis and fibromyalgia that intermittently limits her ability to walk. Since she cannot sit for long periods or drive on a regular basis, she has not been able to hold a steady job. Her ex-husband pays a reasonable level of child support, but he has no health insurance either. Ironically, the child support puts her just over the income level that would make her eligible for Medicaid in her state. She recently enrolled her children in the State Children's Health Insurance Program (SCHIP), but she finds it difficult to drive them to their regular appointments, either for preventive services or to deal with the mild scoliosis (spinal curvature) of her oldest child. Suzanne, a smoker since she was 15, has tried to quit on her own but, like most heavy smokers, has failed repeatedly. As a caring mother however, she is very good about not smoking around her children.

Suzanne's health would be a lot better if she could get to the doctor regularly, get regular medications for her pain, and get medications and support to help her quit smoking completely. Now that her youngest child is in school every day, she really wants to go to work. She is aware that if her pain were controlled she could likely get some kind of job (maybe even one with health care coverage!) that would help her and her family both financially and emotionally. She thinks she might be eligible for at least partial disability benefits and with this Medicaid coverage for people with disabilities, if only she could afford the full diagnostic work-up needed to document her condition. Suzanne lives in a state that is currently considering expanding the SCHIP program to parents of eligible children. This would be a solution that would help Suzanne and her children a great deal.

---

[1] This vignette is a composite of circumstances documented in the research literature and statistics.

5

Family Well-Being and Health Insurance Coverage

Family members' health insurance status, use of health care, and health itself are interrelated. This chapter documents the relationship between *parents'* health insurance coverage, access to, and use of health services and their *children's* coverage and use of health care. Second, it explores the mechanisms by which the health and attitudes of parents can affect the well-being of other family members, specifically their children's health and life chances. The Committee's previous report, *Care Without Coverage,* demonstrates that uninsured parents are likely to have poorer health than they would if insured. Research presented in the second section of this chapter demonstrates the interrelatedness of the health of family members and the effects of stress on the family as a whole.

PARENTS' INFLUENCE ON CHILDREN'S ACCESS TO AND USE OF HEALTH SERVICES

Parent's Role in Obtaining Insurance Coverage for the Family

Finding: Many uninsured children are eligible for, but not enrolled in public programs. More than half of the 8 million children who remain uninsured are eligible for Medicaid or State Children's Health Insurance Program (SCHIP) coverage.

Finding: Extension of publicly supported health insurance to low-income uninsured parents is associated with increased enrollment among children.

Growth in the enrollment of children in Medicaid and SCHIP accounts for most of the increase in the general population insurance coverage rate that occurred between 1999 and 2000 (Hoffman and Pohl, 2002). By December 2001, 3.46 million children were enrolled in SCHIP (Smith and Rousseau, 2002). An estimated 8 million children remained uninsured in 2000 (Urban Institute, 2002a). More than half of those uninsured children, nearly 5 million, were eligible for Medicaid or SCHIP. The potential of these public insurance programs to eliminate much of the problem of uninsurance among children, despite the fact that SCHIP is not an entitlement, has not yet been fully realized.

Overall, if parents are insured, the likelihood is greater that the children will be insured as well (see Chapter 2, Figure 2.7). This pattern holds for lower-income families: if parents are insured children are more likely to be insured (Lambrew, 2001b). Medicaid and SCHIP are more likely to provide coverage for children than for their parents. Thus, lower-income parents have an uninsured rate one and a half times as high (33 percent) as that of lower-income children (Lambrew, 2001b).

Although the simple descriptive information presented in Chapter 2 demonstrates a strong association between parental and child insurance coverage, it does not address whether more low-income children would be insured if coverage were extended to their parents. Very recent studies show that this is likely to be the case. Two studies have examined the coverage rates of children in states that expanded Medicaid coverage to parents. While using different methodologies and different data sets, both studies found that states that had implemented broad coverage expansions to low-income parents had higher child participation rates compared to states that had not expanded coverage to parents (Ku and Broaddus, 2000; Dubay and Kenney, 2002).

One study, based on Current Population Survey (CPS) data examined the coverage of children under age 6 with family income below 133 percent of the federal poverty level (FPL) in three states (Hawaii, Oregon, and Tennessee) that expanded Medicaid eligibility to parents beginning in 1994 (Ku and Broaddus, 2000). The authors report a gain in children's enrollment of 16 percentage points in the expansion states compared to a 3-point gain in the states that did not expand coverage prior to 1998.

The second study found that in states without coverage expansion to parents, 57 percent of the lower-income children who were eligible enrolled in the Medicaid program, compared to 81 percent in states that expanded coverage to parents (Dubay and Kenney, 2002). When differences among states in the characteristics of the eligible population were taken into account in the analysis (using a multivariable model that controlled for age, race, and health status of the child; work status, education, and nativity of the parent; income and welfare history of the family; and number of children in the family), Medicaid participation rates among eligible children in states with family coverage expansions remained more than 20 percentage points higher than in states with no family coverage.

An examination of Medicaid coverage rates for children in Massachusetts before and after expansion to their parents confirms these findings (Dubay and Kenney, 2002). In July 1997, Massachusetts introduced expanded coverage for parents up to 133 percent FPL, and found that not only did adult enrollment increase, but enrollment of children also increased, primarily among those already eligible (Dubay and Kenney, 2002). Researchers contrasted changes in the Medicaid coverage for children in Massachusetts before and after implementation of the family coverage with changes in Medicaid coverage for children over this period in the rest of the nation. They also contrasted changes in private coverage and in the uninsured rate in Massachusetts with comparable changes in the rest of the nation in order to assess whether the observed increases in coverage are due to reductions in the uninsured rate or to substitution of public for private coverage.

The studies to date do not explain how these program expansions to parents led to increased enrollment of children. Studies of why so many eligible children remain uninsured, however, demonstrate that parents' lack of information about the programs, confusion about eligibility, and problems associated with the enrollment process limit children's participation (Cohen and Wolfe, 2001; Kaiser Commission, 2000). When parents themselves have an opportunity to enroll, they may be more likely to learn about and more motivated to pursue coverage for both themselves and their children. The application process for publicly sponsored health insurance is often fraught with delays and barriers that may be particularly burdensome for lower-income parents. Although the process is being simplified in many states, it can still be cumbersome and humiliating (see Box 5.2).

After initial enrollment, public insurance coverage typically lasts for only one year and parents must recertify themselves and their children annually (and sometimes more frequently) to maintain coverage.[1] A survey of more than 3,700 parents in seven states shows that 34 percent of parents of current SCHIP enrollees and 44 percent of families who did not re-enroll thought that too much background paperwork, such as pay stubs or income documentation, was required for renewal (National Academy for State Health Policy et al., 2002).

Care-Seeking Behavior Within Families with Children

Finding: If parents use health care, their children are more likely to use health care as well.

Parents bring their own experiences to bear when making decisions about care for their children, and children's use of health care is highly correlated with their parents' utilization. For example, mothers with high physician use are nearly four times as likely to have children with high physician use, compared to children of mothers with low use (Newacheck, 1992). Parents who have experienced

---

[1]This situation is different from that of most employment-based insurance benefits, in which families simply select a plan type and often remain covered by default if they do nothing during the annual enrollment period.

BOX 5.2
Enrolling in Medicaid and SCHIP[1]

Applying for Medicaid or SCHIP is more difficult than enrolling in a workplace health plan, and enrollment periods are shorter. To qualify for either Medicaid or SCHIP, a child must be in a family with income below a specified level (the level may vary with the age of the child), reside in the state, and in some cases, be a citizen or have resided in the United States before a given date. As part of the application process, families need to fill out an application form and supply proof of family income, child's age, child's residence, and for some children, immigration status. Federal law requires only one document—proof of qualified alien status for individuals applying who are not citizens of the United States.[2] States determine what constitutes proof of meeting the other eligibility requirements and the information that is requested on the application form. States establish the period of enrollment and thus determine how frequently families must document eligibility. They also determine whether applicants must have a face-to-face interview or can apply by mail. Each of these administrative choices affects how burdensome the application process is for enrollees.

Most of the states have simplified enrollment in Medicaid and SCHIP: For example,

- 42 out of 51 states have lengthened the enrollment period to 12 months for Medicaid, and 33 out of 35 states with a separate SCHIP program have established eligibility periods for SCHIP at 12 months or more. This does not eliminate the requirement for families to report changes in circumstances during that period that could affect eligibility.
- In addition, 17 states have established a *guaranteed* 12-month enrollment period for Medicaid children and 11 states have this option only for children in their separate SCHIP program. This provision permits children to retain coverage for a full year, even if family income increases above the eligibility standard. (Under this 12-month guaranteed eligibility provision, families are not required to report changes in income that may occur during the 12-month period, as they are generally required to do under the typical 12-month enrollment.)
- The requirement for a "face-to-face" interview has been eliminated in 47 out of 51 states for Medicaid and 34 out of 35 for SCHIP.
- The asset test for children applying for Medicaid has been eliminated in 45 out of 51 states and 34 of the 35 separate SCHIP programs do not have an asset test.
- In states with separate SCHIP programs, 33 out of 35 have combined the Medicaid and SCHIP application into a single form. This is important because at the time of application, it may not be clear whether family income falls above or below the eligibility threshold for Medicaid and thus whether the child is eligible for Medicaid or SCHIP.

Most states no longer require documentary proof of age (e.g., birth certificate) or residence (e.g., lease). To a lesser extent (a quarter of the Medicaid programs and a third of the separate SCHIP), states are moving away from the requirement for documentary proof of income (e.g., pay stubs) if evidence of income is available elsewhere in the state's records.

---

[1] Material in this box drawn primarily from Ross and Cox, 2002.
[2] Centers for Medicare and Medicaid Services, 2001.

access problems or negative encounters with health care may have less confidence not only in obtaining care for themselves, but also for their children. Further, a parent who does not have a regular source of care or who has problems with access may also have difficulty negotiating the health care system on behalf of their children. This section looks first at studies that relate parental use of care to their children's use and then at subjective experiences with health care.

The Relationship Between Parent's Use and Children's Use

Studies conducted over the past two decades suggest that insuring children without insuring parents may not be enough to ensure that children fully benefit from their coverage. A parent's lack of connection to the health care system may be a more important barrier to care for the child than lack of insurance, as demonstrated by several large studies.

One of the early studies (Newacheck and Halfon, 1986) examined the association between mothers' and children's use of physician services using the 1978 National Health Interview Survey (NHIS) and found that mothers' use of health care was the single best predictor of children's use or nonuse and second only to the child's health status in predicting number of visits.

More recently, other studies have reexamined the link between parents' and children's health care utilization and have reached similar conclusions (Hanson, 1998; Minkovitz et al., 2002). Hanson (1998) analyzed the impact of maternal utilization separately for children with private insurance and children with no insurance, using the 1990 NHIS and found that a primary parent's use of physician services remains the most potent predictor of children's use for both uninsured and privately insured children, when other individual and family attributes are controlled. No other independent variables approached the magnitude of this effect, with the exception of measures of age and health status of the child. Both groups of children are more likely to have a physician visit if their parents do and to have more physician visits if their primary parent also has more visits. Minkovitz and colleagues (2002) used the 1996–1997 Community Tracking Study Household Survey to examine the relationship between maternal use of services and children's use and found a strong relationship for a variety of services, including physician visits, emergency department use, hospitalizations and mental health visits. These authors concluded that the strong associations suggest that patterns of maternal use are important for understanding and improving children's health care utilization.

The association between parental and children's use of care is more substantial in the privately insured group. Uninsured children whose primary parent had a physician visit were twice as likely to have had a visit themselves, whereas privately insured children were three times as likely, compared with children whose parent had no visit. This finding demonstrates that the *combination* of parental experience within the health care delivery system (measured here as at least one physician visit) and financial access for the child (measured here as private health insurance coverage) increases a child's likelihood of having a physician visit over the effect of insurance alone. Hanson (1998) concludes that even if all children were insured, parents' health care utilization would remain a key determinant in children's use of services.

Most recently, the relationship between parental insurance status and children's access to care has been evaluated. Davidoff and colleagues (2002) analyzed the NSAF 1999 data set and found that having an uninsured parent decreased the likelihood that a child would have any medical provider visit by 6.5 percentage points and the likelihood of a well-child visit by 6.7 percentage points, compared with having an insured parent. In addition, this analysis found that a parent without health insurance is less likely to have confidence in the family's ability to get medical care when needed. As would be expected, the effects of having uninsured parents are smaller than the effects of the children themselves being uninsured. Still, they add to the mounting body of evidence that links parents' well-being to that of their children.

The link between parental use of health care and the use of such care for their children possibly is established even before birth. For example, mothers receiving less-than-adequate prenatal care also take their children for well-child visits less often than do women with adequate prenatal care. Also, children of mothers with less-than-adequate prenatal care are less likely to be immunized, even after controlling for a number of important factors, including income and insurance status (Bates et al., 1994; Kogan et al., 1998a; Freed et al., 1999). Further evidence of parental attitudes affecting the care children receive is provided by a study of influenza vaccination rates for children with asthma. It found parental concern to be an important factor in whether or not such children were vaccinated (Szilagyi et al., 1992).

Experiences with the Health Care System

The experiences that parents have when seeking care can affect their decisions about health care for their children. Uninsured adults are more likely to have negative reactions to their encounters with health care institutions and providers than are insured adults. They are more likely than insured adults to rate physician care experiences more negatively and to express dissatisfaction with waiting time and time spent with physicians (Schoen and Puleo, 1998). Finally, uninsured adults are more likely to have negative experiences with the health care system related to bill paying (Duchon et al., 2001).

Racial and ethnic minority families are more likely to be dissatisfied with their experiences seeking health care and they are more likely to be uninsured than are white, non-Hispanic families. Proportionally more Hispanics, African Americans, and Asian Americans than non-Hispanic whites report that they had been treated with disrespect by the health care system. Furthermore, they report that they think they would have received better care or would have been treated with more respect were it not for their race or ethnicity, their language skills, or their ability to pay for their care. They report negative experiences with the health system more frequently than do whites (Collins et al., 2002; Doty and Ives, 2002; Hughes, 2002).[2]

Insurance coverage is an important factor contributing to improved satisfaction with care received:

• Insured Hispanic adults more often report being very satisfied with their care than do uninsured Hispanic adults (62 percent and 42 percent, respectively).
• Uninsured respondents in all racial and ethnic categories are less likely to have confidence in their ability to receive quality care than are insured respondents (35 percent compared to 51 percent) (Collins et al., 2002).

These negative experiences of minority adults may affect their attitudes and behavior in seeking care for their children.

Uninsured adults in poor health are especially likely to encounter access problems in obtaining care for themselves; they are two to three times as likely to go without needed care and are twice as likely to lack a regular source of care as healthier uninsured adults (Schoen and Puleo, 1998; Duchon et al., 2001). Uninsured adults in fair or poor health are more likely to have experienced a time without needed care than are continuously insured adults of comparable health status. Schoen and Puleo (1998) find that the worse the health status, the greater is the likelihood of access problems when insurance status is controlled in the analysis. At the same time, they found that being currently or recently uninsured at least doubles the likelihood of experiencing access problems compared to those with insurance at every level of health (Schoen and Puleo, 1998).

Conclusion

The Committee has previously shown that insured adults are more likely to have a physician visit and use other health services than are uninsured adults (IOM, 2001, 2002a). The weight of the studies just discussed suggest that neglecting financial access to care for adults may have the unintended effect of diminishing the impact of targeted health insurance programs for children. While providing health insurance to parents would not guarantee appropriate health care visits for their children, it is one potential intervention that might help.

EFFECT OF FAMILY HEALTH ON CHILD HEALTH AND WELL-BEING

The previous section demonstrates that parental insurance and use of health care may be important determinants of children's coverage and use of health care,

---

[2]Studies were based on a multilingual random national survey of more than 6,700 adults that oversampled minorities.

which suggests that providing health insurance for children is a necessary, but not sufficient, condition for ensuring appropriate health care for children.

In this section, the Committee extends the discussion of interdependencies within families beyond health insurance and health care use to health itself. Specifically, this section explores the interactions between parental health and family environment and children's health and well-being. Research in this area, too, suggests that parents are critical to the well-being of their children.

Studies to date have not addressed the role of health insurance in these larger complex family health interactions. Nonetheless, family health interdependencies should serve as a backdrop when considering health insurance policy issues. Debates around current policies, which target individuals, often lose sight of the larger family context in which the consequences of policies are actually experienced.

Parents' Health and Children's Well-Being

Finding: The health of one family member can affect the health and well-being of other family members. In particular, the health of parents can play an important role in the well-being of their children.

Finding: Parents in low-income families and families with children have higher rates of poor mental and physical health than do parents in higher-income families. There is substantial overlap between poor parental physical and mental health.

Parents in poor health may have greater difficulty attending to their children's health needs. It is easy to imagine that getting children to a doctor, getting immunizations on schedule, and coping with children's illnesses are likely to be more difficult for parents in poor health, particularly those with impaired mobility or certain mental health conditions. Parents with health insurance are more likely to receive appropriate care for their health conditions and would be expected to experience better health than they would if they lacked coverage (IOM, 2002a).

Much of the research on parental health and its effect on children addresses mental health, particularly depression in mothers. There is a growing body of evidence that parents' mental health strongly affects childrearing practices (Shonkoff and Phillips, 2000). Those parents reporting poor mental health are more likely to yell and feel frustrated with their children and less likely to read, play with, or hug their children or to establish orderly daily routines for meals, naps, and bedtime (Young et al., 1998), as shown in Figure 5.1.

Research also shows that children of depressed mothers display greater social, behavioral, and academic impairment from infancy through adolescence than do children of non-depressed mothers (Hammen et al., 1987; Downey and Coyne, 1990; Nolen-Hoeksema et al., 1995). Studies find that parental depression is reflected in the child, increasing the probability of significantly decreased social

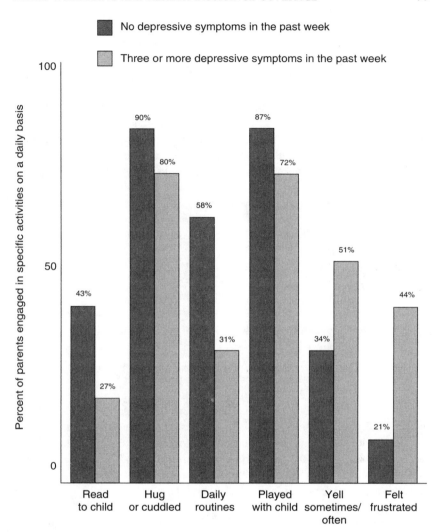

FIGURE 5.1 Depression adversely affects parents' daily child rearing practices.
NOTES: Depressive symptoms included feeling depressed, sad, or disliked, experiencing crying spells, and not finding life enjoyable. Daily routines included naps, meals, and bedtime.
SOURCE: Young et al., 1998.

competence, impaired academic performance, poor school behavior, and relatively chronic, clinically significant problems in psychosocial functioning (Anderson and Hammen, 1993), as well as significantly higher rates of affective disorder (Beardslee et al., 1993; Boyle and Pickles, 1997). In addition, parental depression increases the likelihood of negative maternal behavior and disengagement from the child.

While most research has examined the impact of poor parental health on children's health and well-being, recent studies have investigated the relationship in the other direction. These studies use poor child health as a risk factor for poor parental health (Lyons-Ruth et al., 2000). A very recent study (Bethell et al., 2002) showed this association for a group of Medicaid-insured parents. Specifically, parents of children who are in poor physical health or have special health needs are more likely to be in poor mental health themselves than are parents whose children are not in poor physical or mental health. Of parents who have a child with a special health need or in poor health, 30 percent show symptoms of depression in contrast to 18.6 percent of parents who do not have such children. Because all parents in this study were enrolled in Medicaid, it does not provide comparative information about uninsured and insured parents. Rather, it suggests that the demands on parents of caring for sick children can be severe and place parents' health at risk.

Other studies also find that when children are in poor health, their parents may be adversely affected. For example, the well-being of parents may be affected by having a child with asthma, but other family characteristics such as "coherence" and "hardiness" also play important roles (Svavarsdottir et al., 2000). Stress and negative health outcomes in parents have been found to be associated with the presence of specific chronic conditions in children (Bouma and Schweitzer, 1990; Walker et al., 1992). In low-income households with other stressors in the home, the presence of children in the home may be a contributor to poor parental mental health (Lyons-Ruth et al., 2000). Having an unhealthy child is associated with a greater likelihood that a mother will be single and thus that she and her child will face additional social and economic challenges and obstacles (Corman and Kaestner, 1992).

Studies find that the rates of poor parental health vary by income groups, with the lowest-income groups at greatest risk (Lovejoy et al., 2000). A study of first-time welfare recipients reported that 52 percent were at risk for clinical depression (Kalil et al., 2001). A number of studies and surveys have found that women with young children, those who are low income, and single mothers report high numbers of depressive symptoms (Belle, 1990; Jackson, 1992; Kahn et al., 2000; Siefert et al., 2000; Reading and Reynolds, 2001). It is unclear the extent to which poverty and its related economic effects might contribute to clinical depression in parents, the extent to which depression in parents might limit their earnings, and the impact of health insurance on these circumstances.

The National Survey of American Families also shows high levels of poor physical and mental health, particularly among parents of children at the lowest income levels.[3] One-third of parents with family incomes below 100 percent

TABLE 5.1 Percentage of Parents in Poor Physical and Mental Health Across Income Ranges

Parents	<100% FPL n = 4,889	100-200% FPL n = 7,692	>200% FPL n = 21,651
Fair or poor physical health	27.2	14.6[a]	5.9[a]
Poor mental health	33.1	16.8[a]	10.1
Very poor mental health	22.3	10.8[a]	5.5[a]

[a] $p < .001$.
SOURCE: Analysis of 1999 National Survey of American Families data conducted by Gerry Fairbrother.

FPL report symptoms of poor mental health and more than one-quarter (27 percent) describe their physical health as fair or poor (see Table 5.1). In fact, only 37 percent of parents below 100 percent FPL say that their physical health is either "excellent" or "very good." (This is the income band at which most of the Medicaid expansions that include parents are targeted.) Parents with family incomes between 100 and 200 percent FPL and proportionally more of those with incomes above 200 percent FPL report better physical and mental health than do those in families with incomes below 100 percent FPL. Only 10 percent of parents in the highest-income group and 17 percent of those from 100 to 200 percent FPL report symptoms of poor mental health compared with 33 percent of those in families with incomes below 100 percent FPL.

The physical and mental health of parents serving as the primary child caregiver is related. Forty-three (43) percent of caregivers with poor physical health reported poor mental health as well. Adding together the percentage of caregivers with *either* poor physical *or* poor mental health yields 42 percent of caregivers in families with incomes below 100 percent FPL, compared to 23 percent within families with incomes at 100–200 percent FPL and 10 percent in families with incomes above 200 percent FPL.

The impact of health insurance for either parent or child on the psychological well-being of the other has not been studied. Thus, conclusions about the degree to which health insurance coverage could improve family members' psychological well-being cannot be drawn based on the research conducted so far. However, the Committee's previous report, *Care Without Coverage*, concluded that health insurance was associated with better physical and mental health outcomes for working-age Americans and that adults who do not have health insurance suffer diminished health and experience reduced life expectancy. In addition, the Committee found that having any health insurance, even if it does not specifically cover

---

[3]Analysis of 1999 NSAF data conducted by Gerry Fairbrother, Genevieve Kenney, and Lisa Dubay.

mental health services, increases the likelihood that an adult with a condition such as depression or anxiety will receive some care for that condition (IOM, 2002a). The separate strands of research regarding health interactions among family members and the potential of health insurance to ameliorate these are promising and warrant further investigation.

The Family Environment

> **Finding: Family stress may adversely affect the health of its members and is associated with higher levels of behavioral and emotional problems in children. Lower-income families tend to have higher levels of stress than higher-income families.**

> **Finding: There is some very limited evidence that having health insurance for children may reduce the amount of family stress, enable children to get the care they need, and ease some family burdens.**

Some researchers have moved beyond the health of the parents to examine the health of the family environment and its impact on child well-being (Shonkoff and Phillips, 2000). These researchers have identified linkages between stress in families and adverse physical and psychological effects on children and adolescents (Garmezy, 1983; Johnson, 1986; Compas, 1987).[4] Moore and Vandivere (2000) show that family stress affects the level of children's engagement in their schoolwork and that it is also associated with higher levels of behavioral and emotional problems for both children and youth. Although Moore and Vandivere do not address the possibility of children's behavior or school problems causing family stress, their findings are consistent with other research indicating that maternal psychological distress and high family stress are associated with greater behavioral problems among children (Myers et al., 1992; Resnick et al., 1993). Yager (1982) describes the possible role of family stress patterns in the development of anorexia nervosa in adolescents, and other studies show an association between family stress and the use of mental health services among children (Verhulst and van der Ende 1997). It would be reasonable to expect that families with children suffering the ill effects of stress and in need of mental health services would have easier access to them if their children were insured. This has not been directly examined in empirical studies, however.

Families with incomes below 200 percent FPL experience more stress than do

---

[4]The Committee uses "stress" in its broad, conventional sense, as any kind of mental, emotional, or physical tension or strain. These researchers have operationalized stress in families variously as potentially threatening or challenging situations or specific circumstances to be measured, such as the presence of marital discord, low social and economic status, overcrowding, paternal criminality, and maternal psychiatric disorder.

higher-income families.[5] Forty percent of children in families with incomes below 200 percent FPL live in stressful environments, in contrast to 22 percent of all children (Moore and Vandivere, 2000). Echoing the link between parental health and child well-being, other studies show the effect of family stress on the physical health and well-being of children. Specifically, studies show that high levels of family stress are associated with the poor metabolic control of diabetes in children and adolescents (Viner et al., 1996) and that family stress may play an important role in the development of coronary risk in children (Weidner et al., 1992). The connections between family stress and difficulties for parents in providing good home environments for their children are evident (Straus et al., 1980; Cole and Cole, 1993).

Family stress has many varied dimensions, and health policies may have at least the potential for ameliorating some of them. For example, parents report that having health insurance for their children reduces the amount of family stress, enables children to get the care they need, and eases family burdens (Lave et al., 1998a). Dubay and Kenney (2001) report that parental confidence that family members can obtain needed care is strongest when all family members are insured. There are still too few studies examining the relationship between family stress and health insurance coverage to support definitive conclusions. Nevertheless, the recent studies provide good reason to assess a broader array of phenomena and indicators of personal and familial well-being in considering the effects of the lack of health insurance than has been customary in health services research.

SUMMARY

A family encompasses an array of social, economic, and emotional relationships that are not well studied by health services and health policy researchers. Research that addresses discrete aspects of health, care-seeking behavior, and well-being within families suggests, however, that having the whole family covered by health insurance is important. Because parents are the key decision makers and seekers of care for their children, their own connections to the health care system are important for their children as well as for themselves.

If parents are insured they are more likely to have insured children than are uninsured parents. Medicaid and SCHIP have not yet fulfilled their considerable potential for reducing uninsurance among American children. Some states have found that expanding eligibility for parents is an effective way to promote enrollment of eligible children in Medicaid and SCHIP.

Insured adults have better access to the health care system and are more likely to use services than are uninsured adults. In addition, insured adults are less likely to have unmet health needs, have their health deteriorate, and die prematurely

---

[5]The index of stress uses economic hardship, crowding, and family member health status as components.

than are uninsured adults. Studies show that a mother's use of health services is a strong predictor of her child's use of care. Being uninsured can affect one's attitudes toward and use of the health care system, and for parents this has implications for their children.

Healthier parents are better able to care for their children and have better child rearing practices. The illness of a parent, particularly depression, is associated with poorer psychosocial functioning of the child. The Committee previously found that health insurance is associated with more appropriate care for conditions such as depression.

Stress in the family environment, particularly at higher levels, is associated with physical and behavioral health problems for the children. Lower-income parents are more likely to report higher levels of stress than are parents with higher incomes. Parents also report that having health insurance for their children reduces stress.

Many factors contribute to the health and stability of families. Health insurance is one important factor. Recent studies examining the relationship between family stress and health insurance coverage are suggestive and argue for a more systematic assessment of the impact of health insurance on a broad array of indicators of personal and familial well-being. Providing health insurance to all members of a family is one intervention that could improve the health not only of those who gain coverage but also, through the interdependence of the health and activities of family members, of others in the family as well.

BOX 5.3
Summary of Findings

• Extension of publicly supported health insurance options to low-income uninsured parents can have the additional benefit of increasing enrollment of their children.

• Uninsured parents have poorer health, have poorer access to the health care system, are less satisfied with the care they receive when they gain access, and are more likely to have negative experiences related to bill collection compared with insured parents.

• Parents' use of health care is a powerful predictor of children's use of health care services.

• The health of one family member can affect the health and well-being of other family members. In particular, the health of parents can play an important role in the well-being of their children.

• Parents in low-income families and families with children have higher rates of poor mental and physical health than do parents in higher-income families. There is substantial overlap between poor parental physical and mental health.

• Family stress may adversely affect the health of its members and is associated with higher levels of behavioral and emotional problems in children. Lower-income families tend to have higher levels of stress than higher-income families.

• There is some very limited evidence that having health insurance for children may reduce the amount of family stress, enable children to get the care they need, and ease some family burdens.

BOX 6.1
Summary of Findings

- Uninsured children have less access to health care, are less likely to have a regular source of primary care, and use medical and dental care less often compared with children who have insurance. Children with gaps in health insurance coverage have worse access than do those with continuous coverage.
- Previously uninsured children experience significant increases in both access to and more appropriate use of health care services following their enrollment in public health insurance programs.
- Lower-income, minority, non-citizen, or uninsured children consistently have worse access and utilization than do children with none of these characteristics. These factors overlap to a large extent. However, each exerts its own independent effect on access and utilization.
- Uninsured adolescents are more likely to lack a regular source of care and have unmet health needs than are insured adolescents.
- Uninsured children with special health care needs are more likely than those who have insurance coverage to be without a usual source of health care, to have gone without seeing a doctor in the last 12 months, and to be unable to get needed medical, dental, vision, and mental health care and prescriptions.
- Uninsured children often receive care late in the development of a health problem or do not receive any care. As a result, they are at higher risk for hospitalization for conditions amenable to timely outpatient care and for missed diagnoses of serious and even life-threatening conditions.
- Undiagnosed and untreated conditions that are amenable to control, cure, or prevention can affect children's functioning and opportunities over the course of their lives. Such conditions include iron deficiency anemia, otitis media, asthma, and attention deficit–hyperactivity disorder.
- Uninsured women receive fewer prenatal care services than their insured counterparts and report greater difficulty in obtaining the care that they believe they need. Studies find large differences in use between privately insured and uninsured women and smaller differences between uninsured and publicly insured women.
- Health insurance status affects the care received by women giving birth and their newborns. Uninsured women and their newborns receive, on average, less prenatal care and fewer expensive perinatal services.
- Uninsured newborns are more likely to have adverse outcomes, including low birth weight and death, than are insured newborns. Evidence of improvements in outcomes for newborns as a result of increased population health insurance rates is inconclusive, however.
- Uninsured women are more likely to have poor outcomes during pregnancy and delivery than are women with insurance. Studies have not demonstrated an improvement in maternal outcomes related to health insurance alone.

6

Health-Related Outcomes for Children, Pregnant Women, and Newborns

This chapter examines clinical and epidemiological evidence about the effects of health insurance status on the health of children, pregnant women, and newborns.[1] It extends the assessment of health outcomes that the Committee presented in *Care Without Coverage* to pediatric and pregnancy-related care and outcomes. It places this analysis within the broader context of family interests, behavior, and constraints of this report because, as demonstrated in the previous chapter, children's access to and use of health care is highly dependent on their parents' opportunities and actions. The financially constrained patterns of use by uninsured families, as documented in Chapter 4, can affect the overall health and development of their members, particularly of children. Table 6.1 summarizes the health insurance status of American children by age, race and ethnicity, and family income.

The Committee reviewed studies that compare the access to and use of health care services by insured and uninsured children, pregnant women, and newborns as well as research that relates their insurance status to health outcomes.[2] Only

---

[1]Many studies classify people age 18 and under as children, conforming to the federal Medicaid eligibility standard definition of children; others, however, are based on national surveys that classify people age 17 and under as children. The American Academy of Pediatrics considers people up to age 21 children.

[2]The review draws on studies identified in a MEDLINE search of the English language literature published between 1985 and September 2001. The search terms included "insurance status," "insurance, longitudinal," "insurance, cohort," "uninsured, longitudinal," "uninsured, cohort," "payer status," "payer source," "medically indigent," and "uncompensated care." Studies with fewer than 250 participants, those with unadjusted results, and those from a single institution were excluded, unless broader studies of a particular outcome were unavailable or limited. In addition, more recent

TABLE 6.1 Number of Uninsured Children by Age, Race or Ethnicity, and Family Income, 2000, United States

	Total Number (millions)	Total Uninsured[a] (millions)	Percent Uninsured
All children	72.6	8.4	11.6
Age			
Under 3 years	11.9	1.3	11.3
3–5 years	11.8	1.3	10.8
6–11 years	24.8	2.8	11.5
12–17 years	24.1	2.9	12.2
Race or ethnicity			
Non-Hispanic white	45.4	3.3	7.3
Black	11.6	1.6	13.5
Asian and Pacific Islander	3.1	0.4	14.3
Hispanic origin	12.0	3.0	24.9
Family income			
0–99% FPL	12.2	2.7	22.1
100–149% FPL	7.7	1.5	19.5
150–199% FPL	7.6	1.1	14.5
200% FPL and over	45.0	3.1	6.9

NOTE: FPL = federal poverty level.

[a]The Current Population Survey (CPS) defines uninsured as having no form of health insurance during an entire calendar year.

SOURCES: Census Bureau, CPS Annual Demographic Survey, March Supplement, 2001, Table HI08. Available at: http://ferret.bls.census.gov/macro/032001/health/h08_000.htm. Accessed April 21, 2002; and Fronstin, 2001.

studies that the Committee judged methodologically sound are presented in this chapter. Additional studies reviewed by the Committee and the Subcommittee are included in Appendix C.

Opportunities for low and lower-income children and pregnant women to obtain coverage through public health insurance programs have increased substantially over the past one and a half decades. Many of the studies reviewed in this chapter are evaluations of these program expansions. Others of the studies of access, use and health outcomes pre-date most of these expansions. The Committee believes that the general patterns of utilization and outcomes that are reported for insured and uninsured children, pregnant women and infants remain valid even as

journal articles and unpublished studies brought to the Committee's attention by experts were included if they met the other criteria mentioned above. Appendix C provides brief descriptions of all the studies that met the review criteria.

the relative proportions of insured and uninsured populations have shifted over time.

Appropriate health care interventions for children and pregnant women have been related to educational achievement, exit from welfare or social services, and ultimate employment—all outcomes that extend well beyond traditional health. For children, using health care services routinely and appropriately is considered a positive health outcome in its own right because well-child care is a practice grounded in evidence of its effectiveness in enhancing longer-term health and development. Early intervention, even in the face of severe physical or mental problems, often can minimize long-term health and developmental problems and thus can benefit society overall. Without opportunities for health and developmental assessments, particularly with an ongoing source of care, problems go undetected and children may suffer consequences that limit their life chances in both obvious and less evident ways. Before birth, good prenatal care also provides opportunities to ensure the best possible health for both mother and child. To the extent that having health insurance can remove access barriers and foster timely assessments of development and health, the health of children measured on a population-wide basis will improve.

Of course, health insurance is not the only factor influencing use of health care, and use of health care is but one of many factors that influence health outcomes. For example, poverty, presence of chronic disease, socioeconomic status, educational attainment (and, for children, their parents' educational attainment), and health-related behaviors such as diet, exercise, drug use, and smoking may affect utilization and outcomes as much as health insurance status (Szilagyi and Schor, 1998). Figure 1.1 in Chapter 1 depicts the multiple factors and characteristics that relate health insurance to access, use, and outcomes. A full discussion of the conceptual framework that depicts the relationships among personal characteristics, health care, and outcomes is presented in Appendix A.

Ideally, to answer the question, Does health insurance enhance health status?, one would perform a true experiment, in which some individuals would be randomly assigned to receive insurance and others not. Because of the ethical and practical obstacles to conducting a health insurance experiment that leaves some participants uninsured, none have been conducted.[3] Instead, most of the evidence for the effect of insurance on health outcomes is based on observational studies of insured and uninsured individuals. A few studies with quasi-experimental designs

---

[3]The notable exception to this generalization is the RAND Health Insurance Experiment, conducted between 1974 and 1982, which randomly assigned roughly 2,000 families in six different sites to one of 14 experimental health insurance plans that varied in their cost-sharing arrangements. Cost sharing ranged from none in the free care plan to 95 percent for all health services, limited to a maximum of $1,000 per family per year (in then-current dollars) with reduced amounts for low-income families (Keeler et al., 1985; Newhouse et al., 1993). The study was designed so that no participating family could be made worse off as a result of its participation than if it had not participated. This social experiment did not, however, include a study group without any health insurance at all.

have been conducted within the past decade and a half. These so-called natural experiments are ones in which

- a population of children or pregnant women gains coverage because of policy changes (e.g., as a result of increases in the Medicaid income eligibility standard or the introduction of the State Children's Health Insurance Program [SCHIP]) allowing comparisons of access, use, and outcomes before and after coverage policy changes; or
- differences in income eligibility levels among state Medicaid programs provide an opportunity to evaluate the impact of the different levels.

These quasi-experimental studies allow for greater confidence in the validity of their results than do cross-sectional studies that rely on analytic controls for characteristics that co-vary with health insurance status.[4]

Other factors that can influence health outcomes, such as income, educational attainment, race and ethnicity, or immigrant status, often coincide with lack of insurance. This report relies on studies that account for these factors with analytic adjustments that isolate the effects of health insurance status. Studies report adjusted statistics (e.g., odds ratios [ORs][5]) that account for such characteristics as family income, race or ethnicity, age, gender, and sometimes health status. Quantified study results are presented only if they are statistically significant at the conventional $p = 0.05$ level or at higher significance levels, unless otherwise noted.

The first section of this chapter reviews the link between children's health insurance status and their access to and appropriate use of services. The second section presents empirical studies that examine specific health outcomes for children and youth as related to coverage status. The third section reviews longer-term adverse outcomes for children's health and development for specific conditions that have not been studied in terms of their relationship to health insurance status that merit further investigation. The fourth and last section assesses the evidence regarding the relationship between pre- and perinatal care and birth outcomes for mothers and infants.

---

[4]See Chapter 2 of *Care Without Coverage* (IOM, 2002a) for a fuller discussion of methodological issues.

[5]The odds ratio is the relative odds of having an outcome in the uninsured and insured groups. For example, if the odds of receiving an immunization are 2:1 in a group of uninsured children (i.e., two out of every three children, or 67 percent, receive the immunization) and the odds are 4:1 in a group of children with insurance (i.e., four out of every five children, or 80 percent, receive the immunization), the odds ratio for uninsured compared to insured children is 0.5 (2:1/4:1). The OR is not a good estimate of the relative risk (the probability of being immunized in the uninsured group divided by the probability of being immunized in the insured group) because immunization is not a rare event.

ACCESS TO AND USE OF HEALTH CARE BY CHILDREN

Access is most simply understood as the ability to see a physician or other health care provider when one wants to do so. Access and use of health care services are closely connected. A child without good access is expected to have a harder time using care and thus expected to have fewer visits and more unmet needs than one with good access to care. Research examining the impact of insurance on access employs a variety of measures, such as whether a child or pregnant woman has a regular source of care or a "medical home," a usual physician within a regular place of care (i.e., a medical home), ability to obtain care outside of normal business hours, a regular dentist (for children), and unmet health needs or delays in care due to cost.[6] Measurement of utilization has two aspects, the number of visits and the appropriate use of health care services (e.g., receipt of indicated services on a timely basis or inappropriate use of emergency departments as the site of primary care). Empirical studies support the link between access to care, use, and improved health outcomes (Bindman et al., 1995; Starfield, 1995; Hadley, 2002; IOM, 2002a).

Finding: Uninsured children have less access to health care, are less likely to have a regular source of primary care, and use medical and dental care less often compared to children who have insurance. Children with gaps in health insurance coverage have worse access than do those with continuous coverage.

Studies using databases with national probability samples, such as the National Health Insurance Survey (NHIS), the Medical Expenditure Panel Survey (MEPS), and the National Survey of America's Families (NSAF), consistently report that uninsured children have poorer access to health care and use health services less frequently than their insured counterparts. Insurance status remains a significant factor even after studies control for income, race and ethnicity, and health status.

Children with health insurance are more likely to have a usual source of health care than uninsured children. A study based on the 1993–1994 NHIS reported an odds ratio of 6.1 between insured and uninsured children's likelihood of having a usual source of care (Newacheck et al., 1998b).[7] Among those

---

[6]The American Academy of Pediatrics (AAP) characterizes a "medical home" for infants, children, and adolescents as one that provides continuous, comprehensive, family-centered, coordinated, and compassionate care delivered by well-trained physicians known to the child and family who are able to develop a relationship of mutual responsibility and trust with them (AAP, Medical Home Statement. Available at: http:www/aap.org. Accessed December 28, 2001).

[7]Health insurance is not the only factor in parental decision-making on whether to develop a relationship with a health care provider for their children. An analysis of the 1996 MEPS reports that parents of children who did not have a regular source of care give as the main reasons, that the child is seldom or never sick (66 percent) and, that they cannot afford one (10 percent) (Weinick et al., 1998). Financial reasons do, however, constitute the main barriers to receiving care perceived as needed.

children whose parents reported having a usual site of care, uninsured children were more likely to lack a regular physician and to be unable to obtain medical care after normal business hours. Uninsured children were also more likely than those with insurance to go without care that parents reported they needed (OR = 5.8), to go without any dental care (OR = 4.3), and more likely to have had no contact with a physician during the previous year (OR = 2.1) (Newacheck et al., 1998b). Not surprisingly, the parents of uninsured children were more likely to be dissatisfied with at least some aspect of their child's care. This comprehensive survey analysis adjusted for age, sex, race, family income, family structure and size, region of the country, population density, and health status. These results confirmed those of an earlier study using 1988 NHIS data. Holl and colleagues (1995) reported that uninsured children were more likely than those with insurance *never* to have had a regular source of care (OR = 1.8) and more likely not to meet standards of timeliness for well-child visits (OR = 1.3). Furthermore, uninsured children were more likely to obtain routine and sick care from different sources than were insured children (Holl et al., 1995).

Uninsured children are less likely to have received medical care for common childhood illnesses than are children with health insurance. In a study based on the 1987 National Medical Expenditure Survey (NMES), uninsured children were significantly less likely to visit a physician for pharyngitis, acute earache, recurrent ear infection or asthma, conditions for which medical attention is usually considered necessary (ORs = 1.7, 1.85, 2.1, 1.7, respectively) (Stoddard et al., 1994). The uninsured child's worse odds remained despite extensive sociodemographic and health status adjustments.

Most studies combine both children with private and children with public insurance into a single "insured" category. The impact of insurance on access and utilization differs depending on whether it is private or public insurance, with better access and higher use rates among those with private insurance.[8] However, children with no insurance still have the worst measures of access and utilization, below those of publicly insured poor children. Although not all of the differences in access and use among children of differing health insurance status are due to their coverage status, these differences are pronounced.

Children with private insurance have considerably more medical office visits, dental visits, and filled prescriptions than do both children who have public insurance and those who are uninsured. An analysis of 1996 MEPS data shows the following differences in the use of any service within a year for

---

Among families who reported difficulty in obtaining care or a delay in getting care, 60 percent cited their inability to afford the care as the main reason (Weinick et al., 1998).

[8]See pp. 34 and 100–101 of the Committee's report *Care Without Coverage* for discussions of the factors contributing to systematic differences in use and outcome findings for adults insured by Medicaid and private coverage (IOM, 2002a).

- physician office visits (76, 67, and 51 percent for privately insured, publicly insured, and uninsured children, respectively);
- dental visits (50, 29, and 21 percent, respectively); and
- prescriptions filled (61, 56, and 43 percent, respectively) (McCormick et al., 2001).

Despite being the least likely to have a regular source of care, uninsured children on average receive less care from emergency departments than do children with any kind of coverage (McCormick et al., 2001). Hospitalizations and emergency department visits are highest for children with public insurance, possibly reflecting inadequate access to other ambulatory care providers. Publicly insured children are hospitalized at more than twice the rate of the privately insured and uninsured (5.4, versus 2.4 and 1.9 percent with any hospital stay for publicly insured, privately insured, and uninsured, respectively). Emergency department visits are also highest for the publicly insured (15.5, versus 12.5 and 10.8 percent with a visit for publicly insured, privately insured, and uninsured, respectively) (McCormick et al., 2001).

Finding: Previously uninsured children experience significant increases in both access to and more appropriate use of health care services following their enrollment in public health insurance programs.

Studies that have evaluated Medicaid program expansions since the mid-1980s and, more recently, children's health insurance demonstrations that preceded SCHIP conclude that increased eligibility for and enrollment in public programs results in greater and more appropriate use of health services among children. Between 1984 and 1992, the first period of expansions in Medicaid eligibility and enrollment, Currie and Gruber (1996b) analyzed National Health Interview Survey (NHIS) data as a function of state Medicaid eligibility standards and found that eligibility for Medicaid was associated across the child population with reducing the likelihood that a child would go without any physician visit within a year by half. They also found an association between increases in Medicaid eligibility at the state level and reductions in child mortality after the first year of life.

A second study by Currie (2000) that used NHIS data from 1989 to 1992 (prior to the enactment of Medicaid restrictions on eligibility for immigrants) to compare the effects of Medicaid eligibility on insurance coverage and use of services between children of U.S.-born and immigrant parents found that the effects of increased Medicaid eligibility on utilization of ambulatory care were twice as great for the children of immigrants, whose average use of physician services was lower, as for children of U.S.-born parents. As discussed later in this chapter, a national study of Medicaid eligibility expansions between 1983 and 1996 concluded that these expansions reduced potentially avoidable hospitalizations among children (Dafny and Gruber, 2000).

Enactment of SCHIP in 1997, with implementation beginning the next year, provided the opportunity for states to insure children at higher family income levels than those established for Medicaid. States vary in how much they raised the income eligibility threshold for public health insurance, but expansion to 200 percent FPL was most common. Studies of the earliest state demonstration programs in two states, New York and Pennsylvania, report a significant increase in both access and utilization for previously uninsured children after receipt of health insurance.

The New York program evaluation involved an examination of the state as a whole (Szilagyi et al., 2000c) as well as a focused study on six upstate counties (Rodewald et al., 1997; Holl et al., 2000; Szilagyi et al., 2000a, 2000b). In both cases, the researchers compared children's health care use and health outcomes for the year before they entered the New York program to those for the first year after enrollment. A study of a similar program in 29 counties in western Pennsylvania also used a before-and-after design (and also had a comparison group of later enrollees) and surveyed newly enrolled children at 6 and 12 months following enrollment (Lave et al., 1998a).

The findings of these three evaluations consistently show that the newly insured children had increased access to a medical home, paving the way for more timely and appropriate care and greater satisfaction with services. In Pennsylvania, 12 months after enrollment, 99 percent of the children had a regular source of medical care and 85 percent had a regular dentist, up from 89 and 60 percent, respectively, at baseline. Further, the proportion of children reporting any unmet need or delayed medical care in the previous six months decreased from 57 percent at baseline to 16 percent at 12 months (Lave et al., 1998a). The proportion of children with any physician visit increased from 59 to 64 percent, accompanied by a 5 percentage point decrease in the proportion with an emergency room visit, from 22 percent to 17 percent (Lave et al., 1998a). The proportion of children seeing a dentist increased from 40 percent at enrollment to 65 percent after 12 months (Lave et al., 1998a). Because the separate comparison group of later-enrolling children were similar to those initially enrolling, these changes over time in the insured group can be attributed to the coverage with greater confidence.

In New York State, enrollment in the state insurance program also reduced the number of children without a medical home (from 5 percent before the expansion to 1 percent after enrollment), and one in three parents of newly insured children reported improved quality of care for their children (Szilagyi et al., 2000c). Visits to primary care physicians for preventive, acute, and total care increased markedly (up by 25, 52, and 42 percent, respectively). Visits to specialists following enrollment more than doubled from before enrollment. Emergency department (ED) use did not change significantly, but hospitalization declined by 36 percent statewide (Szilagyi et al., 2000c). In the upstate program, the parents of one-quarter of the enrolled children reported that their children's health had improved as a result of the coverage (Holl et al., 2000).

Tracking specific services and childhood conditions also reveals changes in access and use. For example, throughout New York, use of public health departments for immunizations decreased by 67 percent after implementation of the program, with more immunizations delivered in the medical home during the period of expanded coverage (Rodewald et al., 1997). The upstate evaluation reported that visits to medical homes increased for children with chronic conditions (from 5.7 to 7.1 visits annually), a sign of better care (Szilagyi et al., 2000b). The impact of insurance status on one chronic condition, asthma, was also documented. Following enrollment in the insurance program, parents perceived that their child's severity level and quality of care for asthma had improved, and about half of these parents reported that their asthmatic child's overall health had improved as a result of the program services (Szilagyi et al., 2000a). Primary care visits increased following enrollment; with no significant changes in ED or hospital use for asthma care, suggesting increased access to ambulatory services for these children. The authors hypothesize that uninsured children with asthma who gained health insurance coverage were more likely to receive care both for acute exacerbations of their conditions and for routine services because of reduced financial barriers (Szilagyi et al., 2000a).

The results of these program evaluations suggest that the nation's near-poor children will likely benefit from the recently implemented SCHIP program. The Pennsylvania study did not focus on the urban population, and although the New York statewide study did include New York City and both urban and rural regions throughout the state, low-income urban populations were still underrepresented. Because the problems of poverty and lack of insurance may be distinctive for residents of large cities, the effects of insurance program expansion within major metropolitan areas may be even greater than those noted in the early demonstration programs. For example, the portion of children lacking a medical home in New York City was more than twice that of the state as a whole (11 percent versus 5 percent prior to expansion), and many of the access measures improved most in New York City, where baseline levels of access had been the poorest (Szilagyi et al., 2000c).

In examining children's health insurance expansions and anticipating the impact of SCHIP, it is important to keep in mind that children enrolled in SCHIP are from families with higher income than children enrolled in Medicaid and may have different characteristics and respond to insurance and health care differently. One study based on 1993–1994 NHIS data suggests that SCHIP-eligible children have markedly different socioeconomic and health status characteristics than either Medicaid or privately insured children (Byck, 2000). SCHIP-eligible children more often live with college-educated and employed adults than do Medicaid-eligible children, but less often than privately insured children. SCHIP-eligible children are more likely to be in excellent health than Medicaid children but also are twice as likely to be in fair or poor health than privately insured children (Byck, 2000).

Interactions and Covariance of Race and Ethnicity, Income, Immigrant Status, and Health Insurance

Finding: Lower-income, minority, non-citizen, or uninsured children consistently have worse access and utilization than do children with none of these characteristics. These factors overlap to a large extent. However, each exerts its own independent effect on access and utilization.

The finding that lower-income, minority, and uninsured children have worse access to and lower use of health care services than other children is well established (Newacheck et al., 2000a; Weinick et al., 2000; McCormick et al, 2001). Further, there is high overlap between poverty, minority status, and lack of insurance. Among children in one of these at-risk groups, 40 percent also belong to other at-risk groups (Newacheck et al., 1996).

This high degree of overlap among risk groups means that results from studies on the impact of gaining insurance must be interpreted with caution. For example, when it is found that poor children have fewer physician visits, this result could be attributable partly to lack of insurance but also to the interplay of other characteristics (e.g., a parent's inability to take time off from work or a different conception of the value of medical attention for certain kinds of health problems). The results presented in the preceding sections examine the effect of insurance on access and use that are isolated analytically from the effects of income and race or ethnicity. These adjustments help to measure the impact of health insurance status alone. However, more information would be helpful about the effect on utilization for a child who is *both* uninsured *and* a member of a minority group or who is uninsured *and* poor.

Because these risk factors exert independent effects on access and utilization, children who are members of more than one at-risk group (e.g., African American and uninsured; poor and uninsured) tend to have even more difficulty using medical services than do children who are members of only one at-risk group.

Using 1987 NMES data, researchers report that with few exceptions, being low income (below 100 percent FPL), a member of a minority racial or ethnic group, or uninsured is each independently and significantly related to six different measures of access to or use of primary care (Newacheck et al., 1996). When compared with the reference group of children who are white, not low income, and *in*sured, children in each of these at-risk groups are less likely to have a usual source of care and more likely to not see a specific physician even if they have a usual source of care. They are also more likely to wait 60 minutes or more at their sites of care and more likely to go without after-hours emergency care. Uninsured children are least likely to have a usual source of care than the reference group (OR = 0.47), while low-income and minority children are least likely to see a consistent physician within their care site and are most likely to wait a long time for care at their care site (Newacheck et al., 1996).

Dubay and Kenney (2001) investigated differences in access and use for insured and uninsured children below 200 percent of FPL, a group of special interest because it is the target population for Medicaid and SCHIP. In a cross-sectional analysis with extensive sociodemographic and health status adjustments, they found that lower-income children (in families with income less than 200 percent FPL) who have no insurance had significantly worse access to care and lower utilization than either lower-income children insured privately or those who had Medicaid coverage. Uninsured, lower-income children were more likely to have no usual source of care or to use the emergency department as a usual source of care, and to postpone or forgo medical, surgical, and dental care. Their families were less confident about their ability to obtain needed care and less satisfied with whatever care they did receive. In this study, children insured by Medicaid and private plans had similar access measures (i.e., reporting a regular source of care or delays in care) (Dubay and Kenney, 2001).

Race–Ethnicity and Income

Racial and ethnic disparities in access to health care actually increased between 1977 and 1996, particularly for Hispanic Americans (Weinick et al., 2000). Black and Hispanic children are substantially less likely to have a usual source of care than are white, non-Hispanic children, after controlling for health insurance and socioeconomic status (Weinick and Krauss, 2000). Controlling for language, however, eliminates differences between Hispanic and white non-Hispanic children, suggesting that differences in access may be related to English language fluency. The differences between black and white non-Hispanic children remain.

Low-income children of any race are more likely to experience access problems than those with family incomes above the federal poverty level. Newacheck and colleagues (2000a) used NHIS data spanning 1993 to 1996 to examine unmet health needs of America's children under age 18.[9] They found that overall, 7.3 percent of U.S. children (an estimated 4.7 million) experience at least one unmet health care need, but both children below 100 percent FPL and those with family incomes between 100 and 200 percent FPL were more likely to have an unmet need (medical, dental, medication, or vision) than were higher income children, after controlling for health insurance status.

---

[9]The NHIS for the years covered by this analysis included supplemental questions on unmet health needs. Questions about medical care, dental care, prescription drugs, and eyeglasses were posed to respondents (including parents on behalf of their children) in the following form: During the past twelve months, was there any time that someone in the family needed [e.g., dental] care but could not get it? (Newacheck et al., 2000a).

Immigrant Children

Immigrant children have a high risk of being uninsured and face additional barriers to care resulting from language and cultural differences. Parents' unfamiliarity with U.S. health care, attitudes about accepting public benefits, and fears of challenges to their immigration status all deter immigrants from seeking care for themselves and their children. About 54 percent of non-citizen children with non-citizen parents are uninsured (Ku and Matani, 2001). The Institute of Medicine–National Research Council Committee on the Health and Adjustment of Immigrant Children and Families concluded that health care for children in immigrant families benefits both from insurance coverage and from families' efforts to establish an ongoing connection with the health care system, as is the case for all children (Hernandez and Charney, 1998).

Only 66 percent of foreign-born children of lower-income working families have access to a regular source of care compared with 92 percent of lower-income U.S.-born children (Guendelman et al., 2001). U.S.-born children of immigrants with no regular source of care and no insurance are the least likely to have seen a physician (Hernandez and Charney, 1998). Immigrants are particularly reliant on safety-net health care providers (Ku and Freilich, 2001).

Differences persist between the health care utilization patterns of immigrant children and those of children of citizens, but disparities are less when only those children in both of these groups who have health insurance are compared. Whereas 43 percent of uninsured immigrant children reported having had no physician visit within the previous 12 months in 1996, the comparable proportion was 28 percent for immigrant children with private coverage and 16 percent for those with Medicaid (Brown et al., 1999).

Special Issues for Adolescents

Finding: Uninsured adolescents are more likely to lack a regular source of care and have unmet health needs than are insured adolescents.

Just as access and use are declining, adolescents encounter new and challenging health care needs. Specifically, reproductive health needs may come into play as many high school students report being sexually active. The need for mental health screening and treatment increases as depression, exposure to violence, and risky behaviors including substance abuse rise. Trips to the emergency department tend to double from the preteen to older adolescent years. The seeds of many behaviors that can lead to chronic diseases—obesity, hypertension, diabetes—are set during this formative period (NCHS, 2000). Finally, late adolescence may be the last time for several years that some youths have ready access to regular care within a medical home because more than a quarter of young adults age 18–25 (7.3 million) are uninsured (Mills, 2001).

McCormick and colleagues (2001) report that as age increases, the percentage of children with any office visits generally declines. Adolescents ages 15 to 17 years have the highest uninsured rate of all children (17 percent), due in part to the age-related income eligibility standards in Medicaid (McCormick et al., 2001). In addition to the risk of increasing age, adolescents with minority status, with lower family income, or who live with a single parent have a greater likelihood of being uninsured (Lieu et al., 1993; Newacheck et al., 1999). Higher proportions of African-American and Hispanic adolescents than white non-Hispanics are uninsured (16 and 28 versus 11 percent, respectively) (Lieu et al., 1993).

Older adolescents' risk of being uninsured increases markedly with decreasing family income. Among 16–17-year-olds in families with incomes less than 100 percent of the FPL, 38 percent are uninsured; among those in families with incomes in the range of 100–200 percent FPL, 29 percent are uninsured, whereas just 7 percent of adolescents in higher-income families are uninsured.

The percentage of uninsured teens who do not have a health care visit within a year is 2.6 times higher than that for insured teens (NCHS, 2000). Compared with their insured counterparts, uninsured adolescents are substantially less likely to have a regular source of care (71 percent versus 96 percent) or to have had contact with a physician during the course of the past year (75 percent versus 90 percent) (Newacheck et al., 1999). Adolescents who are uninsured are also more likely to have unmet health needs (24 percent versus 6 percent).

Despite having worse reported health status, African-American and Hispanic adolescents have fewer doctor visits annually than their white non-Hispanic peers (1.8, 1.7, and 2.6, respectively) and are more apt to lack a regular source of care. Having health insurance is associated with relatively higher rates of access and use for minority youth than for white non-Hispanic youth (Lieu et al., 1993). In 1988, African-American adolescents with coverage averaged 2.2 visits annually compared to 1.4 for those who were uninsured. Hispanic adolescents with insurance averaged 2.2 visits compared to 1.1 visits annually for those who were uninsured, while non-Hispanic white adolescents had comparable annual visit rates of 2.8 and 2.0.

Children with Special Health Care Needs

Finding: Uninsured children with special health care needs are more likely than are those who have insurance coverage to be without a usual source of health care; to have gone without seeing a doctor in the last 12 months; and to be unable to get needed medical, dental, vision, and mental health care and prescriptions.

Approximately 18 percent of U.S. children under 18 years of age, or 12.6 million children nationally, have a chronic physical, developmental, behavioral, or emotional condition that causes impairment in a basic function such as hearing, seeing, or learning. These children require health and related services of a type or amount beyond those required by most children (Newacheck et al., 1998a).[10] Children with special needs are disproportionately lower income and otherwise socially disadvantaged. Despite their greater expected use of health care services, one out of every nine children with special needs (roughly the same rate as among all children) remains uninsured (Newacheck et al., 1998a). Uninsured children with special needs also are disproportionately likely to be Hispanic and to have mothers with less than a high school education (Aday et al., 1993).

Although the associations between poverty, minority race or ethnicity, and lack of insurance and diminished access hold true for all children, the consequences for children with special needs are particularly concrete and immediate. Both low-income special needs children and those in families with incomes between 100 and 200 percent FPL are more than four times as likely to be uninsured as are children in families with higher incomes (17, 18, and 4 percent, respectively) (Newacheck et al., 2000b). Not surprisingly, given the association between lack of insurance and poverty, parents cite the high cost of health insurance as the primary reason for being without coverage for three of every four children. Further, uninsured special needs children are far more likely than special needs children who have insurance to be unable to get medical care due to cost (adjusted OR = 11.4), according to their parents (Newacheck et al., 2000b).

As is true for uninsured children generally, uninsured children with special needs are more likely than insured children to

- be without a usual source of health care (OR = 5.8),
- have gone without seeing a doctor in the last 12 months (OR = 2.5), and
- be unable to get needed medical (OR = 5.8), dental (OR = 4.0), prescriptions or vision care (OR = 3.2) and mental health care (OR = 3.4) (Newacheck et al., 2000b).

This analysis adjusted for sociodemographic factors and measures of health status. These findings confirm results of similar examinations using older surveys (Aday, 1992; Newacheck, 1992; Aday et al. 1993).

HEALTH OUTCOMES FOR CHILDREN AND YOUTH

Establishing the links between health insurance status and clinical outcomes and then estimating population-wide health effects involves several analytical steps.

---

[10]This study uses the definition developed by the federal Maternal and Child Health Bureau's Division of Services for Children With Special Health Care Needs, which states: "Children with special health care needs are those who have or are at increased risk for a chronic physical, developmental, behavioral, or emotional condition and who also require health and related services of a type or amount beyond that required by children generally" (Newacheck et al., 1998a).

Population-wide effects may be harder to discern in children than in adults because an even smaller proportion of the child population than the adult population has diagnosed health problems and chronic conditions. Consequently, the immediately apparent effects of health insurance status on health are muted within the largely healthy-child population.

One recent analysis has examined health and functional outcomes for children under age 15 on a broad population basis using the variability among states in instituting Medicaid eligibility expansions to assess the effect of health insurance coverage on episodes of acute illness, restricted activity days, and bed days. Lykens and Jargowsky (2002) combined the NHIS Child Health Supplements data for 1988 and 1991 for children in lower-income families (under 185 percent of FPL) and analyzed these outcomes as a function of the state Medicaid eligibility level. They found a statistically significant decrease for acute illness episodes for non-Hispanic white children and statistically insignificant decreases for non-Hispanic black and Hispanic children. The authors note that these insignificant findings could either be due to small sample sizes or to worse access to care for minority children (Lykens and Jargowsky, 2002). In all cases the findings for restricted activity and bed days were not statistically significant but inversely related to Medicaid income eligibility standards.

It is important also to consider subacute or asymptomatic conditions for which no medical visit is ever sought, particularly as the conditions affect the development of children's physical and mental capabilities. When no care is sought, this introduces a methodological limitation to studies of health outcomes dependent on insurance status: rates of "no shows" can be quantified only indirectly and the attendant health consequence may be difficult to quantify. Pent-up demand for care clearly exists for uninsured children, as illustrated by the evaluation of the Pennsylvania insurance expansion described earlier: the portion of children reporting unmet need dropped from 57 percent to 16 percent 12 months following the program expansion (Lave et al., 1998a).

When uninsured sick children do not receive appropriate care, the consequences may be serious. This section examines the relationship between health insurance and health outcomes, including mortality, disease severity, condition-specific morbidity, and avoidable hospitalizations. Lack of insurance results in poorer access to and use of health care, which in turn leads to delays in seeking care for a serious medical condition and possibly no visits for less serious conditions. Delaying care has several consequences:

- it may be detrimental for the health and survival of a child because the condition or disease can become more advanced;
- this increased severity frequently demands a more intense level of treatment (e.g., hospitalization) when it is finally obtained; and
- any lingering physical and mental health problems may affect a child's chances for success in school and life.

Delays in Care for Uninsured Children and Youth

> **Finding:** Uninsured children often receive care late in the development of a health problem or do not receive any care. As a result, they are at higher risk for hospitalization for conditions amenable to timely outpatient care and for missed diagnoses of serious and even life-threatening conditions.

Parents of uninsured children often opt not to seek care for what appear to be non-life-threatening conditions and for which insured families in otherwise similar circumstances would consider medical attention necessary, as would medical providers. This lack of care can have both physical and psychosocial repercussions. Studies of injuries and mental health problems illustrate diminished care seeking for uninsured children with these conditions. Some conditions (e.g., asthma, ear, nose, and throat [ENT] infections and their complications; vaccine-preventable diseases) respond to timely outpatient care, and without that care, unnecessary hospitalizations frequently follow. In the worst cases of delayed care seeking on the part of families and the failure of the health care system to provide the same intensity of services to uninsured children, the uninsured child has a greater risk of dying.

Uninsured children with certain diagnoses have been found to be more likely to die than insured children, due to failure to reach a hospital or receive appropriate specialized care until late in the course of the illness and to the greater severity of illness at presentation resulting from delayed care. Two studies illustrate worse survival rates for uninsured children, one for coarctation of the aorta and the other for trauma.[11]

In one study, uninsured infants under 1 year of age with coarctation of the aorta were more likely to die than infants with any type of health insurance (33 versus 3.8 percent), controlling for case severity (Kuehl et al., 2000).[12] Fifty-five (55) percent of the deaths occurred prior to surgical treatment, and one-third occurred without diagnoses. The authors report that parents had unsuccessfully attempted to obtain medical care for their children, delaying their diagnosis and an intervention that could improve their chances for survival.

Using data in the National Pediatric Trauma Registry, Li and Davis (2001) report that compared to pediatric trauma patients with commercial insurance, both patients with public insurance and those without any coverage had a significantly increased risk of in-hospital mortality (relative risk [RR] = 1.48 and 2.02, respectively). This increased risk existed in different age groups and for both blunt and penetrating trauma patients, and the increased risk remained statistically significant after adjusting for injury severity.

---

[11] This is a relatively common congenital cardiovascular malformation in which there is a narrowing of the aortic arch. It can be treated through surgical correction or medical management.

[12] This was a population-based study of 103 cases of infant coarctation of the aorta diagnosed before 1 year of age.

Uninsured children are less likely to receive medical attention for their injuries. Overpeck and Kotch (1995) report that children without insurance had lower rates of both total and serious injuries that received medical attention, compared with the rates for children covered by Medicaid or private insurance. They estimated that uninsured children are 30 percent less likely to receive medical attention for their injuries than are insured children and 40 percent less likely to receive medical attention for *serious* injuries than are insured children. Further analysis by these authors found that this experience of lower rates of medically attended injuries for *uninsured* children applied across racial and ethnic groups (African-American, non-Hispanic white, and Mexican-American children) (Overpeck et al., 1997).

Hospitalization for conditions that could have been treated at a less advanced stage, sometimes called ambulatory-care-sensitive conditions (ACSCs), has been used as a population-level indicator of access to appropriate outpatient services. For children, some common, potentially avoidable hospitalizations are for asthma, pneumonia, seizures, and gastrointestinal infections. Prompt and, for chronic conditions such as asthma, regular attention by a primary care provider can better manage the underlying condition and forestall its exacerbation to a point where hospitalization is required.

Lack of insurance is one barrier to timely and appropriate primary care, and several studies have explored ACSCs for child populations and their relationship to insurance status. As in cross-sectional studies of ACSCs for adults, cross-sectional studies of children find that those enrolled in Medicaid have higher population rates of hospitalizations for ACSCs than do either privately insured or uninsured children (Pappas et al., 1997; Parker and Schoendorf, 2000; Shi and Lu, 2000). Some, but not all, studies report higher rates of avoidable hospitalizations among uninsured as compared with privately insured children. These researchers attribute the lower rates of hospitalization for these conditions among uninsured children to access barriers that they face even for exacerbated conditions that often require hospital care. Younger children, children who live in poorer neighborhoods, and African-American children also have higher rates of ACSCs than do older children, children in wealthier areas, and white, non-Hispanic children (Parker and Schoendorf, 2000; Shi and Lu, 2000).

Studies of a population over time, however, suggest that increased Medicaid coverage may have reduced rates of avoidable hospitalizations. Dafny and Gruber (2000) evaluated avoidable hospitalizations among children under age 16 between 1983 and 1996 as a function of state-level Medicaid eligibility standards and found that Medicaid eligibility expansions over this period reduced avoidable hospitalizations on a population basis 22 percent.

Kaestner and colleagues (2001) examined the effect on ACSC hospitalizations by comparing NHIS data before (1988) and after (1992) the Medicaid eligibility expansions initiated in the late 1980s. They report that the incidence of ACSC hospitalizations decreased among children ages 2–6 years living in the lowest-income areas (family income <$25,000 annually), those most likely to have gained

Medicaid coverage following the expansions. However, for children ages 7–9 (the only other group studied) the results were mixed. Children in this older age group were less likely to have been affected by the expanded Medicaid programs, which increased eligibility and enrollment to a greater extent for children under age 6.

Timely receipt of immunizations for childhood diseases is important in its own right and also indicates a population's access to primary health care services. An evaluation of the children's health insurance expansion in New York found that the immunization rate in New York State rose from 83 to 88 percent for all children ages 1 to 5 following the introduction of this program (Rodewald et al., 1997). The increase was greatest among previously uninsured children and among those who had had a gap in insurance coverage longer than six months. As noted previously, visits to health department immunization clinics decreased by 67 percent and visits to primary care providers' offices increased by 27 percent (Rodewald et al., 1997). Thus, insurance coverage for children who were previously uninsured results not only in an improved overall immunization rate but also in a shift in the provision of services from health departments to a medical home.

EFFECT OF HEALTH ON CHILDREN'S LIFE CHANCES

Finding: Undiagnosed and untreated conditions that are amenable to control, cure, or prevention can affect children's functioning and opportunities over the course of their lives. Such conditions include iron deficiency anemia, otitis media, asthma, and attention deficit–hyperactivity disorder.

Adverse impacts on the health of children have special significance because childhood illnesses, left untreated, can affect not only present health but also future development. For example, illnesses may result in absences from school, which may in turn affect learning (Wolfe, 1985). Achievement may also be lowered by moderate or severe psychological problems (Wolfe, 1985). Further, specific illnesses (e.g., untreated and chronic ear infections), can hurt a child's life chances in more direct ways (by impairing hearing). Of course, health is only one in a constellation of factors that affect a child's life chances.

In this section, the Committee examines five conditions or diseases: iron deficiency anemia, dental disease, otitis media, asthma, and attention deficit–hyperactivity disorder. They were selected from among the many conditions that may affect children's life chances because these are very common, have extensive literatures, and most importantly, are amenable to therapy. There is limited or no research that directly connects the evidence about long-term impacts of these untreated health conditions in children to their health insurance status. However, studies of overall access to and utilization of care by children demonstrate that a lack of insurance can lead to delayed therapy or no therapy. Research that evaluates and documents the relationships between particular child health outcomes and health insurance status would help make this argument more definitive.

Iron Deficiency Anemia

Iron deficiency anemia, the most prevalent nutritional deficiency in childhood, has been linked to mental retardation and poor school performance (Dallman et al., 1984; Lozoff et al., 1998). Approximately 9 percent of toddlers, 9–11 percent of adolescent girls, and 11 percent of women of childbearing age in the United States are iron deficient (Looker et al., 1997). There is an increased likelihood of mild or moderate mental retardation associated with anemia, the risk increasing with the severity of the anemia (Hurtado et al., 1999). Academic deficiencies and developmental delays are seen in children who were iron deficient early in life and then followed throughout their school career, as well as in students of all ages whose iron levels are currently too low (Otero et al., 1999; Lozoff et al., 2000; Grantham-McGregor and Ani, 2001; Halterman et al., 2001). Importantly, the long-term health risks of iron deficiency are frequently interrelated with other detrimental environmental exposures and social and economic deprivations, which may intensify the likelihood of poorer outcomes (Lozoff et al., 1998; Shonkoff and Phillips, 2000).

Dental Disease

Dental care is incorporated into employment-based health insurance plans less often than it is excluded (KPMG, 1998). For children, however, dental services have been part of the basic Medicaid benefit package through the Early and Periodic Screening, Diagnosis and Treatment (EPSDT) Program and are frequently included in SCHIP plans as well. Thus, the Committee includes dental services in this review focused on children, while it did not consider dental services in its review of health outcomes for working-age adults. Dental care was recently identified as the most prevalent unmet health need among American children (Newacheck et al., 2000a). Among 5–17-year-olds, dental caries are five times as common as a reported history of asthma (NCHS, 1996). Children in families with incomes below the federal poverty level are more likely not only to have decayed teeth, but also to have them go untreated: 37 percent of poor children (aged 2 to 9 years) compared to 17 percent of non-poor children have one or more untreated decayed primary teeth (Litt et al., 1995; NCHS, 1996; Vargas et al., 1998). Just 20 percent of lower-income children had a preventive dental care visit in 1996, less than half the proportion of children under 18 overall (43%) who had such a visit (DHHS, 2000). Untreated oral disease in children is associated with compromised nutrition (Acs et al., 1999), serious general health problems, pain, problems with eating, overuse of emergency rooms, activity limitation, sick bed days, and lost school time (Brunelle, 1989; NCHS, 1997; Edmunds and Coye, 1998).

Otitis Media

Recurrent otitis media and otitis media with effusion (middle-ear disease) are common in children before 3 years of age and may be associated with hearing loss (Lanphear et al., 1997). A substantial body of research exists demonstrating the negative impact of these conditions on expressive language ability, cognitive ability, auditory perception, school readiness for preschoolers, and school performance for students (Teele et al., 1990; Zargi and Boltezar, 1992; Lous, 1995; Mody et al., 1999; Roberts et al., 2000; Casby, 2001).

Asthma

Asthma is the most common chronic childhood illness (CDC, 1996a). Asthma disproportionately affects poor and minority populations (Gergen and Weiss, 1990; Carr et al., 1992; Lang and Polansky, 1994; Taragonski et al., 1994). Children with asthma miss significantly more days of school than do nonasthmatic children (McCowen et al., 1996; Silverstein et al., 2001). A number of studies suggest that asthmatic children do not do worse academically than their non-asthmatic classmates (Gutstadt et al., 1989; Lindgren et al., 1992; Celano and Geller, 1993; Rietveld and Colland, 1999; Silverstein et al., 2001). However, children with uncontrolled and more severe asthma may be at greater risk for language and/or learning disorders and poor academic performance (Celano and Geller, 1993; Lubker et al., 1999). Children whose asthma is not under control may be either diagnosed and receiving poor medical management or undiagnosed with no proper management.

One multicenter study of children with asthma assessed the quality of asthma care received by uninsured children as significantly worse than that received by insured children (Ferris et al., 2001). As discussed earlier in this chapter, a before-and-after comparison study of an SCHIP prototype program in New York found that asthma care and parent-evaluated health outcomes for children with asthma improved after enrollment in the program (Szilagyi et al., 2000a).

Attention Deficit–Hyperactivity Disorder (ADHD)

ADHD is the most commonly diagnosed behavioral disorder of childhood and is estimated to affect between 3 and 5 percent of school-aged children. Symptoms of ADHD include developmentally inappropriate levels of attention, concentration, activity, distractability, and impulsivity both in early childhood and during the school years. ADHD has been linked to lower school readiness (DuPaul et al., 2001), poorer academic performance (Fischer et al., 1990; Frick et al., 1991; Shelton et al., 1998; Marshall et al., 1999; Willcutt et al., 2000; Merrell and Tymms, 2001), lower vocational attainment (Mannuzza et al., 1997), and less optimal social and emotional development (NIH, 2000). The general incapacity to sustain attention, even in children who are not formally diagnosed with ADHD, is also linked to having to repeat a grade more often than children without behavioral problems (Gordon et al., 1994).

Mannuzza and Klein (2000) examine the developmental course of ADHD and conclude that in adolescence, there remain relative deficits in academic and social functioning for two-thirds to three-quarters of these children. These deficits are manifested in lower grades, more courses failed, worse performance on standardized tests, having fewer friends, and lower psychosocial adjustment.

Lack of insurance is one important barrier to evaluation and treatment of ADHD (NIH, 1998). For those who do have insurance, many families cannot afford out-of-pocket costs for services not covered, and coverage of mental health services in private insurance plans is often very limited. Although evidence of the importance of ADHD as a health and developmental problem is plentiful, the impact of health insurance coverage on receipt of appropriate care for this condition is lacking, as it is for child mental health services in general.

PRENATAL AND PERINATAL CARE AND OUTCOMES

This section examines how health insurance status affects the receipt of health care by uninsured pregnant women and outcomes for both mother and child. The expected relationships between health insurance, health care, and health outcomes for pregnant women and infants are illustrated in Figure 6.1. The section is organized according to the following:

- access to and use of prenatal care,
- hospital-based perinatal care, and
- health outcomes for mother and infant.

Insurance status can affect whether a pregnant woman seeks care and how often, the services and facilities available to her, and ultimately her own health and that of her infant. Both cross-sectional studies and natural experiments provide evidence of the influence of insurance status on prenatal care.[13] Factors that covary with health insurance status and also affect access to and use of care include socioeconomic status, educational attainment, and racial and ethnic identity (IOM, 2002a; IOM, 2002b). These factors are controlled for in the most rigorous studies, although sometimes adjustments for characteristics such as income are imputed from aggregate-level data if this information is not available from individual

---

[13]Expansions of federal income eligibility standards for Medicaid for pregnant women that occurred beginning in the late 1980s have constituted "natural experiments" in population-level analysis of service use and birth outcomes before and after the program expansions and in variations in the rates at which individual states enacted these expansions. For a more extensive review of studies of prenatal care and outcomes, some in the economics literature, see Hadley (2002). The Committee's more limited review here is consistent with the findings in the broader Hadley review paper.

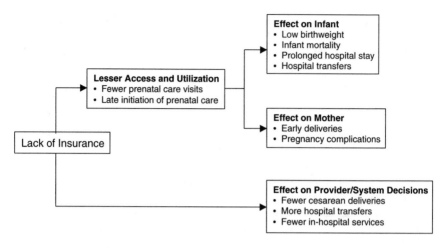

FIGURE 6.1 Effects of having no insurance on outcomes for pregnant women and infants.

records. Even when insurance becomes available, care-seeking patterns are not always optimal.

Access and Use of Prenatal Care

> **Finding: Uninsured women receive fewer prenatal care services than their insured counterparts and report greater difficulty in obtaining the care that they believe they need. Studies find large differences in use between privately insured and uninsured women and smaller differences between uninsured and publicly insured women.**

Box 6.2 summarizes professional standards and national statistics for prenatal care.

A recent study based on the national Community Tracking Study Household Survey conducted in 1996 and 1997 reports that, on average, uninsured women have fewer prenatal care visits that women with health insurance and 15 percent had no prenatal visits, compared to 4 percent of women with private or public coverage (Bernstein, 1999). This same study found that 29 percent of uninsured pregnant women did not have a usual source of care, compared to 14 percent of women with Medicaid and 9 percent of those with private health insurance. Eighteen (18) percent of uninsured women also reported an unmet need for care, more than twice the rate of privately or publicly insured pregnant woman (Bernstein, 1999).

State-specific studies also find less use of prenatal care among uninsured women than among women with insurance. In California, investigators report that uninsured women were more likely than privately insured women to initiate

BOX 6.2
Prenatal Care

- Professional and public health guidelines for prenatal care recommend a first visit for pregnancy-related care in the first trimester and regular visits at increasing frequency throughout the course of the pregnancy (DHHS, 2000; ACOG, 1989).
- The recommended number of visits over the course of pregnancy varies, depending on the source of the recommendation, and ranges from 13 to 14 prenatal visits to as few as 9 visits for low-risk pregnancies (ACOG, 1989; Public Health Service, 1989; McDuffie et al., 1996).
- Fully a quarter of pregnant women receive less than adequate prenatal care as measured by an index that takes both initiation of prenatal care and the number of visits into account (Kogan et al., 1998b; Minino et al., 2002).
- Women who belong to racial and ethnic minority groups on average receive less prenatal care than do non-Hispanic white women. In 1999, 74 percent of African-American and Hispanic women and 88 percent of non-Hispanic white women began prenatal care in the first trimester of pregnancy. 7, 6, and 2 percent of African-American, Hispanic, and non-Hispanic white women, respectively, had their first prenatal visit very late, in the third trimester of their pregnancy, or no prenatal care at all (NCHS, 2001).

prenatal care late (OR = 2.54) and to have too few prenatal visits (Braveman et al. 1993).

A number of studies examine changes in care patterns across entire populations when insurance coverage changes. These studies have taken advantage of the large-scale expansions of Medicaid coverage for previously uninsured women that began in 1986. Prior to these expansions, pregnant women were eligible for Medicaid only if they were single and received income support benefits or if they met very low income thresholds. By 1990, Medicaid eligibility was universal for all pregnant women and newborns in families with incomes below 133 percent of FPL, although states were allowed to raise the income ceiling to 185 percent FPL.

Enrollment grew rapidly and the number of pregnant women with health insurance grew substantially (Howell, 2001).[14] By 1991, 43 percent of women of childbearing age were eligible for Medicaid coverage and about a third of deliveries

---

[14]Howell (2001) reviewed 14 studies examining the impact of these expansions and added a further study of her own. Five (5) of the 14 studies were national in scope, whereas the remaining 9 were conducted in individual states and generally involved linking data from Medicaid files to birth certificates. The methodologies varied. The early studies often used aggregate state or county data, which did not permit analyses by subgroup. Studies using this methodology were not able to examine impact for specific socioeconomic groups or birthweight categories. Nor were they able to examine impact on infant mortality since they did not include death certificates. Later studies linked individual birth and death certificate information to files that contained Medicaid enrollment information.

in that year were covered by Medicaid (Singh et al., 1994; Currie and Gruber, 1996a). However, a significant percentage of pregnant women remained uninsured. In California, for example, 11 percent of births in 1990 were to women who remained uninsured for prenatal care (Braveman et al., 1993).

Some of the studies of the impact of the Medicaid program expansions examine changes in utilization across entire populations, rather than by comparing insured and uninsured groups. In general, these studies have found that among low-income women within a particular state, the timeliness with which prenatal care is initiated and the total number of visits are improved (Cole, 1995; Kenney and Dubay, 1995; Ray et al., 1997; Long and Marquis, 1998; Currie and Grogger, 2002). For example, a study in Florida in 1991 after its Medicaid expansion, found that the percentage of low-income women (including both uninsured and publicly insured women) who received no prenatal care dropped from 2.3 to 1.6, their total number of visits increased on average, and fewer women entered care late than had done so prior to the expansion in 1989 (Long and Marquis, 1998).

Three nationwide studies comparing prenatal care indicators in counties that had expanded coverage to those without expansions report that the rate of timely initiation of prenatal care in counties with expanded programs is slightly higher (Cole, 1995; Kenney and Dubay, 1995; Dubay et al., 2001). Other studies have shown that improvements in prenatal use are limited to certain geographic areas (i.e., South and Midwest) and to some groups of women (e.g., white women, teenagers) (Cole, 1995; Coulam et al., 1995; Howell, 2001).

State-level studies in four states (Tennessee, California, Massachusetts, and Wisconsin) show no difference in prenatal care use before and after expansion (Piper et al., 1990; Braveman et al, 1993; Haas et al. 1993b) whereas studies in three states (a later study in Tennessee, Missouri, and Florida) do find better prenatal care use following expansion (Coulam et al., 1995; Ray et al., 1997; Long and Marquis, 1998). The states with improvements in prenatal care use were those that had the most restrictive eligibility standards for Medicaid prior to the expansions (Howell, 2001).

Several studies have examined the quality of prenatal care used by a cross section of privately insured, publicly insured, and uninsured women at a point in time, controlling for variables such as maternal education, marital status, race and ethnicity.[15] The investigators find large differences in utilization between privately insured and uninsured women and smaller differences or no differences between uninsured and publicly insured women (Braveman et al., 1993; Amini et al., 1996; Bernstein, 1999). The researchers evaluating the California experience with a Medicaid expansion reported that uninsured and Medicaid-enrolled women as a single group are much more likely than those with private insurance to receive *no* prenatal care (OR = 6.7) (Braveman et al., 1993).

---

[15]Even with these analytic adjustments for characteristics other than health insurance status that affect use and outcomes, cross-sectional studies are not as strong a research design as are longitudinal studies.

Hospital-Based Perinatal Care

Finding: Health insurance status affects the care received by women giving birth and their newborns. Uninsured women and their newborns receive, on average, less prenatal care and fewer expensive perinatal services.

At the time of delivery, the care received by uninsured women and their newborns differs from the care received by women and newborns that are covered by health insurance. Studies that have examined providers' and pregnant women's decision making find that uninsured pregnant women and their newborns are less likely to have certain more expensive maternity and neonatal services. Procedures and services such as cesarean sections and neonatal intensive care can have a substantial financial impact on providers. Researchers have also looked at whether patients of lower socioeconomic status have lower expectations for the care that they receive.

Obstetric Services

Insurance coverage affects the services women receive at childbirth. A study based on hospital data over the period 1987–1992 of rates of use of four obstetric procedures: cesarean section, use of fetal monitor, ultrasound, and induction of labor among women covered by Medicaid found that, among those most likely to have been without Medicaid prior to coverage expansions, use of each of these procedures increased. However, among those women who were most likely to have been covered by private health insurance before expanded Medicaid coverage, increased Medicaid coverage resulted in lesser use of these technologies at birth (Currie and Gruber, 2001).

There is a strong relationship between insurance status and cesarean section rates, with uninsured women less likely to receive cesarean sections (Keeler and Brodie, 1993). It is difficult to determine the extent to which the differences in cesarean section rates between insured and uninsured women are due to overuse of the procedure among women with coverage and to underuse of the procedure among uninsured women. Overuse of cesarean section is well documented (ACOG, 2000; DHHS, 2000). Nonetheless, it is apparent that economic incentives are at work in the case of both insured women's rates of cesarean section and uninsured women's rates, incentives that act in opposite directions.

At the time data were collected by Keeler and Brodie (1993), cesarean section charges, including both hospital and physician fees, were 66 percent higher than those for vaginal deliveries. Hospitals are unlikely to recoup fully the costs of care provided to uninsured women, and hospitals lose more money when deliveries are by cesarean section than when they are vaginal.

Financial incentives also exist for the women themselves who are giving birth. Whereas out-of-pocket costs for mothers with fee-for-service insurance may be low, uninsured mothers may face substantial out-of-pocket costs. Because of limited resources to pay for the deliveries of uninsured women, these women, their physicians, and hospitals all have incentives to opt for less expensive alternatives when clinical considerations allow for choice.

Studies of cesarean section rates have the same methodological problem as other outcomes studies; health insurance status is associated with other factors such as age, race and ethnicity, income, and education that also affect these rates. Analyses adjust for at least some of these factors to isolate and measure the contribution of health insurance status to the likelihood of being delivered by cesarean section. Studies in California (Stafford, 1990; Stafford et al., 1993), Ohio, and Maine, New Hampshire, and Vermont (Aron et al., 2000) found substantial differences in adjusted cesarean section rates by payment source, with uninsured women having the lowest rates. The rates for women with public insurance tend to fall between those for uninsured and privately insured women. Haas et al. (1993a) reported an increase in cesarean section rates after expansion of Medicaid in Massachusetts.

Some studies that have examined the relationship between health insurance status and rates of cesarean section have also taken clinical appropriateness into account. One study reported that in cases where cesarean section was more clearly indicated, such as with breech presentation, fetal distress, or failure of labor to progress, uninsured women were still significantly less likely than those with any form of insurance to receive a cesarean section (Stafford, 1990). Aron and colleagues (2000) found that after adjusting for a wide variety of maternal and neonatal risk factors, uninsured women were less likely to receive a cesarean section (OR = 0.65, p = .067). While not statistically significant at the conventional .05 level, this finding was consistent across all levels of clinical risk. Of particular concern is the lower rate of cesarean section among the very high-risk women who were uninsured.

Site of Care

Differences in the care received by low-birthweight babies with differing health insurance status may stem from differences in the resources available to the hospitals that predominantly treat patients with either private, public, or no coverage. A study conducted among maternity patients in San Francisco revealed that privately insured women at high risk for complications were much more likely to deliver at a hospital with neonatal intensive care facilities than were similar women with Medicaid or without insurance (Phibbs et al., 1993). Hospitals with more privately insured patients, especially those with more privately insured low-birthweight newborns, have more neonatal intensive care beds than do those with fewer such patients (Glied and Gnanasekaran, 1996). The result persists within hospital categories (public, private nonprofit, and proprietary) and after adjusting for low birthweight and other measures of patient need.

Uninsured pregnant women and newborns may be more likely to be transferred between hospitals than are those with private insurance. A study conducted in southeastern Pennsylvania found that uninsured newborns were twice as likely (RR = 1.96) to be transferred to another general or specialty acute care hospital than were similar infants with private insurance, after controlling for prematurity, severity of illness, and expertise of neonatal care in the referring hospital (Durbin et al., 1997).

Health Outcomes for Mother and Infant

As depicted in Figure 6.1, health insurance status is hypothesized to affect the extent of premature deliveries and pregnancy complications in mothers and of low birthweight, mortality, and prolonged hospital stays for infants. The benefits of appropriate prenatal care accrue to both the newborn and the mother, resulting in improved birth outcomes, particularly in reduced rates of low birthweight and a subsequent reduction in infant mortality. For the mother, good prenatal care is expected to translate into reduced complications of pregnancy.

Birth Outcomes

Finding: Uninsured newborns are more likely to have adverse outcomes, including low birthweight and death than are insured newborns. Evidence of improvement in outcomes for newborns as a result of increased population health insurance rates is mixed, however.

Box 6.3 presents national statistics on birth outcomes. Investigators have examined the effect of insurance on birth outcomes using measures such as low birthweight, prematurity, prolonged hospital stays, in-hospital services, and infant mortality.

Low Birth Weight and Prematurity. Evaluations of Medicaid expansions to previously uninsured women have yielded mixed results for improvements in birthweight and rates of prematurity. Two of five national studies found no effect of increased insurance coverage of the population overall on these factors (Kenney and Dubay, 1995; Currie and Gruber, 1996a) while the remaining three found improvements only for select subgroups (white women and black teenagers [Cole, 1995]; white women without a high school diploma [Dubay et al., 2001]; white women had a lower incidence of very low birthweight babies [Currie and Grogger, 2002]).

State-level studies also show mixed effects after widening Medicaid eligibility and expanding benefits. In Florida, Long and Marquis (1998) report a reduction in low birthweight for the expansion group relative to low-income women with private insurance. An expansion in Washington that includes supportive services and counseling was associated with a reduction in the ratio of low birthweight infants. Reduction was greatest among high-risk women with preexisting condi-

BOX 6.3
Neonatal Outcomes

- More than 4 million babies were born in the United States in 2000 (Martin et al., 2002).
- Low birthweight babies (less than 2,500 grams or 5.5 pounds) comprise 7.6 percent of all births, and very low birthweights (less than 1,500 grams or 3.25 pounds) account for 1.4 percent of all births (Martin et al., 2002).
- Preterm births account for 11.6 percent of the total number, with preterm births among non-Hispanic black women significantly higher at 17.4 percent of the total (Martin et al., 2002).
- The U.S. infant mortality rate for 2000 was 6.9 deaths per 1,000 live births; the second leading cause (after congenital abnormalities) was disorders related to short gestation and low birthweight: 15.4 percent of all infant deaths (Martin et al., 2002).
- Infant death rates among non-Hispanic whites and Hispanics were roughly the same at 5.6–7 deaths per 1,000 live births and were much higher among African Americans at 14.0 deaths per 1,000 live births (Martin et al., 2002).

tions such as diabetes or hypertension (Baldwin et al., 1998). In Colorado, a state without additional supportive services, the rate of low-birthweight infants among medically high-risk women increased slightly during the same period.

Infant Mortality. Infants of uninsured women are more likely to die than are those of insured women. In one region of West Virginia, the fetal death rate dropped from 35.4 to 7.0 per 1,000 live births after introduction of a prenatal care program for the uninsured (Foster et al., 1992). Despite this decline, the fetal death rate among uninsured women was still twice that among privately insured women, and the rate for the uninsured climbed again to 10.3 after the program was discontinued (Foster et al., 1992).

A nationwide analysis of insurance coverage and Women, Infants, and Children (WIC) program participation based on the 1988 National Maternal and Infant Health Survey (NMIHS) found that despite the more adverse risk profile of infants born to mothers with Medicaid coverage compared to those born to uninsured mothers, uninsured infants had a significantly higher risk of death due to endogenous causes (i.e., those that are closely related to pregnancy and delivery) (OR = 1.42) than did either Medicaid (OR = 1.04) or privately insured infants (the comparison group) (Moss and Carver, 1998).

Two studies of Medicaid expansions examined their impact on infant mortality (Currie and Gruber, 1996a; Howell, 2001). Currie and Gruber calculated an overall population reduction in infant mortality of 8.5 percent associated with a 30 percentage point increase in Medicaid coverage among women 15–44 between 1979 and 1992. The authors acknowledge that they are unable to determine whether the mortality decrease should be credited to better prenatal care or to more intensive hospital care after birth. Howell's original analysis finds no significant differences in the rates of change in infant mortality for unmarried women as a function of the extent of Medicaid expansions between 1985 and 1991. She concludes that the decline in infant mortality found by some investigators after Medicaid expansions is in part a consequence of improvements in the care of fragile infants during the same time period and suggests that the Medicaid expansions provided additional resources to hospitals that allowed them to add, improve, or expand neonatal intensive care services (Howell, 2001).

In Tennessee, no decrease was observed in infant mortality but there was also no increase in the use of prenatal care in the first trimester (Piper et al., 1990). In Missouri, Coulam and colleagues (1995) likewise found no impact on mortality but also report improvements in prenatal care among enrolled low-income teens.

Prolonged Hospital Stays and In-Hospital Services. In the several years before Medicaid expansion (1982 to 1986), the percentage of newborns without health insurance in California increased by 45 percent (from 5.5 to 8.0 percent). Hospital discharge data on births to residents of selected counties show the consequences of this decline in coverage (Braveman et al., 1989). Researchers found that the increasing uninsured rate over time was associated with an elevated and increasing risk of adverse outcomes in newborns (defined as prolonged hospital stay, transfer of the newborn to another institution, or death), after adjusting for race or ethnicity. These results are most marked in African-American (OR = 2.24) and Hispanic populations (OR = 1.56). The authors suggest that inadequate and diminishing access to care accounts for the increased rates of adverse outcomes and that this disproportionately affects minority populations.

Looking at length of hospital stay alone, on average, uninsured infants do not stay as long in the hospital or receive the same scope of services while in the hospital as do privately or publicly insured infants. A retrospective analysis of discharge data from all California acute care hospitals demonstrated a link between newborns' insurance coverage and the allocation of hospital services as measured by total hospital charges and charges per day (Braveman et al., 1991). After controlling for race and ethnicity, diagnoses, hospital characteristics, and disposition, sick newborns without insurance received fewer inpatient services than did comparable privately insured newborns. The mean stay was 15.7 days for privately insured newborns, 14.8 days for Medicaid-covered newborns, and 13.2 days for uninsured newborns. Resources for newborns covered by Medicaid were generally greater than for uninsured and less than for privately insured newborns, despite the fact that both uninsured and Medicaid-covered newborns had more severe medical problems than did those with private coverage.

Maternal Outcomes

Finding: Uninsured women are more likely to have poor outcomes during pregnancy and delivery than are women with insurance. Studies have not demonstrated an improvement in maternal outcomes related to health insurance alone.

Studies find that uninsured women have higher rates of adverse maternal outcomes, such as pregnancy-related hypertension, placental abruption, and extended hospital stays, than do privately insured women (Weis, 1992; Haas et al., 1993a). Despite the greater likelihood of maternal complications, uninsured women have shorter hospital stays than either publicly or privately insured women (Weis, 1992).

Although better prenatal care may be associated with better obstetrical outcomes, insurance coverage alone may not be enough to improve infant or maternal outcomes detectable at the population level (Weis, 1992; Haas et al., 1993b). Smoking, substance use, poor diet, and other health-related behaviors affect birth outcomes and providing health insurance coverage alone is unlikely to change these behaviors (Joyce, 1987). With respect to the use of prenatal care, other factors beyond insurance, such as the mother's level of education, the availability of providers in general and a regular source of care in particular, may also be important determinants (Braveman et al., 2000).

The point at which health insurance becomes available to women of child-bearing age also affects the adequacy and timeliness of prenatal care, which become important when examining the effect of coverage on birth outcomes. Ellwood and Kenney (1995) note that depending on the state, 39 to 54 percent of women enrolled in Medicaid *after* the first trimester of pregnancy. When the State of Washington, in addition to providing insurance coverage, also provided assessment, education intervention, and nutritional and psychosocial counseling to pregnant women and targeted case management to women needing further services, substantial improvements in birthweight were achieved for high-risk mothers (Baldwin et al., 1998). Another study in California reports that provision of at least one nutrition, psychosocial, and health education service session each trimester of care is significantly associated with better birth outcomes, compared to provision of fewer sessions (Homan and Korenbrot, 1998). Nonetheless, insurance remains an important determinant of access to and utilization of health care by low-income women, who have significantly more trouble obtaining care, receive fewer recommended services, and are more dissatisfied with the care they receive than their insured counterparts (Salganicoff and Wyn, 1999).

SUMMARY

Having health insurance increases the chances that infants, children, and pregnant women will receive preventive services when well and timely medical care when sick or at high risk of poor outcomes. These, in turn, help avoid unnecessary hospitalizations, premature births, extended morbidity, or even death.

Less Access and Use

Uninsured children have poorer access to health care, use fewer services, and delay seeking care. This scenario repeats itself for uninsured pregnant women and newborns. Having a medical home is a hallmark of quality pediatric care, and uninsured children are less likely to have a medical home than are children with health insurance of any kind. The deficits in health services for the uninsured extend to

- preventive medical, dental, and mental health care for children and youth;
- care when a child is sick or has special health care needs;
- access to prescription medications;
- prenatal care, more expensive obstetrical procedures, and length of maternal stay; and
- specialized care such as interventions for children with injuries or coarctation of aorta.

Too often uninsured parents do not seek care that insured parents and their providers would consider necessary. Disparities stem from their financial constraints and from providers' decisions to provide less intensive services to uninsured patients or the failure to develop health facilities that are geographically accessible to uninsured populations.

Interplay of Insurance with Race, Poverty, and Immigrant Status

Low-income, minority, non-citizen, and uninsured children and pregnant women fare worse than those with health insurance in access to care. Uninsured children and pregnant women usually have one or more of these additional risk factors. Each characteristic exerts its own independent effect on access and utilization, but insurance remains a significant factor even after controlling in research studies for poverty, race, and ethnicity (Haas and Adler, 2001). Those who are members of more than one risk group have greater difficulty obtaining care and worse health outcomes.

Type of Insurance

Children and pregnant women with private health insurance are most likely to receive adequate health care. Generally, those with no health insurance have the least adequate care, and those with Medicaid coverage have access and utilization experiences intermediate between the privately insured and the uninsured.

Lack of private insurance is a strong risk factor for receiving inadequate medical care for children or inadequate prenatal care. On measures of access and use, generally the uninsured have the least access to and use of health care services, with persons with Medicaid coverage being intermediate between those who are uninsured and those with private insurance. Sometimes, however, there is little difference between having Medicaid coverage and being uninsured. Children insured through public programs are at greater risk than privately insured children of experiencing periods without coverage because of the frequent need to reestablish eligibility. These gaps may interrupt relationships with a usual source of care, resulting in access problems comparable to those faced by the uninsured.

Studies of Expanded Insurance Coverage

Natural experiments that compare the experiences of a population before and after expansion of public insurance coverage demonstrate improvements in access to and use of care for uninsured children and frequently for pregnant women as well. These natural experiments allow assessment of population-wide changes in care patterns when insurance coverage is made available.

In the public program expansions and demonstrations reviewed earlier in this chapter, newly insured children experienced increased access to a medical home and were more likely to visit primary care practitioners, specialists, and dentists. In one state, this increased access was accompanied by a 5 percent decrease in emergency department use and, in the other, by a 36 percent decline in hospitalizations.

Investigators generally, but not always, find that timeliness of initiating prenatal care and the total number of prenatal visits for low-income women are better after the Medicaid expansions. The states with the greatest improvements tended to be those that had the most restrictive eligibility prior to expansion.

Health Impact of Delayed or No Care

When needed care is delayed or nonexistent, health can deteriorate. We have the ability to prevent or control many of the health problems associated with common childhood conditions that can have a long-term detrimental impact on children's development and opportunities in life. This argues for access to well-child care for all children to identify problems early and manage chronic conditions effectively. Delays in receipt of care when acutely ill are also more common for uninsured children than for those with coverage. Uninsured children are more likely to be hospitalized than privately insured children for conditions such as pneumonia or asthma because they are less likely to receive appropriate care early in the course of their illness. Similarly, women with less prenatal care, particularly those at high risk of complications, may have worse obstetrical outcomes. The newborns of uninsured mothers have longer hospital stays and have a higher mortality rate. Uninsured mothers themselves have higher rates of complications of delivery than do privately insured women but have shorter hospital stays despite more maternal complications.

Improving Health Outcomes Through Expanded Insurance Coverage

Evaluations of expansions in health insurance coverage for children and pregnant women indicate that health outcomes improve with coverage. Children's access to and utilization of appropriate health care, a positive outcome in itself, improves with higher rates of insurance coverage. In examining population-wide improvements in birthweight and prematurity due to public insurance expansions, some states found no improvement while others identified progress for selected groups (e.g., white women and black teenagers). Attributing improvements in infant mortality to insurance expansions is complicated by co-occurring improvements in neonatalogy. The population effect of public insurance eligibility expansions on utilization and health outcomes is less than some experts would predict based on the substantial number of pregnant women who are eligible. However, a significant number of eligible women do not enter prenatal care in the first trimester or enroll at all.

This chapter has reviewed the research addressing the impact of insurance status on access to health care, its use, and ultimately, health outcomes for children, pregnant women, and newborns. Although having insurance makes a difference, simply making insurance available may not be enough to improve health care and health outcomes for all of the uninsured. Some high-risk groups may require additional services (e.g., educational interventions, targeted case management) if they are to obtain good preventive and routine care.

BOX 7.1
Conclusions

- The whole family can be affected by any member's lack of insurance. If anyone in the family is uninsured, the financial and emotional well-being of the entire unit is at risk, as well as the health of those who are uninsured.
- Employment-based and public insurance programs leave gaps in coverage for many families. The families in which some or all members lack insurance disproportionately include those with lower income, a single parent, and racial and ethnic minorities.
- Purchasing health insurance for uninsured family members is not practical for most of these families because of their limited incomes and lack of assets.
- Uninsured families are less likely to use any medical services than are insured families and those who do, use fewer services on average. When uninsured families are affected by illness or injury, they are also more likely to have high health expenses relative to income.
- Transitions over the course of a family's life related to aging, employment, and marital status, such as job changes, divorce, retirement, or death of the insured member, may disrupt health coverage. Many of the transitions are unavoidable or unpredictable and result in loss of coverage.
- Parents' insurance status is an important determinant of their children's insurance and health care. Federal programs have expanded coverage to children, but insuring children may not be enough. Insuring parents is an important part of the process of bringing health care to children.
- Uninsured parents are more likely to suffer poor mental and physical health than are insured parents and their health can play an important role in their children's well-being.
- Uninsured women and their newborns receive, on average, less prenatal care and fewer expensive perinatal services. Uninsured women are more likely to have poor outcomes during pregnancy and delivery than are insured women.
- Evidence of improvements in outcomes for newborns based on measures of overall population insurance coverage is mixed.
- Children with insurance have better access to and use more health care services than uninsured children. The parents of insured children are also less likely to delay seeking care for their children for conditions that require it, and illnesses or conditions are not as severe when they do seek care. Uninsured children are less likely to receive important preventive services that can have beneficial long-term effects.

7

Conclusions

The Committee's overarching conclusion is that insurance coverage within a family concerns and may affect the entire family unit. The lack of insurance of any family member has the potential to affect the financial and emotional well-being of all members of the family. This suggests that we focus not only on the more than 38 million uninsured adults and children in the United States, but also on the 17 million *families* in which some or all members are uninsured.[1]

A FAMILY PERSPECTIVE

Of the 85 million families in the United States, 17 million have one or more members who lack health insurance. Narrowing the focus to the roughly 38 million families with children, in 3.2 million of these families *all* members lack insurance and in an additional 4.3 million families some but not all members are uninsured (see Chapter 2, Table 2.1). Together these uninsured families with children account for about one-fifth of all families with children. Among married, childless couples, an additional 3.7 million family units have one or both members uninsured. More than 38 million uninsured people live in the 11.1 million family units mentioned above, with relatives other than their own children under age 18, with people other than conventionally recognized kin, or alone. Because of family relationships—financial responsibilities, psychosocial ties, and traditional child rearing obligations—an uninsured individual may affect the lives of other immediate family members, even if they have coverage. Thus, the consequences of not

---

[1]The CPS estimates those who have been uninsured for the complete year.

having health insurance may intimately touch the lives of more than 58 million of the 276.5 million people in this country.

FINANCIAL AND HEALTH CONSEQUENCES FOR FAMILIES

Many of these 58 million feel the impact of living with uninsured family members as merely an insecurity or worry about the possibility of a very large health-related expense. Fortunately, very serious and expensive illnesses and accidents occur relatively rarely, although chronic and expensive conditions are more common. Uninsured families do have reason to worry. More than 15 percent of families with all members uninsured for the full year experience health expenditures that exceed 5 percent of their family income in a year compared with 9 percent of families in which all members are either privately insured or covered by Medicaid. Expenditures are also higher for families whose members are uninsured for the full year than for those who may have lacked coverage for a shorter period. Because families with at least one uninsured member tend to have lower incomes than do fully insured families, along with very few assets, they generally have fewer financial resources to help cope with these higher expenses. This may financially destabilize the entire family. The Committee recognizes, however, that high out-of-pocket medical bills can be damaging to families at almost any income level, whether or not they are insured.

For uninsured families, what is more common than ruinous health costs is the likelihood that they will go without needed care. Although uninsured people tend to have poorer health status than otherwise comparable insured people, they are less likely to visit a physician, fill prescriptions, and obtain preventive care and other services. Chapter 6 of this report presents strong evidence that insured children have better access to and use more health care services than do uninsured children. Uninsured children are less likely to receive the routine medical attention that is considered necessary for quality preventive care than are insured children. Low-income, minority, non-citizen, or uninsured children consistently have worse access and use than do children without those characteristics. Uninsured adolescents are more likely than those with insurance to have no regular source of care, fewer visits, and unmet health needs. Similarly, uninsured children with special health care needs, whose medical conditions require significantly more than routine well-child care, also have less access to a usual source of care, are less likely to have seen a doctor in the past year, and are less able to get needed medical, dental, prescription, and other care compared to children with special health care needs who do have insurance.

Many of the health and developmental implications of the reduced access to and use of services by uninsured children may not become apparent on a population-wide basis, at least not for many years, because most children tend to be healthy and have many fewer chronic conditions than their elders. Nonetheless, studies demonstrate that parents delay seeking care for their uninsured children until the symptoms are more severe. These delays may result in unnecessary hospitalizations for conditions that could have been treated on an ambulatory basis and, in some cases, place uninsured children at a higher risk of premature death. If left untreated, some of the common childhood illnesses that can be detected and treated with routine care can also have long-term negative impacts on children's development, including middle-ear infections, asthma, and iron deficiency. To the extent that timely and appropriate medical care might ameliorate or even prevent these conditions, insurance contributes to better future functioning and life chances for children. Further, provision of preventive care to children can have beneficial long-term effects that extend beyond health, so that society can reap the rewards in the future. The Committee recognizes, however, that there are many factors in addition to medical care that influence children's health and development.

IMPLICATIONS OF PARENTAL COVERAGE

The Committee's second report, *Care Without Coverage: Too Little, Too Late,* shows that the 30 million adults without coverage, many of whom are parents, are less likely to receive appropriate, timely care, particularly for chronic illnesses and certain life-threatening conditions, such as cancer, than are insured adults. Health policy researchers and health care professionals understand the financial and health risks of having family members without insurance. The public also appreciates these risks by showing a strong preference for insuring their families, when given a realistic and affordable option for family coverage. The Committee's analyses in this report reveal another, more insidious and subtle consequence of uninsurance, namely that if a parent is uninsured, the children in the family may be less likely to get the medical care they need, even if the children *have* coverage.

Because children depend upon their parents and guardians as decision makers as well as caregivers, parents' experiences with the health care system and their beliefs about health care are important. Parents' ability to negotiate that system on behalf of their children affects how children benefit from their insurance eligibility and coverage. In Chapter 5, the Committee shows that parents' own use of health care, including whether they have a usual source of care and are connected to the health care system, are powerful predictors of their children's use of services. Compared to insured adults, uninsured adults are more likely to have no doctor visit in the previous year, to use fewer medical services, and to have negative experiences when they finally obtain health care. The evidence suggests that children of uninsured parents may be less likely to get the full benefit of their own coverage than are children whose parents are also insured.

Not only may parental coverage be an important determinant of children's access to care, it also can affect the parents' health. The mental and physical health of parents plays an important role in child well-being. Being in poor physical or mental health, which is more likely for those of low income and those without insurance, has a bearing on a parent's child rearing practices and ability to cope with the stresses of raising a family. The physical and emotional health and development of their children may suffer as a result of parents' poor health.

A key example of a parent's health affecting that of the child can be seen during pregnancy. Providing public health insurance to previously uninsured pregnant women increases the use of prenatal care but not to the level seen with privately insured women. Uninsured women and their newborns receive less prenatal care and fewer expensive perinatal services than do insured women. Uninsured newborns are more likely to have adverse outcomes than are their insured counterparts. The evidence to date on whether expanding coverage improves an outcome such as low birthweight is not definitive, however.

POPULATIONS AT RISK

Families having some or all members with no insurance for extended periods are at greater risk of adverse consequences than are those with brief gaps in coverage. The Committee has shown that families with members uninsured for long periods are more likely to incur substantial health care costs for services and to suffer adverse consequences to health. These risks have added significance because of the types of families most likely to have some or all members uninsured.

The families in which some or all members lack insurance disproportionately are low income, single parent, immigrant, and racial and ethnic minorities. They face multiple barriers to care—of culture, education, and language—in addition to lack of financial means. The percentage of families with children in which no members are insured increases as family income declines. Also, minority population families are more likely to be wholly uninsured or have some members without coverage than are other families. The uninsured rate for immigrants and naturalized citizens has been significantly higher than that of U.S.-born residents.

In addition, there are families more likely to suffer negative consequences of having uninsured members, even though they are relatively more likely to have insurance than are the populations above. These families have members in late middle age, approaching retirement. Their increased risk comes from the fact that their health care needs and costs are likely to be higher than those of younger families. The limitations of employment-based insurance and the frequency of retirement before the age of Medicare eligibility put both the early retiree and the dependent spouse in danger of losing coverage. In fact, some health conditions and certain chronic illnesses can precipitate early retirements, either for the worker to care for an ill spouse or because work is no longer possible for the ill member of the family.

A PUBLIC POLICY PERSPECTIVE

Public policies that affect opportunities for and the structure of health insurance coverage have great societal significance, given the harmful impacts on families as well as on individuals that are associated with the lack of insurance.

What can the Committee's analysis in this report on families contribute to policy makers dealing with issues related to health insurance coverage?

In its previous report, the Committee highlighted the importance of ease of access to a regular and continuing relationship with a health care professional, which is associated with better health outcomes and is usually facilitated through insurance. In this study the evidence demonstrates that uninsured children are less likely than insured children to have a usual source of health care or a regular physician. For children, gaps in coverage are associated with health access and use that resemble those of chronically uninsured children. There are several limitations of current insurance arrangements that hinder ease of access to a usual source of care for families. There is also evidence that expanding public programs to previously uninsured children brings a significant increase in access to and use of health services.

The nature of private and public health insurance means that transitions over the course of family life—job changes, divorce, retirement, death of an insured member—often disrupt health coverage for those who had it. Eligibility for private insurance may exclude some family members because they do not meet specific legal definitions or because a child ages beyond a specified limit. Definitions of eligibility and requirements for re-enrollment in public programs may also contribute to gaps in coverage. While some rules for insurance programs are unavoidable, from the family perspective, some of these definitions and limits may cause disruption and discontinuities that are counterproductive to promoting healthy families. Policy efforts targeted at expanding the limits and definitions of insurance eligibility and smoothing the discontinuities will be examined further in the Committee's sixth report.

Approximately 20 million children are currently covered by Medicaid and the State Children's Health Insurance Program (SCHIP) program expansions. Nonetheless, almost 5 million children who are potentially eligible for these programs remain uninsured (Urban Institute, 2002a). Recent efforts to simplify the application and re-enrollment processes in many states have contributed to increased coverage. The Committee's evidence-based review shows clearly that lack of insurance for children reduces access, appropriate utilization, and some health outcomes. In addition, lack of coverage for parents means they are less likely to obtain care or to have positive experiences with the health care system and that this is likely to have a negative impact on their seeking care for their children.

The perspective of this report on coverage of families also highlights the importance of the interdependence of individuals within families, the shared health and economic consequences of uninsurance, and the importance of stronger efforts to view the family in its entirety and to consider health insurance for the whole family. Among private, employment-based insurance plans there has been a small but promising trend to expand the definition of family to include both partners in a relationship, for example, unmarried couples, both mixed sex and same sex. This development increases the opportunity for some adults to receive coverage as dependents.

OUTLOOK

While enrollment in the employment-based insurance market grew during the strong economy of the past decade, continuing growth in enrollment seems less promising now. Recent economic trends relating to recession, a soft labor market, an increasing rate of health cost inflation, and resulting premium increases all support the expectation that employers will be shifting more costs onto their employees. Higher premiums, copayments, and deductibles are likely to result in fewer employees deciding they can afford to take up the offer of coverage for themselves and their families. There are also indications that the trend for employers to reduce the amount of health insurance they offer to their retirees will continue.

The Committee notes the recent policy discussions regarding subsidizing Consolidated Omnibus Budget Reconciliation Act (COBRA) coverage for workers who lose their jobs under particular circumstances.[1] The discussions recognize the value of health insurance and the need to make it more affordable for workers and their families to keep. Although many workers cannot benefit from COBRA protections (e.g., those whose jobs do not offer health benefits), it could help some workers and their families through some employment-related transitions if it were affordable. The limited real opportunities for coverage available to uninsured workers has recently become more widely understood by the public, but political solutions are yet to be found.

The outlook for continuing expansions of Medicaid and SCHIP may also be affected by the recession. Eligibility for Medicaid coverage is likely to grow as unemployment rises. Most state budgets are feeling the constraints of lower-than-forecasted revenues and some may be tempted to cut back on public coverage rather than to expand it (Kaiser, 2001a). Even without formal changes in eligibility, there has been discussion in some states to stop aggressive campaigns to enroll currently eligible children in their SCHIP program because the campaigns are perceived as sufficiently successful that they are increasing program costs. Such cutbacks might mean that fewer of the millions of eligible children will enroll than might have done.

The Committee's final report will examine in further depth both the implications for public policy of the consequences of uninsurance on families and the impact of various programs and policies designed to counteract the negative effects.

---

[1]See footnote 4, Chapter 3, for a brief description of the recently enacted P.L. 170-210, which provides for federal tax credits for health insurance for displaced workers.

A

Conceptual Framework for Evaluating the Consequences of Uninsurance for Families

The conceptual framework used in this report, and the variations on this framework as described in Chapter 5, are closely related to the conceptual framework introduced in the Committee's first report, *Coverage Matters* (IOM, 2001). In the paragraphs that follow, the Committee's initial framework is described and its modification for use in this report is clarified.

Figure A.1 depicts the conceptual framework used in *Coverage Matters*. The framework is based on Andersen's model of access to health services, which incorporates ideas from the behavioral sciences to understand the process of health services delivery and health-related outcomes for individuals (Andersen and Davidson, 2001). In addition, it draws on an economic model of insurance status and the impact of out-of-pocket costs on health care demand.

To describe the roles of factors at the individual, family, and community levels (e.g., an individual's health insurance status) that influence both the process of services delivery and the consequences of health care experiences, the framework uses Andersen's grouping of variables into three categories: (1) resources that foster or enable the process of obtaining health care; (2) personal or community characteristics that favor or predispose action related to obtaining health care; and (3) needs for health care, as articulated by those in need, determined by health care providers, or identified by researchers and decision makers. Arrows and spatial relationships among the boxes indicate hypothesized causal and temporal relationships. For example, the young child of a lower-income, uninsured parent may be eligible for Medicaid, but if the parent does not enroll him or her, the family may not be able to afford health care for the child, and the child's health and psychosocial development may suffer as a result. This case can be followed through the model in Figure A.1.

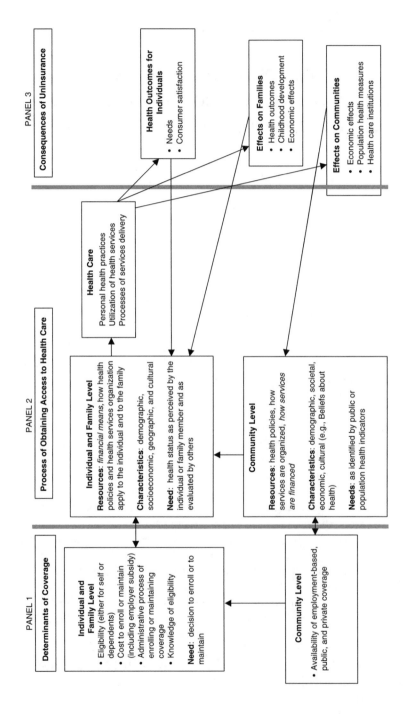

FIGURE A.1 A conceptual framework for evaluating the consequences of uninsurance—a cascade of effects.

NOTE: Italics indicate terms that include direct measures of health insurance coverage.

To depict the economic consequences of uninsurance, the Committee creates links within Andersen's framework among determinants of health insurance and such factors as family economic well-being, the institutional viability of health services, and community-level socioeconomic conditions. This expansion allows the Committee to assess hypothesized interactions between economics and health and, in particular, the growing literature on the psychosocial dimensions of family well-being and childhood development. The Committee recognizes that insurance is one of many factors that can influence the health of an individual and that of the family unit.

CONCEPTUAL FRAMEWORK INTRODUCED IN COVERAGE MATTERS

The left panel of Figure A.1 addresses the main economic forces affecting the insured or uninsured status of individuals and families. Individual- and family-level characteristics include financial resources, categorical eligibility for public health insurance, labor market determinants of employment-based insurance, and the requisite skills to enroll and maintain coverage. In the example mentioned above, the differing eligibility of child and parent for public insurance would together function as a determinant of coverage, the top box in Panel 1. Community-level factors include public program eligibility standards, labor market characteristics that determine the availability of employment-based health insurance, and the commercial market for individual health insurance.

The center panel of Figure A.1 is based almost directly on Andersen's model of access to health care (Andersen and Davidson, 2001). The boxes labeled "individual and family level" and "community level" each contains individual- and aggregate-level variables, respectively, believed to influence how people obtain access to health care. Community-level variables are ecologic or aggregate measures to describe the context or environment within which individuals and their families seek and use health care. For example, the community's morbidity rate for whooping cough might indicate the need for an immunization campaign. Because health care services are provided and consumed locally, the term community refers to a residential or geographic grouping. For example, the family of mixed insurance status described earlier may be more likely to seek health care for its child for immunization, if it lives in an area with low-cost services available through a community health clinic or public health department program, factors that would be included in the lower left box of Panel 2.

Implicit in the categories of resources, characteristics, and needs are judgments about how much a particular variable may be susceptible to change. Variables labeled "resources" are considered, at least theoretically, to be more open to change. Those termed "characteristics" are considered less flexible or manipulable, and those called "needs" comprise a mixed or heterogeneous grouping, with some needs being more changeable than others.

As a whole, community-level and individual- and family-level variables describe many *potential* scenarios for accessing health care. The variables within the box labeled "health care" describe how these potentials may be realized, with particular attention to the role of health insurance coverage. The process of health care delivery is characterized in terms of three types of variables; (1) personal health practices (e.g., dietary habits, physical exercise); (2) use of health services (e.g., number and kind of physician visits within a year); and (3) processes of care (e.g., adherence to clinical practice guidelines). In the example given, the child's lack of immunization could be described as underutilization of health services, a variable related to processes of care. The Committee focuses most of its attention on the literature concerning the processes of services delivery and the utilization of health services while recognizing that personal health practices may be influenced by insurance coverage and access to care.

The right panel of Figure A.1 describes the ways in which the Committee anticipates that health insurance status may affect the health, economic, and social characteristics of individuals, families, and communities by means of access to and the process of health care delivery. These effects of *realized access* to health care cascade from the smallest unit of analysis, the individual, to increasingly larger units, first the family and then the community. The consequences linked to health insurance influence community-level and individual- and family-level variables that describe the process of obtaining access to health care and also of gaining or losing health insurance coverage. This last panel should make it clear that the process is dynamic with multiple feedbacks. For example, employment status and income affect family insurance status, which affects current and future health status. Health status, in turn, can influence future employment status, bringing us full circle.

CONCEPTUAL FRAMEWORK FOR THIS REPORT

Figure A.2 depicts a version of Figure A.1 modified to reflect the focus of the Committee in this report. The modified version draws on the same theories and conceptual approaches to health insurance as does the initial version in Figure A.1. Figure A.2 also shares the same overall structure of three panels, with a first panel depicting determinants of coverage (left side of diagram), a second panel depicting the process of obtaining access to health care (center of diagram), and a third panel depicting selected consequences of uninsurance (right side of diagram). Where both frameworks are similar, the text description is shortened in Figure A.2, for example, in the individual- and family-level and community-level boxes where the same variables are used in Figures A.1 and A.2.

Key differences between the two frameworks are as follows:

• Rather than treat the resources, characteristics, and needs of individuals and their families as a whole, Figure A.2 acknowledges the differences between the situations of children and those of their parents or, alternatively, between those

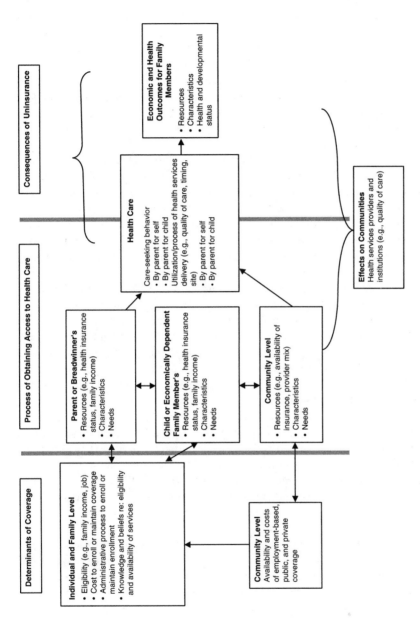

FIGURE A.2 Conceptual framework for evaluating the consequences of uninsurance on the family.

of a breadwinner and those of family members who depend economically on the breadwinner. In the example described above, the differing coverage status of child and parent may translate into different experiences with the health care system, and different consequences of being uninsured for families with at least one uninsured member, than if both child and parent were covered by public insurance. Likewise, parents' knowledge of both their children's and their own eligibility for insurance and their beliefs about the value of coverage may affect whether they enroll themselves and their children. Their knowledge of and beliefs about health care and the availability of services may influence whether they seek care for themselves and their children. The availability and costs of coverage at the community-wide level (lower left box) may influence aggregate enrollment and use of health care in the community.

• Within the box labeled "health care," Figure A.2 merges the three categories listed in Figure A.1 (i.e., personal health practices, utilization of health services, processes of services delivery) into two categories that highlight the influence of a parent or family breadwinner's decision making on the process of obtaining access to health care. The quality, quantity and continuity of the services obtained can affect the box labeled health outcomes for families in the right panel on consequences as well as the community level in the box effects on communities.

• In Figure A.2, the box labeled economic and health outcomes for family members is roughly equivalent to the box in Figure A.1 labeled effects on families. These consequences include effects on family resources (e.g., current and anticipated future income, economic status, long-term asset accumulation), some of the family's characteristics (e.g., decisions about marital status and childbearing), and the health of all family members (e.g., health status, family stress and well-being, childhood development). These consequences may have different effects on the family as a unit from those on individual members.

• The "effects on communities box" in Figure A.2 reflects the influence on communities of the aggregate efforts of families to obtain access to health care. A community's uninsured rate may influence the configuration of services, providers, and institutions and their costs and revenues. The uninsured rate in the community also may influence the quality of care that providers and institutions deliver, the health care needs of its residents, and their use of care. These community-level effects will be examined in detail in the next report of the Committee.

To tailor the conceptual framework for use in assessing the literature on health outcomes for pregnant women and newborns (in Chapter 6), Figure 6.1 reflects the specific processes and outcomes studied in the literature reviewed. Figure 6.1 emphasizes the role of health insurance for pregnant women in obtaining access to health services and enumerates specific health outcomes for both women and their newborn infants that may be consequences of the mother having been uninsured. It makes linkages between the process of health services delivery and the care received to decisions of providers of care that reflect health insurance status.

B

Overview of Public Health Insurance Programs

MEDICARE

Background. Medicare is the federal health insurance program for the elderly and disabled—Part A for hospital care, Part B for medical services. It is run by the Centers for Medicare and Medicaid Services. The program was created in 1965 by Title XVIII of the Social Security Act. The end-stage renal disease (ESRD) program has been in operation since 1973 and covers more than 90 percent of the population that suffers from this disease. The Balanced Budget Act of 1997 extended Medicare coverage to include annual mammograms, Pap smears, prostate and colorectal cancer screenings, diabetes management, and osteoporosis diagnosis.

Eligibility. Individuals (or their spouses) who have paid into the Social Security system for a total of 10 years, qualify for Medicare if they are

- aged sixty-five and older; or
- disabled and eligible for Social Security benefits or have ESRD (permanent kidney failure requiring dialysis or transplant).

Enrollment. Medicare covers 34 million Americans ages 65 and older, 5 million younger adults with permanent disabilities, and about 250,000 Americans who suffer from permanent kidney failure. Almost all Part A beneficiaries enroll in Part B, an estimated 37 million in 1999 (Century Foundation, 2001). Most beneficiaries (76 percent) are ages 65 to 84, but the beneficiaries under age 65 that are disabled (13 percent) and those 85 and over (11 percent) are growing more rapidly than the largest age group (Kaiser Family Foundation, 2001). Seventy-eight percent of beneficiaries have incomes below $25,000, and about one in four has an income of less than $10,000 (Century Foundation, 2001). More than half of the disabled beneficiaries reported incomes of less than $10,000.

Program Characteristics. The Medicare program has two components:

1. Part A (Hospital Insurance):
• Enrollment occurs automatically at age 65 with no premium charges, except for those individuals who did not pay Medicare taxes while employed. They can receive Part A by paying premiums.
• Part A provides coverage for care in hospitals as an inpatient, critical access hospitals, skilled nursing facilities, hospice care, and some home health care.
• It does not require periodic re-enrollment.

2. Part B (Medical Insurance):
• Part A beneficiaries may enroll and may sign up anytime during a seven-month period beginning three months before turning 65.
• Enrollees pay premiums of $54 a month for calendar year 2002 (CMS, 2002a).
• Part B covers physician and outpatient services, including the services of physical and occupational therapists, and some home health care.

Revenue and Expenditures. Part A is financed by a 1.45 percent payroll tax paid equally by employees and their employers (Kaiser Family Foundation, 2001). Part B is financed with premiums and deductibles paid by beneficiaries and from general revenues. Premiums are designed to cover about a quarter of total Part B spending. Medicare Part A accounts for 45 percent of program expenditures and Part B accounts for 33 percent (Kaiser Family Foundation, 2001). Medicare+Choice plans contract with Medicare to provide both Part A and B services to enrolled beneficiaries and account for an estimated 18 percent of Medicare spending (Kaiser Family Foundation, 2001). About 5 percent of the Medicare budget goes to the ESRD program, although only about 0.5 percent of Medicare beneficiaries are ESRD patients (Century Foundation, 2001).

Medicare benefit payments totaled $237 billion in 2001, accounting for 12 percent of the federal budget and 19 percent of total national spending for personal health services (Century Foundation, 2001). In 1999, Medicare financed 31 percent of the nation's hospital services and 20 percent of physician services, but only 2 percent of outpatient prescription drugs (Kaiser Family Foundation, 2001).

MEDICAID

Background. The Medicaid program was created in 1965 as Title XIX of the Social Security Act. It was designed as a federal–state partnership to provide public funding of health care for low-income children and adults. Initially, Medicaid was a medical care extension of federally funded programs for the poor, with an emphasis on the aged, the disabled, and dependent children and their mothers. Legislation in 1987 and 2000 further expanded Medicaid coverage to low-income pregnant women, more poor children, and some Medicare beneficiaries who were not eligible for any cash assistance program and had not been eligible previously for Medicaid. Most significant has been the increase of coverage for children. The latest census data show that one out of five children in the country and a quarter of all children under age 6 were enrolled in Medicaid in 2000. Enrollment grew from less than 10 million children in 1980 to over 21 million children in 1999 (Kaiser, 2002a).

Eligibility. The following groups are entitled to enroll in Medicaid:

- federal required minimum: children under age 6 and pregnant women whose family income is below 133 percent of the federal poverty level (FPL) ($19,977 for a family of three in 2002) (DHHS, 2002b);
- federal required minimum: children ages 6–18 with family incomes at or below 100 percent FPL ($15,020 for a family of three in 2002) (DHHS, 2002b);
- no federal minimum: states set income standards for adults without children; parents of children are categorically eligible if they meet income and asset tests. On average, the states' income eligibility level for parents is 41 percent of FPL ($6,158 for a family of three in 2002), varying from a low of 21 percent ($3,048 for a family of three) in Alabama to a high of 275 percent ($40,224 for a family of three) in Minnesota (Kaiser, 2002b; Broaddus et al., 2002);
- Supplementary Security Income (SSI) recipients or those aged, blind, and disabled individuals who qualify in states that apply more restrictive eligibility requirements;
- recipients of adoption assistance and foster care as designated by Title IV-E of the Social Security Act;
- special protected groups (typically individuals who lose their cash assistance from SSI due to earnings from work or increased Social Security benefits but may keep Medicaid for a period of time); and
- qualified Medicare beneficiaries, specified low-income Medicare beneficiaries, and disabled-and-working individuals who previously qualified for Medicare but lost their coverage because of their return to work.

States also have the option of expanding Medicaid coverage to other "categorically needy" groups beyond the minimum federal requirements. Over the years, many states have broadened the reach of their programs to cover a greater portion of their low-income populations than federally required. As of January 2002, state-initiated Medicaid expansions have raised eligibility for children to levels above federal minimum standards in all but nine states (Kaiser, 2002b). The most common expansions covered by federal matching funds for coverage under the Medicaid program include the following:

- infants up to age 1 and pregnant women not covered under the mandatory rules whose family income is up to 185 percent of FPL;
- recipients of state supplementary income payments;
- certain aged, blind, or disabled adults who have incomes above those requiring mandatory coverage but below the FPL;
- persons receiving care under home and community-based waivers;
- persons infected with tuberculosis (TB) who would be financially eligible for Medicaid at the SSI income level (eligibility is only for TB-related ambulatory services and for TB drugs);
- institutionalized individuals with income and resources below specified limits;
- medically needy—persons who meet categorical requirements and have significant health care expenses with incomes in excess of the mandatory or optional levels; these individuals may "spend down" to Medicaid eligibility by incurring medical and/or remedial care expenses to offset their excess income, thus reducing it to a level below the maximum income allowed by that state's Medicaid plan; and
- legal resident aliens and other qualified aliens who entered the United States on or after August 22, 1996, made ineligible for Medicaid for five years because of the 1996 welfare reform law.

Enrollment. Medicaid is the largest program providing medical and health-related services to America's poorest people. Medicaid provided coverage to approximately 44 million Americans in 2001 (Kaiser, 2002a). Medicaid eligibility expansions and enrollment simplification efforts have led to increased health coverage of the low-income population. The number of individuals covered by Medicaid has risen from 42 million in 1999 (Kaiser, 2002a). The recent economic downturn is likely to bring renewed pressure to the Medicaid program. This enrollment growth and the accompanying additional costs during a recession come at a time when states are facing mounting budgetary pressures as tax revenues decline and demand on public programs increases (Kaiser, 2002a).

Medicaid enrollment among nonelderly adults and children declined after 1995, following a decade of steady increase. Many studies suggest that Medicaid enrollment fell as an unintended consequence of the 1996 state and federal welfare reforms that changed eligibility for family cash assistance and "delinked" the two forms of assistance. Previously, families who received cash assistance had automatically been eligible for Medicaid as well. Total Medicaid enrollment of adults and children fell by 1.5 million from 1995 to 1997 as a strong economy and state and federal welfare reform efforts decreased participation in cash assistance programs (Bruen and Holahan, 2002; Urban Institute, 2002b). Several of the biggest declines in total Medicaid enrollment occurred in states with the largest percentage drops in welfare caseloads, such as Idaho, Kansas, and Wisconsin (Ku and Bruen, 1999).

The Medicaid enrollment decline that occurred following welfare reform has now moderated. States have made significant efforts to increase enrollment of those who remained eligible but lost coverage due to confusion on the part of Medicaid eligibility staff or beneficiaries themselves. In addition, section 1931 provisions allow states to extend coverage to parents at much higher income levels than previously available, new opportunities for coverage expansions of which states have taken advantage. Additional growth in Medicaid enrollment has also occurred as the economy experienced a downturn, and more people now meet the current eligibility standards.

Financing. Medicaid funding and administrative responsibilities are shared by both federal and state governments. The federal funding share, known as the Federal Medical Assistance Percentage (FMAP), is determined annually by a formula that compares the state's average per capita income level with the national income average. States with a higher per capita income level are reimbursed a smaller share of their costs. By law, the FMAP cannot be lower than 50 percent or higher than 83 percent. In 2001, the FMAPs varied from 50 percent in 10 states to 76.8 percent in Mississippi and averaged 57 percent overall (DHHS, 2002a). States also can receive federal matching payments to cover additional groups of individuals and provide additional services. These optional groups and benefits account for 65 percent of all Medicaid spending (DHHS, 2002a). As of 2001, more than $200 billion in federal and state funds were spent annually on the Medicaid program (Kaiser, 2002a).

Medicaid spending accelerated rapidly between 1999 and 2000 following a period of relatively slow increase. Spending grew by 7.1 percent in 1999 and by 8.6 percent in 2000, compared to an average of 3.6 percent annually from 1995 to 1998 (Bruen and Holahan, 2002). The Congressional Budget Office projects Medicaid spending growth to average 9 percent per year through 2012 (CBO, 2002). These high spending rates are further intensified by the national economic recession that has led to decreasing revenues and tighter budgets in many states (Bruen and Holahan, 2002).

Program Characteristics. In exchange for federal financial participation, states agree to cover certain groups of individuals and offer a minimum set of services. Each state decides how to structure eligibility, benefits, service delivery, and payment rates within guidelines established by federal law. The state must enroll all people who apply and are eligible under either a mandatory or an optional group. Enrollment caps and waiting lists are not permitted. States, however, can scale back or eliminate optional eligibility and optional benefits, and they may set limits on the amount, scope, and duration of benefits (e.g., limits on doctor visits). Most elderly individuals who receive nursing home care financed by Medicaid are covered by state option. Federal law, however, does not give states the option to cover childless adults with federal matching payments unless they fit into one of the other eligibility groups (e.g., they are elderly or disabled) except with special waivers. The extent to which states exercise the option to cover low-income groups varies widely. In Massachusetts and Vermont, 41 percent of low-income nonelderly residents are eligible for Medicaid, compared to Virginia, which covers just 14 percent (Kaiser, 2002b).

States receive federal Medicaid matching payments for a broad array of mandatory and optional services. The following services must be provided for individuals who are enrolled in Medicaid:

- inpatient and outpatient hospital services,
- physician services,
- early and periodic screening, diagnostic, and treatment services for individuals under 21,
  - nursing facility services for individuals ages 21 years and older,
  - home health care for people eligible for nursing home services,
  - family planning services and supplies,
  - rural and federally qualified health clinic services,
  - laboratory and X-ray services,
  - pediatric and family nurse practitioner services, and
  - nurse midwife services.

Specific Medicaid benefits for children were established in 1967, with the creation of the Early and Periodic Screening, Diagnosis, and Treatment (EPSDT) program. EPSDT is a comprehensive package providing periodic evaluations of health and developmental history, as well as vision, hearing, and dental screening services.

Revenue and Expenditures. Under federal law, premiums are not allowed except in limited situations and certain groups of individuals and some services are fully or partially exempt from cost sharing. Copayments and deductibles are not allowed for services provided to children or for pregnancy-related, emergency, and family planning services and supplies. In most other cases, minimal cost sharing is permitted. Deductibles cannot exceed $2 per month per family, copayments may range from $0.50 to $3.00 depending on the cost of the service, and co-insurance requirements cannot exceed 5 percent of the service cost (Kaiser, 2002b).

Average program costs vary by type of beneficiary. Medicaid payments for services for children average about $1,150 per enrolled child. For adults under age 65, who comprise 21 percent of recipients, payments for services average about $1,775 per person enrolled (DHHS, 2002a). Certain other specific groups have much larger per-person expenditures. Medicaid payments for services for 4 million elderly, constituting 11 percent of all Medicaid recipients, average about $9,700 per person; for 7.2 million disabled, who make up 18 percent of beneficiaries, payments average about $8,600 person (DHHS, 2002a). The combined total of all expenditures averaged about $3,500 per person in 1998 (DHHS, 2002a).

STATE CHILDREN'S HEALTH INSURANCE PROGRAM

Background. The Balanced Budget Act of 1997 created the State Children's Health Insurance Program (SCHIP) and provided new funds for states to cover uninsured children. Nearly $40 billion in federal matching funds over fiscal years 1998 to 2008 were allowed for states to offer coverage to children in families with incomes up to 200 percent of the FPL, who do not qualify for Medicaid (GAO, 2000). This program represents the largest single expansion of health insurance coverage for children in more than 30 years. Under the new Title XXI of the Social Security Act, states were given the option to set up a separate child health program, expand Medicaid coverage, or have a combination of both a separate child health program and a Medicaid expansion.

Enrollment. In 2001, 4.6 million children were enrolled in SCHIP. Of the total number of children enrolled, 18 percent were enrolled in separate child health programs (S-SCHIP), 13 percent were enrolled in Medicaid expansion programs (M-SCHIP), and 69 percent were enrolled in combination programs (CMS, 2002b). Throughout 2001, SCHIP enrollments grew nationally at a steady pace and decreased in only six states. Fourteen states at least doubled the number of children enrolled between 1999 and 2001 (CMS, 2002b). In 2001, more than 75 percent of children ever enrolled in SCHIP were between 6 and 18 years of age. Almost 2 million were 6- to 12-year-olds and 1.5 million were 13- to 18-year-olds.

However, there are still significant barriers to obtaining coverage through SCHIP. A recent Urban Institute study found that complicated enrollment procedures continue to be at the core of difficulties in getting eligible children covered. Thirty-eight (38) percent of low-income families that inquired about Medicaid and SCHIP alluded to administrative obstacles as the major reason for not applying (Kenney and Haley, 2001). For example, many states require families to provide numerous documents verifying information on their applications, despite the fact that such verification is not required under federal law (Maloy et al., 2002).

Program Characteristics. While states with SCHIP Medicaid expansions must provide the same benefits available to other children enrolled in Medicaid, states with SCHIP stand-alone programs have a wide range of options to use in designing their benefit packages, including the benefits available under a state's Medicaid program. SCHIP stand-alone components must cover basic benefits such as physician services, inpatient and outpatient hospital services, and laboratory and X-ray services. However, states have discretion to provide optional benefits such as prescription drugs and hearing, mental health, dental, and vision services on a more limited basis or not at all.

Patient out-of-pocket costs are allowed but limited. Total out-of-pocket costs (premiums, copayments, deductibles, enrollment fees) for children covered in separate SCHIP programs cannot exceed 5 percent of family income (Kaiser,

2002b). In addition, for children with family incomes below 150 percent FPL, premiums and cost-sharing charges cannot exceed nominal amounts prescribed by the Centers for Medicare and Medicaid Services.

Eligibility. In the SCHIP program, states may either cover children in families whose incomes are above the Medicaid eligibility threshold but less than 200 percent of FPL or use their SCHIP funds to cover children at higher income levels (Kaiser, 2002b). Most states provide SCHIP coverage for children in families up to or above 200 percent of the poverty level. Seventeen states set lower income or age standards, which is the major reason that 6 percent of lower-income children (<200 percent FPL) are not eligible for SCHIP (Broaddus and Ku, 2000). A number of lower-income children are also ineligible because of their immigration status.

Program Expansion. States are starting to expand SCHIP to cover uninsured populations other than children. In 2001, four states (Minnesota, New Jersey, Rhode Island, and Wisconsin) received approval for section 1115 waivers to enroll parents of children in SCHIP. New Jersey and Rhode Island will also enroll eligible pregnant women. These four states enrolled more than 230,000 adults in 2001 (CMS, 2002b).

In August 2001 a new initiative was announced to expand coverage to uninsured populations through the Health Insurance Flexibility and Accountability (HIFA) initiative and two states have received approval of their applications:

1. Arizona expects to eventually enroll 50,000 adults. The plan will expand access to health coverage to parents with children enrolled in Arizona's Medicaid program or SCHIP with family incomes between 100 percent and 200 percent of FPL and to childless adults with family incomes up to 100 percent of FPL.

2. California plans to expand coverage to 300,000 uninsured people, including 275,000 parents of SCHIP children with family incomes at or below 200 percent FPL.

In addition, there are currently seven states with approved premium assistance programs: Maryland, Massachusetts, Mississippi, New Jersey, Virginia, Wisconsin, and Wyoming. Premium assistance programs allow states to subsidize health coverage for low-income residents whose employers offer health insurance. Applicants and enrollees are screened for access to employer-sponsored health coverage. The state requests detailed information from potentially participating employers regarding costs, benefit package, employer share of costs, and employee eligibility. If the employer responds and the coverage meets state and federal standards for both benefits and costs, individuals are enrolled in their employer's plan. The state pays the consumer, insurer, and/or employer a subsidy. States may also apply for family coverage waivers, which allow the state to purchase coverage for the entire family if it is cost-effective. The states with family coverage waivers are Maryland, Virginia, and Wisconsin (CMS, 2002b).

C

Research Review: Health Care Access, Utilization, and Outcomes for Children, Pregnant Women, and Infants[1]

---

[1]This appendix provides brief synopses of the studies that were reviewed for and presented in Chapter 6. The table is organized according to the four major sections in Chapter 6: "Access to and Use of Health Care by Children," "Health Outcomes for Children and Youth," "Effect of Health on Children's Life Chances," and "Prenatal and Perinatal Care and Outcomes," Studies are listed alphabetically within each section.

	Sample Size/ Data Source	Outcome Measures

Access to and Use of Health Care by Children

	Sample Size/ Data Source	Outcome Measures
Aday (1992) Health Insurance and Utilization of Medical Care for Chronically Ill Children with Special Needs. *Advance Data*	Data from the NHIS Child Health (CH) Supplement, 1998	Chronic illness and special needs children
Aday et al. (1993) Health Insurance and Utilization of Medical Care for Children with Special Health Care Needs. *Medical Care*	Data from 1988 NHIS, Child Health Supplement; 9.6 million U.S. children with special health care needs	Utilization of physicians, hospitals, and prescribed medicine
Bindman et al. (1995) Preventable Hospitalizations and Access to Health Care. *JAMA*	Data from California hospital discharge records; 6,674 English- and Spanish-speaking adults aged 18–64	Reports of access to medical care
Brown et al. (1999) Access to Health Insurance and Health Care for Children in Immigrant Families. In *Children of Immigrants: Health, Adjustment, and Public Assistance*	March 1996 CPS survey and 1994 NHIS (n = 35,600 children 0–17 and n = 32,000 children 0–17, respectively)	Access to health care services; health insurance coverage; and citizenship status

Findings

The highest-prevalence conditions included in the 1988 NHIS–CH included hay fever and respiratory allergies, frequent or repeated ear infections, and asthma. About 9.6 million children under 18 years of age were estimated to have special needs: 76% of the children had insurance coverage, 11% had Medicaid, and 13% had neither. Black and Hispanic children were two times as likely to be uninsured. The proportion of uninsured children who had seen a physician was lower than the proportion of those with private insurance.

There is substantial variation in access to routine medical care among these children. In general, poor minority children living with their mothers or someone other than their parents, or those without insurance or a regular medical provider, were more likely to experience financial barriers to access or less apt to seek care than other children with comparable needs. Children with Medicaid coverage were more than three times as likely to see a doctor than those who were uninsured. Those who were insured as well as those who had coverage that was not known were more likely to be hospitalized than the uninsured.

Access to care was inversely associated with hospitalization rates for the five chronic medical conditions (asthma, hypertension, congestive heart failure, chronic obstructive pulmonary disease, and diabetes). Self-rated access to care and the prevalence of the condition remained independent predictors of cumulative hospitalization rates for chronic medical conditions. Communities where people perceive they have poor access to medical care have higher rates of hospitalization for chronic diseases. Improving access to care is more likely to reduce hospitalization rates for chronic conditions than changing patients' propensity to seek care or eliminating variations in physician practice style.

The immigration status of both the child and the primary breadwinning parent has an independent effect on the child's risk of uninsurance, even controlling for the parent's educational attainment and residency of 10 years or more. Non-citizen children have the greatest risk of being uninsured. Non-citizen Latino and Asian children have a higher risk of being uninsured than their U.S.-born counterparts or white children with U.S.-born parents. U.S. citizen children with immigrant parents have a greater risk of uninsurance than those with U.S.-born parents. These children have an even greater risk if their families immigrated on or after 1984. Uninsured rates are higher among children in immigrant families from Korea and Central America than those from other regions. Immigrant children and U.S.-born children with immigrant parents are more likely to have difficulty accessing health care services than nonimmigrant children. Immigrant children are less likely to have had a physician visit in the past year than nonimmigrant children. For those who have insurance (immigrant children and citizen children), the disparities are not large: 43% of uninsured immigrant children report having no physician visit in the last 12 months, compared to 28% of immigrant children with private coverage and 16% with Medicaid.

	Sample Size/ Data Source	Outcome Measures
Byck (2000) A Comparison of the Socioeconomic and Health Status Characteristics of Uninsured, State Children's Health Insurance Program-Eligible Children in the United States with Those of Other Groups of Insured Children: Implications for Policy. *Pediatrics*	Data for 50,950 children 0–8 years of age included in the 1993 and 1994 NHIS	Socioeconomic and demographic characteristics of children
Currie and Duncan (1995) Medical Care for Children: Public Insurance, Private Insurance, and Racial Differences in Utilization. *J Hum Resources*	Child–mother module of National Longitudinal Survey of Youth; longitudinal data from 1986 and 1988 waves for children born between 1979 and 1985, repeated observations for same child	Physician checkups; physician illness visits
Currie and Gruber (1996b) Health Insurance Eligibility, Utilization of Medical Care, and Child Health. *Quarterly Journal of Economics*	NHIS sample of children <15; 30,000 each year between 1984 and 1992; CPS for Medicaid coverage rates and eligibility	Any ambulatory visits in year; recent visit; hospitalizations in year; site of care; mortality
Currie (2000) Do Children of Immigrants Make Differential Use of Public Health Insurance? In *Issues in the Economics of Immigration*	NHIS sample of children <15; 1989–1992	Insurance coverage; probability of no visits in past year; number of physician visits annually; hospitalizations annually
Dubay and Kenney (2001) Health Care Access and Use Among Low-Income Children: Who Fares Best? *Health Affairs*	Data from the 1997 NSAF; sample: 12,680 low-income (<200% FPL) children	Access to care and use of services based on insurance coverage

Children in SCHIP differ socioeconomically and by health status from those on Medicaid and those that are privately insured (however, they differ to a lesser extent from those that are privately insured). SCHIP children live with college-educated individuals (39.4%) and employed adults (91.2%) versus 23% and 53.9%, respectively, for Medicaid children and 66.7% and 96.9% for those privately insured. Parents of SCHIP children are disproportionately self-employed or in industries and occupations in which health insurance coverage is less available or affordable. Compared to privately insured children, SCHIP-eligible children are three times more likely to be Hispanic and nearly two times more likely to be rated in fair or poor health.

White children with Medicaid have more checkups than black children with Medicaid. Black children with Medicaid have more checkups than uninsured black children. White children with Medicaid or private insurance have more illness visits than uninsured white children. Black children with Medicaid or private insurance do not have more illness visits than uninsured black children. Over time, the same child receives more services when insured than when uninsured.

Eligibility for Medicaid lowers the probability of no visits within a year by 10–13% (1/2 of baseline probability) and increases the probability of hospitalization by 14%. It also substantially increases the chances of being seen in a physician's office relative to other sites. Between 1984 and 1992, increases in the proportion of children eligible for Medicaid reduced child mortality by an estimated 5%.

Children of immigrants are less likely to take up Medicaid than are children of U.S.-born parents. Becoming eligible for Medicaid increased immigrant children's use of physician visits more than it did for nonimmigrant children. Only children of U.S.-born parents had increased hospital use with greater Medicaid eligibility.

Uninsured children, other things equal, were 8.8 percentage points (p <.01) more likely to rely on the ED or to have no usual source of care than those covered by Medicaid. They were also 2.8 percentage points (p <.01) more likely to have an unmet need for medical or surgical care and 7.4 percentage points (p <.01) more likely to have an unmet need for dental care. The families of uninsured children were 9.2 percentage points (p <.01) more likely to not feel confident that they could get the care they needed and 4.4 percentage points (p <.01) more likely to not feel satisfied with care than those in private and public insurance programs. Uninsured children were less likely than Medicaid-covered children to have at least one physician visit (regression adj. difference = 25.6; p <.01), one visit for well-child care (regression adj. difference = 25.6; p <.01), and at least one visit to a dentist of dental hygienist (regression adj. difference = 29.4; p <.01).

	Sample Size/ Data Source	Outcome Measures
Guendelman et al. (2001) Unfriendly Shores: How Immigrant Children Fare in the U.S. Health System. *Health Affairs*	Data from 1997 NHIS ($n = 14,290$)	Access and use of care
Hernandez and Charney (1998) Health Status and Adjustment. In *From Generation to Generation: The Health and Well-Being of Children in Immigrant Families*	1994 NHIS; 1996 NHANES III	General health status; chronic and acute health conditions
Holl et al. (1995) Profile of Uninsured Children in the United States. *Arch Pediatr Adolesc Med*	1988 Child Health Supplement of the NHIS ($n = 17,110$)	Utilization of medical services and health status; also an assessment of factors associated with lack of health insurance among children
Kogan et al. (1995) The Effect of Gaps in Health Insurance on Continuity of a Regular Source of Care Among Preschool-Aged Children in the United States. *JAMA*	Sample—8,129 children whose mothers were interviewed in the 1991 Longitudinal Follow-up to the National Maternal and Infant Health Survey	Gap in health insurance, length of the gap, and continuity of care
Ku and Freilach (2001) *Caring for Immigrants: Health Care Safety Nets in Los Angeles, New York, Miami, and Houston*	Case study site visits with clinic and hospital administrators, doctors and nurses, local Medicaid and health officials, community-based organizations, and immigration and health experts and advocates: Los Angeles, New York, Houston, and Miami.	The response of local providers and agencies to changes in state and local policies and practices affecting the access to insurance and health care services for immigrants in these areas

Findings

Of the children not born in the United States, 52% were uninsured and 66% had a usual source of care compared to 20 and 92%, respectively of those that were native born. Of foreign-born children, 51% had their usual source of care at a doctor's office or HMO, compared to 68% of U.S.-born children. Of those who were in less than excellent health, 39% of foreign-born children had not seen a doctor in the past year compared to 17% of U.S.-born children. Health insurance and immigrant policies should act to increase health care access for this population.

Children in immigrant families tend to be healthier than children in U.S.-born families. Immigrant children have fewer acute and chronic health problems than U.S.-born children, including acute infectious and parasitic diseases; ear infections; acute accidents; chronic respiratory conditions; and chronic hearing, speech, and deformity impairments. However, over time, immigrant children lose this health advantage concordant with the length of residence in the United States. Children in immigrant families also have a high risk of certain health problems. Mexican immigrant children are more likely to be reported by their parents as being in fair or poor health and having teeth in only fair to poor condition. The report theorizes that these paradoxical findings suggest that strong family bonds among immigrants may act to sustain cultural orientations leading to healthful behavior or that there are other unknown factors at work serving as protection. The subsequent deterioration in the health of children from immigrant families the longer they reside in the United States suggests that with assimilation into American culture the protective aspects of immigrant culture diminish, allowing the harmful effects of low socioeconomic status, high poverty, and racial or ethnic stratification to emerge.

Residence in the South (OR = 2.3) and West (OR = 1.9) and being poor, <100% FPL (OR = 2.2), or nearly poor, 100–200% FPL (OR = 2.1), are independently associated with being uninsured. Being uninsured was independently associated with having different sources for routine and sick care (adj. OR = 1.7; 95% CI = 1.5–2.0). There was also an independent association between never having routine care (adj. OR = 1.8; 95% CI = 1.2–2.7) and being uninsured, as well as an association between not having had a physician visit in the last 12 months and being uninsured (adj. OR = 1.5; 95% CI = 1.3–1.8).

About $1/4$ of children were without health insurance for at least one month during their first three years of life. More than half of these children had a gap of more than six months. Less than half had only one site for care during the first three years of life. Those with a gap longer than six months had an increased chance of having more than one site for care (OR = 1.52; 95% CI = 1.19–1.96). This chance increased when emergency treatment was discounted as a multiple site of care.

All cities reported a sharp decline in enrollment, but these could not be documented because most systems did not indicate if enrollees were immigrants. Data from Los Angeles indicated that the number of non-citizen immigrants and their children on Medicaid fell more than 50% between 1996 and 1998, but some believe that it has begun to climb again. More than half of low-income immigrants are uninsured and are particularly reliant on safety-net providers. Immigrants also tend to use alternative sources of care and delay or go without care. In every city, language barriers were viewed as the most serious threat to medical care quality. The access problem seemed to be the most severe for undocumented aliens who held an additional fear of being reported to the Immigration and Naturalization Service.

	Sample Size/ Data Source	Outcome Measures
Ku and Matani (2001) Left Out: Immigrants' Access to Health Care and Insurance. *Health Affairs*	Data from the NSAF; $n = 109{,}992$	Access to care
Lave et al. (1998a) Impact of a Children's Health Insurance Program on Newly Enrolled Children. *JAMA*	Data for 887 families of newly enrolled children in 29 counties of western Pennsylvania	Access to care and use of care
Lieu et al. (1993) Race, Ethnicity, and Access to Ambulatory Care Among US Adolescents. *Am. J Pub Health*	Data on 7,465 10–17-year-olds included in the Child Health Supplement to the 1998 NHIS	Health care access and use
McCormick et al. (2001) Annual Report on Access to and Utilization of Health Care for Children and Youth in the United States—2000. *Ambulatory Pediatrics*	Data on insurance coverage, utilization, and expenditures from MEPS. (1996, $n = 6{,}735$; 1997, $n = 11{,}278$; and 1998 $n = 7{,}839$); data on hospitalization from the Database for Pediatric Studies	Use of health care services and health expenditures for children and youth in the United States
Newacheck et al. (1998b) Health Insurance and Access to Primary Care for Children. *N Engl J Med*	Sample of 49,367 children under 18 from the 1993–1994 NHIS	Access to care, use of care, satisfaction with care, and unmet needs

Findings

Recent policy changes have limited immigrants' access to insurance and health care. Fewer non-citizen immigrants and their children have Medicaid or job-based insurance, and many more are uninsured than native citizens or children of citizens. Of the non-citizen adults with incomes under 200% FPL, 58% were uninsured, and of the non-citizen children with non-citizen parents, 54% were uninsured. Overall, 41% of non-citizen adults, 38% of non-citizen children, and 21% of citizen children with non-citizen parents had no doctor, nurse, or ED visits in a year, while 21% of native adults and 13% of children of citizens had no doctor, nurse, or ED visits in a year. Even though insured noncitizens had less access to care than citizens, they had better access than uninsured noncitizens. The disparity in access to care has two components. First, noncitizens and their children are much more likely to be uninsured, which reduces the ability to access care. Secondly, even insured noncitizens and their children have less access to medical care than insured native-born citizens. There are nonfinancial barriers that they face such as language difficulties and lack of translations.

Access to services improved after enrollment in the program. At 12 months of enrollment, 99% of the children had a regular source of care (vs. 89% prior to SCHIP) and 85% had a regular dentist (vs. 60% prior to SCHIP). The number of children reporting unmet needs or delayed care in the past six months decreased from 57% to 16%. The proportion of children seeing a physician increased from 59% to 64%, and the proportion visiting an ED decreased from 22% to 17%.

Higher proportions of blacks and Hispanics than whites are uninsured (16% blacks, 28% Hispanics, 11% whites). Blacks and Hispanics reported poorer health status, made fewer doctor visits in the past year, and were more likely to lack a usual source of care than whites. Health insurance was associated with a greater increase in access to and use of care for minority youth than for white youth. After adjustment for health insurance, family income, need and other factors, racial differences persisted.

About 2/3 of Americans are covered by private insurance, 19% by public, and 15% uninsured. Children with any private insurance were found more likely to have office visits than those on public insurance only or those that were uninsured (76% for those with private insurance vs. 67% for those with public insurance only and 51% for the uninsured). Dental visits and prescriptions filled showed the same pattern. Of those with some private insurance, 51% had dental visits, while 29% of those with only public insurance and 21% of those who were uninsured had dental visits. Of those with some private insurance, 61% had their prescriptions filled, while 56% of those with only public insurance and 43% of those that were uninsured had theirs filled. Publicly insured children were more likely to be hospitalized than those who had some private insurance or were uninsured. Of publicly insured children, 5.4% had hospital stays and 15.5% visited the ED. Of those with any private insurance, 2.4% had hospital stays and 12.5% of them visited the ED. For those that were uninsured, 1.9% had hospital stays and 10.8% visited the ED.

An estimated 13% of U.S. children did not have health insurance in 1993–1994. Uninsured children were less likely to have a usual source of care (adj. OR = 6.1; 95% CI = 5.2–7.2). The uninsured were also more likely to have no regular physician (adj. OR = 1.7; 95% CI = 1.4–1.9), to be without access to care after hours (adj. OR= 1.6; 95% CI = 1.3–2.0), and to have families that were dissatisfied with at least one aspect of care (adj. OR = 1.4; 95% CI = 1.1–1.9). Uninsured children were more likely to have gone without needed medical (adj. OR = 5.8; 95% CI = 4.6–7.5), dental (adj. OR = 4.3; 95% CI = 3.7–4.9), or other health care. The uninsured were also less likely to have contact with a physician during the previous year (adj. OR = 2.1; 95% CI = 1.9–2.3).

	Sample Size/ Data Source	Outcome Measures
Newacheck et al. (1996) Children's Access to Primary Care: Differences by Race, Income, and Insurance Status. *Pediatrics*	Data from 7,578 1–17-year-old children of families responding to the 1987 NMES	Measures of access to and use of care
Newacheck et al. (2000a) The Unmet Health Needs of America's Children. *Pediatrics*	NHIS data from 1993 to 1996, 97,206 children <18 years old	Used measures of unmet need for medical care, dental care, prescription medications, and vision care
Newacheck et al. (1999) Adolescent Health Insurance Coverage: Recent Changes and Access to Care. *Pediatrics*	Data on 14,252 adolescents, ages 10–18, from the 1995 NHIS	Assess health insurance status, trends in health care coverage, demographic and socioeconomic correlates of coverage, and role of insurance in influencing use of and access to care
Newacheck et al. (1998a) An Epidemiologic Profile of Children with Special Health Care Needs. *Pediatrics*	Data from 1994 NHIS Disability. Sample based on 30,032 completed interviews for children <18 years old	Characteristics of special needs children such as health status, access to care, satisfaction, and demographics

Results are presented in four subgroups compared to children generally: poor children, minority children, uninsured children, and white non-poor insured children (reference group). Poor, minority, and uninsured children fared consistently worse on all indicators than children in the reference group, and of the children in at least one risk group, 40% are in another risk group as well. Children in all of these risk groups were less likely to have a usual source of care (OR = 0.76; 95% CI = 0.57–1.02 for poor children; OR = 0.56; 95% CI = 0.43–0.73 for minorities; and OR = 0.47; 95% CI 0.35–0.64 for the uninsured). These groups were more likely not to see a specific physician (OR = 1.88; 95% CI = 1.46–2.41 for the poor; OR = 2.44; 95% CI = 1.86–3.19 for minorities; and OR = 1.30; 95% CI = 1.01–1.67 for the uninsured) and were more likely to go without after-hours emergency care (OR = 1.30; 95% CI = 0.99–1.70 for the poor; OR = 1.77; 95% CI = 1.38–2.27 for minorities; and OR = 1.35; 95% CI = 1.03–1.77 for the uninsured). These groups were also more likely to have to wait 60 minutes or more at their site of care (OR = 2.03; 95% CI = 1.52–2.72 for the poor; OR = 2.12; 95% CI = 1.52–2.94 for minorities; and OR = 1.52; 95% CI = 1.14–2.03 for the uninsured). These individuals were more likely to be inadequately vaccinated for measles (OR = 1.40, 95% CI = 1.11–1.79 for the poor; OR = 2.66; 95% CI = 2.18–3.25 for minorities; OR = 1.09; 95% CI = 0.86–1.39 for the uninsured) and more likely to not have seen a physician for selected symptoms (OR = 1.25; 95% CI = 0.90–1.73 for the poor; OR = 1.54; 95% CI = 1.21–1.95 for minorities; OR = 1.65; 95% CI = 1.26–2.16 for the uninsured).

Of children overall, 7.3% experience at least one unmet need. After adjusting for confounders, children who were near poor or poor were both about three times more likely to have an unmet need as non-poor children (adj. OR = 2.89; 95% CI = 2.52–3.32 for near poor adj. OR = 3.0; 95% C I = 2.53–3.56 for poor). Uninsured children were three times as likely to have an unmet need as an insured child (adj. OR = 2.92; 95% CI = 2.58–3.32). The unmet need for dental care was the most prevalent form of unmet need; 5.3% of children reported an unmet need for dental care in the last year during 1993–1996. An unmet need for medical care in the past year during 1993–1996 was experienced by 1.6% of children.

In 1995, 14% of adolescents were estimated to be uninsured. Risk of being uninsured was higher for older adolescents, minorities, those in low-income families, and those in single-parent households. The uninsured were less likely to have a usual source of care (71% vs. 95.6%), more likely to have unmet needs (23.1% vs. 6.2%), and less likely to see a physician during the course of a year (74.9% vs. 89.8%). Between 1984 and 1995 the percentage of adolescents with some sort of insurance remained unchanged; however those with private insurance decreased and those with public insurance increased.

Among U.S. children under 18 years, 18% were classified as a special needs. Of these children, 11% were uninsured, 6% were without a usual source of care, 18% were reported as dissatisfied with one or more aspect of care received at their usual source, and 13% had one or more unmet needs in the past year. Children with existing special needs are disproportionately poor and socially disadvantaged, and many of these children face significant barriers to health care.

	Sample Size/ Data Source	Outcome Measures
Newacheck et al. (2000b) Access to Health Care for Children with Special Health Care Needs. *Pediatrics*	Data on 57,553 children, <18 years old in the 1994–1995 NHIS Disability Survey	Access to and use of care
Newacheck (1992) Characteristics of Children with High and Low Usage of Physician Services. *Med Care*	Data from the Child Health Supplement of the 1998 NHIS (*n* = 17,110).	Use of care (physician services)
Starfield (1995) Chapter 3 in *Health Care for Children: What's Right, What's Wrong, What's Next*	Literature review	Environmental factors, social and economic factors, and medical and health system factors
Stoddard et al. (1994) Health Insurance Status and Ambulatory Care for Children. *N Engl J Med*	Data from a subsample of 7,578 children and adolescents 1–17 years of age included in the 1987 NMES	Medical attention by a physician for pharyngitis, acute earache, recurrent ear infection, or asthma
Szilagyi et al. (2000a) Evaluation of New York State's Child Health Plus: Children Who Have Asthma. *Pediatrics*	187 children (2–12) who had asthma and enrolled in CHPlus between Nov. 1, 1991 and, Aug. 1, 1993	Rates of primary care visits, ED visits, hospitalizations, number of specialists seen, and quality-of-care measures

Of U.S. children, 18% were defined as having special health care needs (based on the Maternal and Child Health Bureau definition) and 89% of these had health insurance. Socioeconomic characteristics were related to insurance coverage: 16.7% of those <100% FPL were uninsured, while 18.1% of those 100–199% FPL were uninsured, and 4.1% of those ≥200% FPL were uninsured. Uninsured children were less likely to have a usual source of care (adj. OR = 5.8; 95% CI = 4.4–7.6) and more likely to have gone without seeing a doctor in the last 12 months (adj. OR = 2.5; 95% CI = 2.0–3.1). The uninsured were more likely to go without or delay care due to cost (OR = 11.4; 95% CI = 6.9–18.9) than the insured. Uninsured children were more likely to report unmet needs in medical care (adj. OR = 5.8; 95% CI = 4.4–7.6) in dental care (adj. OR = 4.0; 95% CI= 3.2–5.0), in prescriptions, and/or eyeglasses (adj. OR = 3.2; 95% CI = 2.4–4.3), and in mental health care (adj. OR = 3.4; 95% CI = 1.7–6.9). Data showed that cost was the primary barrier to obtaining health insurance (74.1% said it was too expensive and they could not afford health insurance).

Children averaged three contacts with doctors; however 21% of children did not use physician services, and 7% had 10 or more contacts (accounting for 37% of the total number of contacts in 1998). Age and ethnicity of the child; family income, health insurance status, size and area of residence, and mother's educational attainment were important sociodemographic correlates of low usage.

Social, environmental, and medical or health system factors promote and inhibit children's health. Social conditions such as poor living conditions and inadequate income are factors that predispose individuals to disease (poverty is an important correlate of disease). On the other hand, good nutrition and good housing counteract disease. Physical factors in the environment have effects on health that are specific to developmental stages for children. Medical care and health system factors can improve health, prevent disease, and reduce the impact of disease. Children in the United States are at a disadvantage compared to those in other industrialized countries due to the lack of guaranteed access to health services.

Uninsured children were more likely to not receive care for all four conditions than those with insurance (unadjusted ORs, 2.83 for pharyngitis; 2.04 for acute earache; 2.84 for recurrent ear infections; and 1.87 for asthma). After adjustment, significant differences remained (for pharyngitis, adj. OR = 1.7; 95% CI = 1.1– 2.7; for earache, adj. OR = 1.85; 95% CI = 1.2– 3.0; for recurrent ear infections, adj. OR= 2.1; 95% CI = 1.28–3.51; and for asthma, adj. OR = 1.7; 95% CI = 1.1–2.8).

Visit rates to primary care providers were significantly higher during CHPlus than before for chronic illness (0.995 visit before and 1.34 visits per year during). The increase was seen in follow-up visits (0.86 vs. 1.32), total visits (5.69 vs. 7.11), and visits for acute asthma exacerbations (0.61 vs. .84) as well. There was no significant association between CHPlus coverage and ED visits or hospitalizations, however specialty utilization increased (30% vs. 40%; p = .02). Parents felt that CHPlus reduced asthma severity for 55% of children. CHPlus was also reported to have improved overall health status for 45% of children, attributed primarily to coverage for office visits and asthma medication. There was no statistically significant effect of CHPlus on several other quality-of-care measures such as follow-up after acute exacerbations, receipt of influenza vaccination, or use of bronchodilators or antiinflammatory medications.

	Sample Size/ Data Source	Outcome Measures
Szilagyi et al. (2000b) Evaluation of Children's Health Insurance: From New York State's Child Health Plus to SCHIP. *Pediatrics*	1,828 children who enrolled in CHP between Nov. 1, 1991, and Aug. 1, 1993, in a six-county region of upstate NY	To measure the association between CHP and access to care, utilization of care, quality of care, and health care costs
Szilagyi et al. (2000c) Evaluation of a State Health Insurance Program for Low-Income Children: Implications for State Child Health Insurance Programs. *Pediatrics*	2,126 children (0–12 years of age) enrolled in Child Health Plus (CHP) in 1992–1993 within New York State. (response rate in New York City was particularly low [33%] due to various barriers, including language)	Access to care, utilization of care, and quality measures
Weinick et al. (1998) Children's Health Insurance, Access to Care, and Health Status: New Findings. *Health Affairs*	MEPS data from 1996	Access to care, use of care, and perceived health status
Weinick and Krauss (2000) Racial/Ethnic Differences in Children's Access to Care. *Am J Pub Health*	Data from the 1996 MEPS	Usual source of care
Weinick et al. (2000) Racial and Ethnic Differences in Access to and Use of Health Care Services, 1977 to 1996. *Med Care Res Rev*	Data from three surveys: the 1977 NMCES ($n = 38{,}336$), the 1987 NMES ($n = 33{,}536$), and the 1996 MEPS ($n = 20{,}793$)	Usual source of care; the probability of having at least one ambulatory care visit; and the average number of visits for those who have used any ambulatory care services

Health Outcomes for Children and Youth

Dafny and Gruber (2000) *Does Public Insurance Increase the Efficiency of Medical Care? Medicaid Expansions and Child Hospitalizations*	NHDS data for four age groups: <1, 1–5, 6–10, and 11–15, 1983–1996	Avoidable hospitalizations for children <16

Utilization of primary care increased after enrollment in SCHIP. However, there was no association between SCHIP and changes in utilization of ED specialty services or inpatient care. SCHIP was associated with improvements in many measures involving quality of primary care, including preventive care and immunization rates. Enrollment was associated with a modest increase in expenditures, $71.85 per child per year.

Enrollment in CHP resulted in fewer children lacking a medical home (5% before vs. 1% during enrollment), with the largest change in New York City (11% vs. 1%). There was also an increase of 42% in total visits for care: 25% of an increase for preventive visits and 52% for acute visits. The number of specialists seen during CHP was more than twice as high as before. CHP was not associated with changes in ED utilization, but hospitalization was lower by 36% (even though this was not covered by CHP). Use of public health departments for immunizations decreased by 64%, and more immunizations were delivered in the medical home. One-third of parents also reported improved quality of health care for their children because of CHP.

Hispanic children are more likely to be uninsured (27.7%), to lack a usual source of care (17.2%), and to be in fair or poor health (7.8%), compared to all other racial and ethnic groups. The main reasons reported by parents for children being without a usual source of care were that the child was seldom or never sick (65.9%), they could not afford it (10.0%), they recently moved or did not know where to go (7.8%), and various other reasons (16.3%). About 11.6% of families had difficulty or delays in obtaining care or did not receive needed care. Of these families, 59.9% stated that they were unable to afford care, 19.5% gave insurance reasons, and 20.7% said there were other problems.

Black and Hispanic children were substantially less likely than white children to have a usual source of care. Differences persisted after controlling for health insurance and socioeconomic status. Controlling for language ability eliminated differences between Hispanic and white children.

The proportion of Americans without a usual source of care had not changed much from 1977 to 1996; however, the proportion of Hispanics without a usual source of care increased from 19.9 in 1977 to 29.5 in 1996, while the proportion for whites and blacks remained fairly stable. Blacks and Hispanics were more likely to lack a usual source of care than whites. Overall, the probability of Americans using ambulatory care increased over the years, but there are differences in this probability based on racial and ethnic groups. Black and Hispanics were less likely to use ambulatory care services over all three years, and the average number of visits for both groups was less than that for whites in all three years.

Over 1983–1996, child hospitalizations increased by 10% due to Medicaid expansions. Avoidable hospitalizations fell 22% due to Medicaid eligibility expansions. Treatment intensity per day increased with an increasing proportion of Medicaid hospital stays, but there were fewer days per stay.

	Sample Size/ Data Source	Outcome Measures
Kaestner et al. (2001) Medicaid Eligibility and the Incidence of Ambulatory Care Sensitive Hospitalizations for Children. *Social Science Medicine*	Nationwide inpatient sample of the Healthcare Cost and Utilization Project (HCUP-3) for 1988 and 1992 (before and after Medicaid expansions)	Difference in ACSC hospitalizations between low-income and high-income groups
Kuehl et al. (2000) Insurance and Education Determine Survival in Infant Coarctation of the Aorta. *J Health Care Poor Underserved*	Data from 1981 to 1989 for 103 cases of infant coarctation of the aorta diagnosed before 1 year of age	Coarctation of the aorta
Li and Davis (2001) Insurance Status and Survival Outcome in Pediatric Trauma Patients. *Academic Emergency Medicine*	National Pediatric Trauma Registry (23,135 patients)	Survival status at discharge in relation to insurance status, demographic characteristics, injury circumstances, and injury severity
Lykens and Jargowsky Forthcoming (2002) Medicaid Matters: Children's Health and Medicaid Eligibility Expansions. *J Policy Analysis Manage*	NHIS Child Health Supplement, 1988 and 1991 combined; children <15 years in families ≤185% FPL	Number of acute illness episodes; bed days; school loss days; restricted activity days reported for two-week period before interview
McInerny et al. (2000) Uninsured Children with Psychosocial Problems: Primary Care Management. *Pediatrics*	235 pediatric and family practice clinicians from 90 practices in 38 states and the Commonwealth of Puerto Rico; each clinician enrolled an average sample of 55 consecutive children (4–15 years old)	Clinician-reported items: insurance status, clinician identification of a psychosocial problem, visit characteristics; parent- or guardian-reported items: psychosocial problems, family functioning
O'Toole et al. (1996) Insurance-Related Differences in the Presentation of Pediatric Appendicitis. *J Ped Surgery*	Retrospective chart review of all cases of confirmed acute appendicitis ($n = 288$) presenting to Children's Hospital of Buffalo, Jan. 1990–Dec. 1993	Rate of appendiceal perforation

Findings

Results of the analyses were mixed. There was "relatively robust" evidence that Medicaid expansions decreased the incidence of ACSC hospitalizations among children aged 2–6 from very low income areas. For other groups of children, results were less consistent. There was some evidence that Medicaid expansion reduced ACSCs in children age 2–6 from near-poor areas (areas with a family income between $25,000 and $30,000). Among older children (from 7 to 9), there was little evidence that Medicaid expansion reduced rates of ACSCs.

Coarctation of the aorta is associated with greater maternal education and having any health insurance but not with measures of severity. Infants without health insurance are 12.8 times more likely to die than infants with any health insurance. Of the infants with coarctation whose mothers were uninsured, 33% died compared to 3.8% of infants with mothers who had health insurance. Of all deaths in infant coarctation, 55% occur prior to surgical treatment. One-third of deaths occur without diagnosis.

The case fatality rate for patients with commercial insurance was 2.06%, increasing to 2.86% for patients with government-assisted insurance (RR: 1.48, 95% CI 1.22, 1.76), and to 4.17% for the uninsured (RR: 2.02, CI 1.69, 2.42). Uninsured and underinsured pediatric trauma patients were at significantly elevated risk of in-hospital mortality. Association with insurance status and likelihood of survival are independent of injury severity and demographic characteristics.

In aggregated analysis, for non-Hispanic whites, both Medicaid eligibility and private insurance reduces the number of acute illness episodes. A 10-percentage point increase in the level of Medicaid eligibility reduced acute episodes 12% from the overall mean for 1991. Although significant, the confidence interval was large. Results for Hispanic and non-Hispanic black children were in the same direction but not statistically significant. Results for bed days, restricted activity days, and school absences as a function of area Medicaid eligibility level did not reach statistical significance for any ethnic group, but the direction of the effect went toward fewer functional limitations at higher Medicaid eligibility levels.

Of the 13,401 visits to clinicians, 93.4% were insured and 6.6% were uninsured. A higher percentage of adolescents, Hispanic children, those with unmarried parents, and those with less educated parents were uninsured. According to clinicians, uninsured children and insured children had similar rates of psychosocial problems (19%) and severe psychosocial problems (2%). No difference was found in clinician reported counseling, medication use, or referral to mental health professionals for children with identified psychosocial problems. A greater percentage of uninsured children are rated as having behavioral problems by their parents; however there is no difference in the rates of clinicians' identifying psychosocial problems for uninsured versus insured children. This implies that clinicians are not recognizing behavioral problems as much in the uninsured. This discrepancy may be explained by the fact that uninsured children have fewer clinician visits than insured children, especially for well-child care. Of these children, 50% had been uninsured before enrollment in CHP and 16% previously had received Medicaid.

All children ($\leq$16) were categorized as Medicaid or uninsured, HMO, or private FFS insurance. Rate of appendiceal perforation was significantly higher among Medicaid or uninsured vs. HMO and private FFS (44%, 27%, 23%; p <.05); duration of symptoms before presentation was longer (47.3, 29.3, and 23.1 hours, respectively p <.01); and their hospital stay was longer (7.9, 4.8, and 4.6 days, respectively; p <.01).

	Sample Size/ Data Source	Outcome Measures
Overpeck and Kotch (1995) The Effect of US Children's Access to Care on Medical Attention for Injuries. *Am J Pub Health*	Data from the NHIS 1988 Child Health Supplement (*n* = 17,110)	Injury rates, severity of injuries, and medical attention
Overpeck et al. (1997) Socioeconomic and Racial/Ethnic Factors Affecting Non-fatal Medically Attended Injury Rates in US Children. *Injury Prevention*	1988 Child Health Supplement to the NHIS (*n* = 17,110)	Injury rates, severity of injury, and medical attention for injury
Pappas et al. (1997) Potentially Avoidable Hospitalizations: Inequalities in Rates Between US Socioeconomic Groups. *Am J Pub Health*	1990 NHDS, NHIS, census (474 hospitals submitted records of which 192,734 were used for study)	Hospital discharge rates (by age, race, median income of zip code, and insurance status)
Parker and Schoendorf (2000) Variation in Hospital Discharges for Ambulatory Care-Sensitive Conditions Among Children. *Pediatrics*	1990–1995 NHDS, U.S. census, NHIS (survey collected 15,000 medical records for children per year)	Hospital discharge rates
Rodewald et al. (1997) Health Insurance for Low-Income Working Families: Effect on the Provision of Immunizations to Preschool-Age Children. *Arch Pediatr Adolesc Med*	1,730 children younger than 6 years who were enrolled in CHP. (for all of the upstate NY area served by CHP)	Number of immunization visits; types of providers (public health department clinics or primary care providers [pediatricians and family physicians]); and series-complete immunization coverage

Findings

Of the serious medically attended injuries, 17% of children had no medical care coverage, 6.5% had no place for sick or injured care, and 2.5% had neither coverage nor a place for care. Adjusted relative rates (uninsured to insured) of total medically attended injuries ranged from 0.70 at ages 12 through 17 years to 0.80 at ages younger than 6 without coverage. Serious injury relative rates for those with no coverage ranged from 0.57 at ages younger than 6 to 0.84 at ages 12 through 17. All relative rates showed that children without medical care coverage were significantly less likely to have injuries attended (except for serious injuries at ages 12–17 (RR: 0.84, 95% CI = 0.061-1.16). The relative rates show that for those without coverage, between 20 and 30% of total injuries in 1988 may not have been attended, and at least 40% of serious injuries occurring to children aged 11 years and younger without coverage may not have been attended.

Lack of coverage was consistently associated with lower medically attended injury rates in non-Hispanic blacks or whites and Mexican Americans. The total rates of medically attended injuries for each group reflected that population's uninsured rate. Injuries occur about 40% more frequently to children and adolescents living in singe-adult households for all injury categories except those occurring in schools.

Children under 15 had 439,000 avoidable hospitalizations, which represented 19% of all discharges (adjusted) for this age group. Avoidable conditions accounted for 27% of all adjusted discharges for children 1–4 years of age compared to 11% for children under 1 year and 19% for those age 5–14. Most of the potentially avoidable hospitalizations for this group were for two conditions: pneumonia (43%) and asthma (39%). A smaller proportion of patients with private insurance (10%) experienced a potentially avoidable hospitalization than patients who are uninsured (13%) or on Medicaid (15%).

Hospitalization rates were significantly higher among children who were younger, were black, had Medicaid insurance, and lived in poorer areas. Hospital discharge rates for ACSCs (per 1,000 children) were 10.5 for uninsured, 25.8 for Medicaid, and 13.3 for private or other insured children. The proportion of discharges attributed to ACSCs was similar for those who were uninsured and those with private or other insurance but higher for those on Medicaid. The authors state that if the assumption is made that uninsured children are disadvantaged within the health care system and may have a higher percentage of discharges for ACSCs, it is likely that some of the findings for the uninsured could be attributed to misclassification of insurance status.

There was a decrease in immunization visits to public health department clinics by 37% for infants and an increase in immunization visits to primary care providers' offices by 15% due to CHP. There was an increase in immunization coverage by 7%. For children aged 1–5 there was a decrease in visits to public health department clinics by 67% and an increase in visits to primary care providers' offices by 27%, with an increase in immunization coverage by 5%. The greatest effect was seen among those who were uninsured and those who had a gap in coverage longer than six months.

	Sample Size/ Data Source	Outcome Measures
Shi and Lu (2000) Individual Sociodemographic Characteristics Associated with Hospitalization for Pediatric Ambulatory Care Sensitive Conditions. *J Health Care Poor Underserved*	Data from 1994 NHDS (478 out of 512 hospitals responded to the survey)	Hospital discharge rates for ACSCs
Spivak et al. (1995) The Relationship Between Insurance Class and Severity of Presentation of Inflammatory Bowel Disease. *Am J Gastroenterology*	20 underinsured (uninsured + Medicaid) children matched with 20 children with private insurance from a pool of 63 with inflammatory bowel disease at a pediatric GI service	Delayed presentation; disease severity at presentation

Effect of Health on Children's Life Chances

Acs et al. (1999) The Effect of Dental Rehabilitation on the Body Weight of Children with Early Childhood Caries. *Pediatr Dent*	Percentile weight categories of children with noncontributory medical histories	Weight percentile
Brunelle (1989) *Oral Health of United States Children: The National Survey of Dental Caries in U.S. Schoolchildren, 1986–1987*	National Survey of Oral Health by the National Institute of Dental Research (NIDR) of children ages 5–17 in 1986–1987; survey was the second in a series (the first was in 1979–1980)	Dental caries
Carr et al. (1992) Variations in Asthma Hospitalizations and Deaths in New York City. *Am J Pub Health*	Data on asthma hospitalizations (1982 to 1986) and deaths (1982 to 1987) among persons aged 0–34	Hospitalization for asthma, death from asthma
Casby (2001) Otitis Media and Language Development: A Meta-Analysis. *Am J Speech-Language Pathology*	Literature review and meta-analysis of existing research	Language development outcomes

Findings

In a logistic regression, children with Medicaid were more likely than privately insured children to be hospitalized for an ACSC (adj. OR = 1.1; CI = 1.04–1.20). Younger children were more likely than older ones to have an ACSC hospitalization (adj. OR = 0.95; CI = 0.95–0.96), and black children were more likely to have an ACSC hospitalization than white children (adj. OR = 1.7; CI = 1.0–1.7).

Underinsured children had more weight loss (20.9 vs. 8.6l; p <.005) and longer delay in months (10.3 vs. 2.7; p <.005) before diagnosis was made. Laboratory data indicated that underinsured children were more ill at presentation than insured (hemoglobin: 10.5 vs. 12.5; erythrocyte sedimentation rate: 59 vs. 21; p <.05) and had higher platelet count and depressed alkaline phosphatase levels.

Before the dental rehabilitation test the percentile weight categories were significantly lower than those of the comparison counterparts. Of the early childhood caries patients, 13.7% weighed less than 80% of their ideal weight. After intervention, these children showed significant weight increases through the course of follow-up. At the end of the follow-up period (1.58–1.36 years) there were no significant differences noted in percentile weight categories.

For the 41.3 million school children aged 5–17 in the United States who have at least one permanent tooth, the mean number of decayed, missing, and filled permanent teeth was estimated at 3.07 per child (CI 2.93–3.21). The caries level in permanent teeth increased with age, and females had slightly higher levels than males.

The average annual hospitalization rate was 39.2 per 10,000, and the mortality rate was 1.2 per 100,000. Death rates and hospitalizations were higher among blacks and Hispanics than among whites (3–5.5 times higher). There were geographic variations in hospitalization and mortality. Hospitalization and mortality rates were highly correlated (r = .67), with the highest rates in the city's poorest neighborhoods. Household income and percentage of blacks and Hispanics in the population were predictors of the areas' hospitalization rates.

The magnitude of the statistical population effect of otitis media with effusion on language development is low. However, it should be acknowledged that the findings of low population effects might be related to vicissitudes of the primary research. Among these are failure to determine research participants' hearing levels, other intrinsic and/or extrinsic individual differences among research participants, and sensitivity of language measures.

	Sample Size/ Data Source	Outcome Measures
Celano, and Geller (1993) Learning, School Performance, and Children with Asthma: How Much at Risk? *J Learn Disabil*	Research review	School functioning
CDC (1996a) *Asthma Surveillance Programs in Public Health Departments—United States*	Data from survey conducted by Council of State and Territorial Epidemiologists and the CDC during March and April 1996 ($n = 48$ states and 3 territories)	Existence of asthma surveillance program
Dallman et al. (1984) Prevalence and Cause of Anemia in the United States, 1976 to 1980. *Am J Clin Nutr*	Data from the second NHANES ($n = 15,093$)	Anemia
DuPaul et al. (2001) Preschool Children with Attention-Deficit/ Hyperactivity Disorder: Impairments in Behavioral, Social, and School Functioning. *J Am Acad Child Adolesc Psychiatry*	Data from children between age 3 and 5 years ($n = 58$ with ADHD and $n = 36$ normal controls)	Parent or teacher ratings of problem behavior and social skills, parent ratings of stress and family functioning, medical functioning, observations of parent–child interactions, classroom behavior, and test of preacademic skills
Edelstein and Douglass (1995) Dispelling the Myth That 50 Percent of U.S. Schoolchildren Have Never Had a Cavity. *Pub Health Rep*	Literature review	Dental caries

Findings

There is not sufficient evidence to suggest that children with asthma are at significantly higher risk for poor school performance than children without asthma. Factors that may contribute to poor school performance include iatrogenic effects of oral steroids, poor medical management of disease, and psychological problems.

Asthma affects more than 14 million persons in the United States. Asthma is the most common chronic disease of childhood, affecting approximately 5 million children aged less than 18 in the United States. Of the respondents, 43 reported no state or territorial-level asthma control programs. When asked why states may not have asthma programs, the most important reasons included lack of funds and shortage of staff. Ten states reported that asthma was not a public health priority, but 86% of the states or territories showed an interest in starting an asthma control program.

Anemia is often defined in terms of individuals with Hb values below 95% of the reference range. Anemia can also be considered in terms of the depression of Hb concentration. The highest prevalence of anemia for all races was in infants 1–2 years of age (5.7%), girls 15–17 years of age (5.9%), young women (4.5%), and elderly men (4.8%). The lowest prevalence of anemia was in children 6–8 years old (2.3%) and in males 12–44 years old (2.6%–2.9%). The prevalence of depression in Hb concentration due to anemia and inflammatory disease was highest in infants between the age of 1 and 2 (6.8%) and declined in children between 3 and 5 years (5.3%), 6 and 8 years (5.5%), and 9 and 11 years of age (4.6%).

Young children with ADHD exhibited more problem behavior and were less socially skilled than their normal counterparts. Parents of children with ADHD experienced greater stress and were coping less adaptively than parents of non-ADHD children. These children show more noncompliant and inappropriate behavior than normal controls particularly during task situations. Parents of ADHD children were more likely to show negative behavior toward their children. Children with ADHD exhibited more negative social behavior in preschool settings and scored lower on tests for preacademic skills. Preschool-age children are at risk for behavioral, social, familial, and academic difficulties relative to normal preschool-age children.

The article reviews the underreporting of children's caries in policy documents and dental literature. The article also review epidemiological studies of caries reported in U.S. dental literature since 1985. Dental caries remain the single most common disease of childhood that is not self-limiting or amenable to a course of antibiotics. The belief that many children do not suffer from this has resulted in inappropriate policy and funding decisions.

	Sample Size/ Data Source	Outcome Measures
Edmunds and Coye (1998) *America's Children: Health Insurance and Access to Care*	CPS, literature review, publicly available information on state and federal programs, other published reports, and papers presented to the committee by various organizations	Multiple measures of access, use, and health status.
Fischer et al. (1990) The Adolescent Outcome of Hyperactive Children Diagnosed by Research Criteria: II. Academic, Attentional, and Neuropsychological Status. *J Consult Clin Psychol*	100 hyperactive children and 60 control children followed prospectively over an eight-year period into adolescence	Academic skills, attention and impulse control, and select frontal lobe functions
Frick et al. (1991) Academic Underachievement and the Disruptive Behavior Disorders. *J Consult Clin Psycol*	177 clinic-referred boys diagnosed as having ADHD or conduct disorder (CD)	Academic underachievement
Gergen and Weiss (1990) Changing Patterns of Asthma Hospitalization Among Children: 1979 to 1987. *JAMA*	NHDS for 1979–1987 (a randomized sample of 181,000 to 227,000 discharges collected per year)	Asthma hospitalization
Gordon et al. (1994) Sustained Attention and Grade Retention. *Percept Mot Skills*	Data from children involved in a project designed to standardize the Gordon Diagnostic System ($n = 83$ students who failed a grade; $n = 93$ normal)	Scores on the Continuous Performance Test, the Peabody Picture Vocabulary Test, the Child Behavior Checklist, and the Child Behavior Checklist Teacher Report Form

Findings

The Committee concluded that health insurance coverage was a major determinant of whether children have access to health care. Access to care can influence children's physical and emotional growth, development, and overall health and well-being. Uninsured children are the least likely population group to have routine access to a physician. Among American children, 20% have chronic problems that could impose on their ability to function effectively in school and at home; 10% of children have one or more severe chronic conditions and account for 70–80% of all medical expenditures for children. The most prevalent chronic conditions are dental conditions, mental health and substance abuse problems, and developmental disabilities. Tooth decay is the single most common chronic disease of children. Access to coordinated, efficient, effective, and cost-effective health care for all American children should be a national goal.

At follow-up, hyperactive children demonstrated impaired academic achievement, impaired attention and impulse control, and greater off-task, restless, and vocal behavior during an academic task. Frontal lobe measures did not differentiate between those who were hyperactive and the control group. Several measures showed age-related declines in both groups, and it was concluded that hyperactive children may remain chronically impaired in academic achievement, inattention, and behavioral disinhibition into late adolescence.

Academic underachievement was associated with both ADHD and CD when the disorders were examined individually. The percentage of children underachieving who had ADHD, was higher in both reading and mathematics than for the control group. However, when examined together, the relationship between CD and academic underachievement was found to be due to its comorbidity with ADHD. When boys with ADHD were divided into those with attention deficit only and those with co-occurring hyperactivity, findings did not support the hypothesis that academic underachievement has a stronger association with attention deficit without co-occurring hyperactivity.

From 1979 to 1987, asthma hospitalizations among children aged 0–17 increased 4.5% per year. The increase was the greatest among 0–4-year-olds, 5.0% per year, vs. 2.9% per year for 5–17-year-olds. For children aged 0–4, blacks had about 1.8 times the increase of whites. Total hospitalizations decreased −4.6% during this time, while admissions for lower respiratory tract infections had a statistically insignificant decrease, −1.3%. Acute and chronic or unspecified bronchitis hospitalizations decreased −6.1%, but this decrease did not begin until 1983.

89 children, who had been retained at some point in school, had a higher frequency of abnormal scores on a sustained attention index than 93 children who had never repeated a grade. Those who had a history of grade retention in a sample of children that had been referred for an evaluation for ADHD had lower scores on the same measures of sustained attention.

	Sample Size/ Data Source	Outcome Measures
Grantham-McGregor and Ani (2001) A Review of Studies on the Effect of Iron Deficiency on Cognitive Development in Children. *J Nutr*	Seven studies in which Hb levels in early childhood were linked to cognitive development or school achievement	Studies were reviewed looking for causal relationship between iron deficiency and children's cognition and behavior
Gutstadt et al. (1989) Determinants of School Performance in Children with Chronic Asthma. *Am J Dis Child*	99 children with moderately severe to severe chronic asthma	Performance on standardized achievement tests
Halterman et al. (2000) Health and Health Care for High-Risk Children and Adolescents. *Pediatrics*	Data from the NHANES III 1988–1994 for children 2 months to 16 years old. (n = 40,000)	Adequate treatment for asthma
Halterman et al. (2001) Iron Deficiency and Cognitive Achievement Among School-Aged Children and Adolescents in the United States. *Pediatrics*	Data from NHANES III 1988–1994. (sample: 5,398 children ages 6–16)	Iron deficiency and cognitive test scores
Hurtado et al. (1999) Early Childhood Anemia and Mild or Moderate Mental Retardation. *Am J of Clin Nutr*	Data from Special Supplemental Program for Women, Infants, and Children (WIC) (1979 to 1980) and school records (from 1990 to 1991) in Dade County, FL (n = 5411)	Special education placement and mild or moderate retardation
Lang and Polansky (1994) Patterns of Asthma Mortality in Philadelphia from 1969 to 1991. *N Engl J Med*	Data from Philadelphia Department of Public Health on deaths from asthma between 1969 and 1991	Death from asthma

---

Findings

Most correlation studies found associations between iron deficiency anemia and poor cognitive and motor development and behavioral problems. Longitudinal studies showed that children anemic in infancy continue to have poorer cognition and school achievement and more behavior problems in middle childhood. Possible confounding of poor socioeconomic status prevents a causal relationship from being determined. In children that are anemic and less than 2 years of age, short-term trials of iron treatment have generally failed to benefit development. Only one trial has shown benefit, and it remains unclear whether poor development of iron-deficient infants is due to poor social background, represents irreversible damage, or is remediable with iron treatment.

Test scores and intelligence tests showed that overall academic capabilities of children with asthma are average to above average. Factors associated with low performance scores were low socioeconomic status, older age, history of continuous oral steroids, and presence of emotional and behavioral problems. Investigation of poor classroom performance of a child with chronic asthma should include investigation of the roles of socioeconomic status, oral steroid therapy, and emotional and behavioral problems.

9.4% of the children had physician-diagnosed asthma. Overall, 74% of the children with moderate to severe asthma had inadequate therapy. Of those with moderate asthma, 26% had taken maintenance medication during the past month. Among children who had two or more hospitalizations in the last year, only 32% had taken maintenance medications. Factors found to be associated with inadequate therapy include ≤5 years old, Medicaid insurance, and Spanish speaking.

Children with iron deficiency had greater than two times the risk of scoring below average in math than did children with normal iron status (OR: 2.3; 95% CI = 1.1–4.4). This elevated risk was present even for iron-deficient children without anemia (OR: 2.4; 95% CI = 1.1–5.2).

There was an increase in the likelihood of mild or moderate mental retardation associated with anemia, independent of birthweight, maternal education, sex, race or ethnicity, the mother's age, or the child's age at entry into the WIC program. In addition, for each decrease in quantity of hemoglobin, the risk of mild or moderate mental retardation increased by 1.28 (adj. OR = 1.28; 95% CI: 1.05–1.60).

Death rates from asthma decreased from 1.68 per 100,000 people in 1969 to 0.68 per 100,000 in 1977. However, there was an increase to 0.92 per 100,000 in 1978 and to 2.41 per 100,000 in 1991. From 1965 to 1990, the concentration of major air pollutants decreased. Between 1985 and 1991, 258 people were identified with asthma as the primary cause of death. These death rates were significantly higher where there was a higher percentage of blacks, Hispanics, females, and people with incomes in the poverty range.

	Sample Size/ Data Source	Outcome Measures
Lanphear et al. (1997) Increasing Prevalence of Recurrent Otitis Media Among Children in the United States. *Pediatrics*	Data from Child Health Supplement to 1981 and 1988 NHIS (n = 5,189 [1981] and n = 6,209 [1988])	Changes in the prevalence of otitis media and associated risk factors for recurrent otitis media
Lindgren et al. (1992) Does Asthma or Treatment with Theophylline Limit Children's Academic Performance? *N Engl J Med*	In Iowa, 255 children with asthma who had taken nationally standardized scholastic achievement tests; matched sibling controls were used for 100 of them	Performance on scholastic achievement test
Litt et al. (1995) Multidimensional Causal Model of Dental Caries Development in Low-Income Preschool Children. *Pub Health Rep*	Data from assessment of 184 low-income preschool children	Dental caries and *mutans Streptococcus*
Looker et al. (1997) Prevalence of Iron Deficiency in the United States. *JAMA*	Data from NHANES 1988–1994 (n = 24,894 aged 1 year or older)	Iron deficiency and iron deficiency anemia
Lous (1995) Otitis Media and Reading Achievement: A Review. *Int J Pediatr Otorhinolaryngol*	Literature review of 19 studies	Reading achievement
Lozoff et al. (1991) Long-Term Developmental Outcome of Infants with Iron Deficiency. *N Engl J Med*	191 participants in San Jose, Costa Rica, follow-up to original study (age 5)	Cognitive, socioemotional, and motor tests, and measures of school functioning

Findings

The number of visits for otitis media, the most common diagnosis among preschool children, increased in the past decade. Recurrent otitis media among preschool children increased from 18.7% in 1981 to 26% in 1988 (OR: 1.6; 95% CI 1.4–1.7). The greatest increase occurred in infants (OR: 0.9; CI 1.3– 2.9). Factors associated with otitis media were allergic conditions (OR: 1.9; CI 1.7– 2.2), survey year (OR: 1.7; CI 1.5–1.9), black race (OR: 0.6; CI 0.5–0.7), Hispanic ethnicity (OR: 0.8; CI 0.6–0.9), day care (OR: 1.5; CI 1.3–1.7), out-of-home care by an unrelated sitter (OR: 1.3; CI 1.1–1.6), and male gender (OR: 1.2; CI 1.1–1.3).

Academic achievement among the children with asthma was similar to normative standards for Iowa and higher than national standards. For the 101 children with control siblings, the composite test score for children with asthma was 58.3 and for siblings 57.5. None of the differences between the children with asthma and their siblings were statistically significant. Achievement among children with asthma, at least for those whose status is closely monitored in structured treatment programs, appears to be unaffected.

Results confirmed that caries development at a one-year follow-up was strongly dependent on earlier caries development. Early caries in this sample was determined in part by mutans levels and by dental health behavior. Historically, blacks had a lower percentage of dental caries than whites. Recently, Hispanics and blacks have been found to have a higher percentage of caries. This has been attributed to socioeconomic status in terms of risk of caries. It is likely that socioeconomic status has more of an indirect effect in that it affects social norms (i.e., tooth brushing, dental services, consumption of sugar).

In the United States, 9% of toddlers aged 1–2 years old and 9–11% of adolescent girls and women of childbearing age were iron deficient. In these individuals, iron deficiency anemia was found in 3% of toddlers and in 2–5% of adolescents and women. Iron deficiency occurred in no more than 7% of older children or those older than age 50 and in any more than 1% of teenage boys and young men. Iron deficiency is more likely to occur in minority, low-income, and multiparous women of childbearing age. Iron deficiency and anemia are still common in toddlers, adolescent girls, and women of childbearing age.

Children catch up in their cognitive development when their ears and hearing become normal. A correlation has been found between secretory otitis media (SOM) and reading, but the correlation is small. Reading achievement was more closely correlated with cognitive, language, and linguistic factors as well as socioenvironmental classroom factors. The high frequency of hearing loss resulting from SOM and the rate of OM in those who are prone to otitis underlie the need for more research.

All children had excellent hematologic status and growth at 5 years. Children who had had moderately severe iron deficiency anemia as infants had lower scores on tests of mental and motor functioning at school entry than the rest of the children. Statistically significant differences were found on all tests except verbal IQ. This difference remained significant after controlling for socioeconomic status. Children who have iron deficiency anemia in infancy are at risk for long-lasting developmental disadvantages compared to their peers.

	Sample Size/ Data Source	Outcome Measures
Lozoff et al. (1998) Behavior of Infants with Iron-Deficiency Anemia. *Child Dev*	191 participants in San Jose, Costa Rica (n = 52 iron deficient infants, n = 139 comparison infants)	Increased proximity to caregivers, increased wariness or hesitance, and decreased activity (mental and motor testing)
Lozoff et al. (2000) Poor Behavioral and Developmental Outcomes More Than 10 Years After Treatment for Iron Deficiency in Infancy. *Pediatrics*	191 participants in San Jose, Costa Rica, follow-up to original study (age 11–14)	Cognitive, socioemotional, and motor tests, and measures of school functioning
Lubker et al. (1999) Chronic Illnesses of Childhood and the Changing Epidemiology of Language-Learning Disorders. *Topics in Language Disorders*	Reviews evidence on chronic childhood illness and psycho-educational and language-learning disorders	Language-learning disorders
Mannuzza et al. (1997) Educational and Occupational Outcomes of Hyperactive Boys Grown Up. *J Am Acad Child Adolesc Psychiatry*	Prospective follow-up of white boys who were diagnosed, at approximately age 7 with ADHD (*n* = 104 of the 207 original boys were evaluated)	Long-term educational achievement and occupational rank
Mannuzza and Klein (2000) Long-Term Prognosis in Attention-Deficit/ Hyperactivity Disorder. *Child Adolesc Psychiatr Clin N Am*	Review of three studies	School achievement, social skills, and self-esteem
Marshall et al. (1999) Arithmetic Disabilities and ADD Subtypes: Implications for DSM-IV. *J Learn Disabil*	20 students aged 8–12 with attention deficit disorder with hyperactivity and 20 students with attention deficit disorder without hyperactivity	Academic deficit

Findings

Infants with iron deficiency and anemia remained in closer contact with caregivers; showed less pleasure and delight; and were more wary, hesitant, and easily tired. They were less playful, made fewer attempts at test items, and were less attentive to instructions or demonstrations. These results indicated that iron deficiency anemia in infancy was associated with alterations in affect and activity.

Children with severe chronic iron deficiency in infancy scored lower on measures of mental and motor functioning even after controlling for background factors. More of the formerly iron-deficient children had repeated a grade and/or been referred for special services or tutoring. Parents and teachers rated their behavior as more problematic in several areas and had increased concerns about anxiety or depression, social problems, and attention problems.

Children with a number of chronic illnesses are at increased risk for language-learning disorders as a result of the conditions themselves and iatrogenesis.

Those with ADHD completed significantly less schooling (about two years less on average) than controls. These individuals also had lower-ranking occupational positions than controls. This study suggested that childhood ADHD predisposes individuals to disadvantages that continue to affect functional domains unrelated to current psychiatric diagnosis.

Among children in early and middle adolescence with lower levels of academic and social functioning, 2/3–3/4 have ADHD symptoms. Many of the same behaviors continue through late teen years, and deficits continue to be present in academic and social areas, compared to control groups (lower grades, more courses failed, worse performance on standardized tests, few friends, and rated less adequate in psychosocial adjustment). About 2/5 continue to experience symptoms to a clinically significant degree; 1/4–1/3 have a diagnosed antisocial disorder, and 2/3 of these individuals are arrested. When individuals were evaluated in their twenties, dysfunctions are apparent in the same areas. Compared to controls, these individuals complete less schooling, hold lower-ranking occupations, and continue to suffer from poor self-esteem and social skill deficits.

Students did not differ in age or grade; however there were significant differences in Full Scale IQ and Performance IQ. Students in the ADD/H group had higher scores than the ADD/noH groups on both tests. No significant difference was found between groups on the achievement measures. Significant differences did appear in within-group comparisons, involving lower performance on the math calculation subtest. Students with ADD/noH had significantly lower scores on the calculation subtest compared to all other achievement

	Sample Size/ Data Source	Outcome Measures
McCowan et al. (1996) School Absence— A Valid Morbidity Marker for Asthma. *Health Bull*	773 children with asthma or related symptoms and 773 controls from school registers in the Tayside, Scotland region	School absences and days absent per term
Merrell and Tymms (2001) Inattention, Hyperactivity, and Impulsiveness: Their Impact on Academic Achievement and Progress. *Br J Educ Psychol*	Data from 4,148 children from a nationally representative sample of schools in England	Behavior and reading and mathematics achievement
Mody et al. (1999) Speech Perception and Verbal Memory in Children With and Without Histories of Otitis Media. *J Speech, Language, Hearing Res*	Data from the participants in the Longitudinal Infant Follow-up and Evaluation program ($n = 14$)	Speech perception and verbal short-term memory tasks
NIH (2000) Consensus Development Conference Statement: Diagnosis and Treatment of Attention-Deficit/ Hyperactivity Disorder (ADHD). *J Amer Acad Child Adolesc Psychiatry*	Literature review	Diagnosis of ADHD
Otero et al. (1999) Psychological and Electroncephalographic Study in School Children with Iron Deficiency. *Int J Neurosci*	Two groups selected randomly from a group of 100 6–12-year-old primary school children	Test outcomes for WISC-R, a computerized test of learning (DEL), and a qEEG
Rana et al. (2000) Asthma Prevalence Among High Absentees of Two Philadelphia Middle Schools. *Chest*	Data from 5th and 6th graders who were absent 25 or more days in two Philadelphia middle schools during spring 2000 ($n = 176$)	Diagnosis of asthma

subtests. These results provided support for the hypothesis that inattention exerts a specific and deleterious effect on the acquisition of arithmetic computation skills.

When the control group and the children taking asthma medication were compared, there were significant differences in the days absent and episodes of absence. The increase in absences was about one school day each term. Severity of asthma was not related to increase in absence. Those who were not receiving asthma medication but had related symptoms were absent more than their matched controls.

The reading and mathematics attainment and value-added for children with high scores on the behavior rating scale were found to be educationally and statistically significantly lower than for children with scores of zero on the rating scale.

The otitis media group performed less accurately than the otitis-free group. However the pattern of errors was the same for each group. The children with and without positive histories of otitis media were negatively affected by an increase in phonetic similarity of the stimulus item. The two groups did not differ on identification or on temporal order recall when multiple features differentiated speech sounds. Findings suggested that long-term effects of early episodes of otitis media on phonological representations and on working memory do exist.

ADHD is the most commonly diagnosed behavioral disorder of childhood estimated to affect 3–5% of school-age children. Symptoms include developmentally inappropriate levels of attention, concentration, activity, distractibility, and impulsivity. Children with ADHD usually have functional impairment in a number of settings including home, school, and peer relationships. This disorder has also been shown to have long-term adverse effects on academic performance, vocational success, and social–emotional development. The lack of insurance coverage and disconnect between medical and educational services are substantial barriers for assessment and follow-up.

The WISC-R showed that iron-deficient children had lower values in WISC item of information, comprehension, and verbal, performance, and full-scale IQ than control children. The EEG power spectrum showed more theta energy in all leads using Laplacian montage and more delta energy in frontal areas using referential montage in iron-deficient children than in the control group. Aside from the well-known effect of iron deficiency on intellectual performance during childhood, the EEG power spectrum of iron-deficient children had a slower activity than that of control children suggesting a developmental lag and/or CNS dysfunction.

High-absentee children were compared to low-absentee children from the same grades. The prevalence of self-reported asthma was 34.9% for high-absentee children and 25.2% for low-absentee children. Diagnosis of asthma through the ISAAC (International Study of Asthma and Allergies in Children) survey showed that 48.3% of high-absentee children and 36.7% of low-absentee children had asthma. Among high-absentee children with asthma, 43% were not aware of the diagnosis, and among low-absentee children, 51.9% were unaware.

	Sample Size/ Data Source	Outcome Measures
Rietveld and Colland (1999) The Impact of Severe Asthma on School Children. *J Asthma*	25 children with severe asthma, aged 10–13 years, compared to 25 matched controls	Normal daily functioning
Roberts et al. (2000) Otitis Media in Early Childhood in Relation to Preschool Language and School Readiness Skills Among Black Children. *Pediatrics*	Data from a prospective study of 85 black children examined from 6 months to 5 years of age	Language skills, school readiness
Shelton et al. (1998) Psychiatric and Psychological Morbidity as a Function of Adaptive Disability in Preschool Children with Aggressive and Hyperactive Impulsive Inattentive Behavior. *J Abnorm Child Psych*	Data from 154 children with aggressive-hyperactive-impulsive-inattentive behavior (AHII); of these, 38 had adaptive disability and 116 did not; 47 control children were also used	ADHD, oppositional defiant disorder, conduct disorder, symptoms of general psychopathology, social skills deficit, parental problems, lower levels of academic achievement
Silverstein et al. (2001) School Attendance and School Performance: A Population-Based Study of Children with Asthma. *J Pediatr*	A cohort of children with asthma and a matched group without asthma in Rochester, MN (*n* = 92 children with asthma)	School attendance and performance
Silverstein et al. (2001) School Attendance and School Performance: A Population-Based Study of Children with Asthma. *Pediatrics*	Data from a cohort of children in Rochester, MN, with asthma and age- and sex-matched children without asthma (*n* = 92 with asthma)	Days absent, achievement test scores, grade point average, grade promotion, and class rank or graduating students
Taragonski et al. (1994) Trends in Asthma Mortality Among African Americans and Whites in Chicago 1968 Through 1991. *Am J Pub Health*	Death certificates among African Americans and whites aged 5–34 in Chicago from 1968 through 1991 (*n* = 340 deaths)	Asthma mortality rates

Findings

Children with asthma did not vary significantly from controls. They reported more dyspnea after physical exercise, which could not be attributed to lung function. Differences in school performance were not significant. It was concluded that children may generally adapt well to living with asthma.

Otitis media and associated hearing loss were significantly positively correlated with measures of expressive language at 3 and 4 years of age. However, this relationship did not remain significant when the child's gender, socioeconomic status, maternal educational level, and the responsiveness and support of the home and child care environments were accounted for. Both otitis media and hearing loss were moderately correlated with school readiness skills at entry. Children with more otitis media scored lower in verbal math problems. Children with more hearing loss scored lower in math and recognizing incomplete words. These associations remained after accounting for background factors.

Children with AHII have greater risk for a variety of psychological, academic, emotional, and social difficulties than children with either behavior pattern alone. Both AHII groups were more likely to have ADHD, oppositional defiant disorder, and conduct disorder than the control group. These children also had more symptoms of general psychopathology, greater social skill deficits, more parental problems, and lower levels of academic achievement.

Children with asthma had 2.21 (95% CI = 1.41–3.01) more days absent than children without asthma. There was no significant difference in standardized achievement scores: reading percentile difference 1.22%; 95% CI = -3.68–6.12; mathematics percentile difference 2.36%; 95% CI = -2.89–7.60, and language percentile difference 2.96%; 95% CI = -4.03–7.15. There was also no significant difference in grade point average, grade promotion, or class rank for graduation.

Children with asthma had 2.21 (95% CI = 1.41–3.01) more days absent than those without asthma. There was no significant difference in the achievement test scores. There was also no significant difference in grade point average, grade promotion, or class rank between the two groups.

African Americans had consistently higher asthma mortality throughout the period. Asthma mortality remained stable for whites, but increased by 337% among African Americans from 1976 through 1991. The increase was greatest among 20–34-year-olds. Outpatient and ED deaths increased during this period, while the proportion of dead-on-arrival cases remained stable. This shift to non-inpatient deaths suggests that lack of access to health care may play a role in asthma mortality.

	Sample Size/ Data Source	Outcome Measures
Teele et al. (1990) Otitis Media in Infancy and Intellectual Ability, School Achievement, Speech, and Language at Age 7 Years. *J Infect Dis*	Data from a randomly selected group ($n = 207$) of 7-year-old children from a larger cohort ($n = 498$) were followed prospectively since birth	Assessment of hearing, cognitive, speech, and linguistic data
Vargas et al. (1998) Sociodemographic Distribution of Pediatric Dental Caries: NHANES III 1988–1994. *J Am Dent Assoc*	Data from the third NHANES 1988–1994 ($n = 10,332$)	Dental caries
Wolfe (1985) The Influence of Health on School Outcomes. *Med Care*	Data used is part of the child health survey conducted over a period of years in the early 1970s in Rochester, NY; sample of chronically ill school-age children and a matched sample of well children ($n = 248$)	School outcomes (achievement and attendance)
Zargi and Boltezar (1992) Effects of Recurrent Media in Infancy on Auditory Perception and Speech. *Am J Otolaryngol*	33 children with a history of at least three episodes of acute otitis media before age 2; a control group of 29 children with fewer episodes of otitis media. All children from 8 to 10 years old	Speech ability

Prenatal and Perinatal Care and Outcomes

Amini et al. (1996) Effect of Prenatal Care on Obstetrical Outcome. *J Matern Fetal Med*	A seven-year computerized perinatal database with 29,225 consecutive deliveries from a single inner city tertiary medical center; data from 23,181 women who had documented prenatal visits	Access and use of services and outcomes from prenatal testing as well as scores at birth

Findings

The time spent with a middle-ear effusion during the first three years of life was significantly associated with lower scores on tests of cognitive ability, speech and language, and school performance at 7 years of age (after controlling for confounding variables). The adjusted mean full-scale WISC-R scores were 113.1 for those with least time with middle ear effusion, 107.5 for those with moderate time, and 105.4 for those with the most time. Significant differences were also seen for verbal and performance IQ scores. It was found that for the Metropolitan Achievement Test, middle-ear disease in the first three years of life was associated with lower scores in mathematics and reading. Similar differences were found for articulation and use of morphologic markers.

Lower-income children and Mexican-American and African-American children are likely to have a higher prevalence of caries and more unmet treatment needs than their higher-income and non-Hispanic white counterparts.

Children with certain health problems, such as those creating problems with strenuous activities and difficulties with physical activities and peer communication, have lower school outcomes compared to children with other health problems. Health problems that are likely to interfere with school interactions such as communication in the classroom or physical activities significantly increase days absent. Severe psychological discomfort has the largest direct negative impact on achievement. On the other hand, health problems that interfere with ordinary activities do not affect attendance, and children with these problems seem to be able to compensate for their health.

Of the children who had a history of at least three episodes of otitis media, 88% had auditory perception disorders. Decreased auditory stimulation during the time of auditory maturation could have prevented the development of these functions completely. Statistically significant differences were not observed in the development of articulation.

Overall, 90.6% of the mothers had at least three prenatal visits (C), while 9.4% had two or fewer visits (NC). The NC group was 2.3 times more likely to be unmarried (80% vs. 59%; $p < .001$), 6.3 times more likely to be staff patients (no private insurance), and 1.5 times more likely to be black. NC mothers delivered at an earlier gestational age (37.3 ± 3.3 vs. 39.0 ± 2.6 weeks; $p < .001$), had lower birthweights (BWs) (2810 ± 743 vs. 3,203 ± 607 g for singleton births; $p < 0.001$), and their infants had longer neonatal hospital stays (8.4 ± 17.3 vs. 4.8 ± 10.4 days; $p < .001$) compared with C mothers. After adjustment, C mothers delivered infants who were on the average 550 g heavier than those of NC mothers. The neonates of NC mothers had consistently lower Apgar scores and were more likely to be breech (5.7% vs. 3.1%) and to be transferred to the ICU (11.6% vs. 5.2%; $p < .001$). The NC group had fewer cesareans (94% vs. 14.2%; $p < .001$), but thicker meconium fluid (12.4% vs. 8.9%; $p < 0.001$). Neonatal outcomes were all uniformly worse in the NC group. Incidences of low birthweight, low Apgar scores, and admissions to the neonatal ICU were all higher compared to the C group.

	Sample Size/ Data Source	Outcome Measures
Aron et al. (2000) Variations in Risk-Adjusted Cesarean Delivery Rates According to Race and Health Insurance. *Med Care*	Data from 25,697 women without prior cesarean deliveries admitted for labor and delivery Jan. 1993– June 1995 (Cleveland, OH)	Cesarean sections
Baldwin et al. (1998) The Effect of Expanding Medicaid Prenatal Services on Birth Outcomes. *Am J Pub Health*	Vital records data linked with Medicaid files and AFDC-enrolled women in Colorado and Washington State	Use of prenatal care and low birthweight
Bernstein (1999) *Insurance Status and Use of Health Services by Pregnant Women*	Data from Community Tracking Study Household Survey, 1996–1997 (*n* = 60,000 individuals)	Access to and use of pregnancy or birth services and subsequent maternal and pediatric outcomes
Braveman et al., (1989) Adverse Outcomes of Health Insurance Among Newborns in an Eight-County Area of California, 1982 to 1986. *N Engl J Med*	Hospital discharge data on births to residents of an eight-county region of California from the Office of Statewide Health Planning and Development for the last half of 1982, all of 1984, and 1986	Adverse outcomes among newborns; transfer to another acute care hospital or to a long-term care facility; death
Braveman et al. (1991) Differences in Hospital Resource Allocation Among Sick Newborns According to Insurance Coverage. *JAMA*	In California civilian acute care hospitals, a population-based sample, including all newborns discharged in 1987 with evidence of serious problems (*n* = 29,751)	Length of stay, total charges, and charges per day

Overall rates for cesarean deliveries were similar among whites and nonwhites (15.8% and 16.1%, respectively). The rates based on insurance status varied according to insurance, with 17.0% for those with commercial insurance, 14.2% for those with government insurance, and 10.7% for those without insurance. After adjusting for clinical factors the adjusted OR for nonwhites was higher (adj. OR = 1.34; 95% CI = 1.14–1.57; p <.001), similar for those on government insurance (adj. OR = 1.01; 95% CI = 0.90–1.14; p = 0.84) and lower for uninsured patients (adj. OR = 0.65; 95% CI = 0.41-1.03; p = 0.067) although not statistically significant. After stratification for predicted risk of cesarean delivery, racial differences were limited to patients who had lower risks. Differences in the odds ratios were seen in all risk categories (odds ratios were not statistically significant).

There was a clinically significant reduction in the overall low-birthweight rate, from 7.1% in 1989 to 6.4% in 1992 in Washington, which provided enhanced prenatal services. This change was greatest among high-risk women, 90% of whom had diabetes or chronic hypertension. The low-birthweight rate for Colorado's population (the control group) increased slightly from 10.4 to 10.6%

Among pregnant women, 17% of the uninsured reported fair or poor health status compared to 6.8% of privately insured patients. In addition, 29% of the uninsured pregnant women reported not having a usual source of care compared to 14% of Medicaid-enrolled patients and 9% of privately insured women. This group also made fewer visits to the doctor (7.9% for the uninsured, 10.3% for Medicaid enrolled, 10.1% for the privately insured). Lastly, uninsured women had greater perceived unmet medical needs (18% of uninsured pregnant women reported they did not receive some needed medical care vs. 7.6% of privately insured and 8.1% of Medicaid-enrolled pregnant women).

Between 1982 and 1986 the percentage of newborns without health insurance increased by 45% (from 5.5 to 8.0%; p <.001); the increases were larger among Asians (54%, from 7.8 to 12.0%; p <.001) and Latinos (140%, from 8.2 to 19.7%; p <.001). By 1986 the adj. OR for an adverse hospital outcome (prolonged hospital stay, transfer, or death) was 1.31 (95% CI 1.17–1.46) in uninsured compared with privately insured controlled for race. The comparable adj. ORs in 1982 and 1984 were 1.11 (95% CI = 0.93–1.33) and 1.19 (95% CI = 1.05–1.35). In 1986 the adj. ORs for uninsured vs. insured among blacks and Latinos were 2.24 (95% CI = 1.60-3-13) and 1.56 (95% CI = 1.26-1.94). The elevated and increasing risk for uninsured newborns may be partly explained by inadequate and diminishing access to care, and this burden was disproportionately borne by blacks and Latinos.

Sick newborns without insurance received fewer inpatient services than comparable privately insured newborns with either indemnity or prepaid coverage. The pattern was observed across all hospital ownership types. Mean stay was 15.7 days for all privately insured newborns (15.6 for those with indemnity and 15.7 for those with prepaid coverage), 14.8 days for Medicaid, and 13.2 for uninsured (p <.001). Length of stay, total charges, and charges per day were 16, 28, and 10% less, respectively for the uninsured than for all privately insured newborns (p <.001). Resources for newborns covered by Medicaid were generally greater than for the uninsured and less than for the privately insured. Both uninsured and Medicaid-covered newborns were found to have more severe medical problems than the privately insured.

	Sample Size/ Data Source	Outcome Measures
Braveman al. (1993) Access to Prenatal Care Following Major Medicaid Eligibility Expansion. *JAMA*	Single live births to California residents occurring in state in 1990 ($n = 593,510$)	Untimely initiation of care, too few visits, and no prenatal care
Braveman et al. (2000) Barriers to Timely Prenatal Care Among Women with Insurance: The Importance of Prepregnancy Factors. *Obstet Gynecol*	Postpartum survey conducted in California during 1994–1995, focusing on 3,071 low-income women with Medi-Cal or private coverage throughout pregnancy	Timely prenatal care
Bronstein et al. (1995) Access to Neonatal Intensive Care for Low-Birthweight Infants: The Role of Maternal Characteristics. *Am J Pub Health*	Alabama vital statistics records between 1988 and 1990 for infants weighing 500–1,499 g	Transfer to hospitals with neonatal ICUs
Cole (1995) *Increasing Access to Health Care: The Effects of Medicaid Expansions for Pregnant Women*	Census data, state-level aggregate birth certificates for all states (1983–1990)	Prenatal care use and low birthweight and/or prematurity
Coulam et al. (1995) *Final Report of the Evaluation of the Medicare Catastrophic Coverage Act: Impacts on Material and Child Health Programs and Beneficiaries*	Birth certificates linked to Medicaid enrollment files for Missouri	Pregnant women eligible for Medicaid or deliveries covered by Medicaid; prenatal care use; low birthweight or prematurity; infant mortality
Currie and Gruber (1996a) Saving Babies: The Efficacy and Cost of Recent Changes in the Medicaid Eligibility of Pregnant Women. *J Political Econ*	CPS state-level aggregate birth and death statistics, United States	Pregnant women eligible for Medicaid, deliveries covered by Medicaid, and infant mortality

Findings

Despite Medicaid expansion, nearly 11% of live births were uninsured for prenatal care. Compared to women with private FFS coverage, uninsured women had a higher risk of untimely initiation (adj. OR = 2.54; 95% CI = 2.47–2.60) and too few visits (adj. OR = 2.49; 95% CI = 2.44–2.55). Those on Medi-Cal also had a high risk of untimely care (adj. OR = 3.33; 95% CI = 3.26–3.40) and too few visits to the doctor (adj. OR = 1.63; 95% CI = 1.60–1.66). Lack of private insurance was also a strong risk factor for no care (adj. OR = 6.70; 95% CI = 6.0–7.47).

Factors associated with untimely initiation of prenatal care among low-income women with continuous prenatal coverage included the following: unwanted or unplanned pregnancy (affecting 43 and 66% of women, respectively), no regular provider before pregnancy (affecting 22% of women), and no schooling beyond high school (affecting 76% of women). Assistance with transportation could contribute to more timely care for some low-income women, but programs focusing primarily on other noninsurance barriers during pregnancy might not substantially improve the timeliness of care, at least among low-income women with third-party coverage.

Non-white mothers with early prenatal care were more likely than white mothers to deliver low-birthweight infants in hospitals with neonatal ICUs without transfers (after adjusting for other factors). In hospitals without such facilities, those with late prenatal care were less likely to be transferred to hospitals with neonatal ICUs before delivery. Medicaid coverage increased the likelihood of antenatal transfer for white women.

An increase in the Medicaid-eligible population was associated with a reduced percentage with late prenatal care; results were more pronounced for white women (those with late prenatal care declined from 22.3% to 21.8%). An increase in the Medicaid-eligible population was associated with reduced rates of low birthweight and prematurity for white women and black teenagers; changes were slight (from 5.5% premature to 5.4% premature) among white women, after controlling for other characteristics.

Medicaid enrollment grew in the AFDC and expansion groups; Medicaid covered 13% of all live births in 1987 and 23% in 1989. Expansion group teenagers had lower rates of inadequate care (27.4%) than non-Medicaid low-income teenagers (32.0%). Significant results were not found for low birthweight, prematurity, or infant mortality.

There was a dramatic increase in the eligibility of pregnant women for Medicaid, but there were different rates of increase across states. The percentage of pregnant women eligible for Medicaid rose from 12% in 1979 to 43% in 1991. A 30% rise in the percentage of pregnant women eligible for Medicaid was associated with an 8.5% decline in state-level infant mortality. In addition, it was found that targeted changes in Medicaid eligibility, restricted to low-income groups, had much greater effects on birth outcomes than broader expansions of eligibility to women of higher income levels.

	Sample Size/ Data Source	Outcome Measures
Currie and Gruber (2001) Public Health Insurance and Medical Treatment: The Equalizing Impact of the Medicaid Expansions. *J Pub Econ*	U.S. birth certificate data 1987–1992	Use of four obstetrical procedures: cesarean delivery, fetal monitor, induced labor, and ultrasound
Currie and Grogger (2002) Medicaid Expansions and Welfare Contractions: Off-setting Effects on Prenatal Care and Infant Health. *J Health Econ*	U.S. birth certificate data 1990–1996	Use and timeliness of prenatal care; low and very low birthweight
Dubay et al. (2001) Changes in Prenatal Care Timing and Low Birth Weight by Race and Socioeconomic Status: Implications for the Medicaid Expansion for Pregnant Women. *Health Serv Res*	Data on 8.1 million births from the National Natality Files, 1980, 1986, and 1993. Births in all areas of the United States except CA, TX, WA, and upstate NY	The rate of late initiation of prenatal care and the rate of low birthweight
Durbin et al. (1997) The Effect of Insurance Status on Likelihood of Neonatal Interhospital Transfer. *Pediatrics*	Southeastern Pennsylvania, five-county general acute care nonpediatric hospitals, 56,789 infants (0–28 days of age) admitted or born in a study hospital between Jan. and Dec. 1991	Transfer to another general or specialty acute hospital
Ellwood and Kenney (1995) Medicaid and Pregnant Women: Who Is Being Enrolled and When. *Health Care Financ Rev*	Medicaid enrollment and claims files for CA, GA, MI, and TN	Women covered by Medicaid and/or deliveries covered by Medicaid

Findings

Among younger and less educated women, Medicaid eligibility expansions were associated with *increased* use of each of the procedures. Among college-educated women for whom higher Medicaid eligibility may have resulted in higher rates of Medicaid coverage relative to private health insurance, higher Medicaid eligibility levels were associated with *decreased* use of these procedures.

Increases in Medicaid eligibility had statistically significant effects on use of prenatal care: reducing the probability of inadequate care for both white and black women; increasing the proportion of each group getting care in the first trimester; and reducing late initiation of care by both groups of women. Increases in Medicaid eligibility slightly reduced the probability of very low birthweight babies to white mothers. No comparable effect was found for black women.

From 1986 to 1993, rates of late initiation of prenatal care decreased by 6.0 to 7.8 percentage points beyond the estimated changes for the 1980–1986 period for white and African-American women of low socioeconomic status. The rate of low birthweight was reduced by 0.26 to 0.37 percentage point between 1986 and 1993 for white women of low socioeconomic status. Other white women and all African-American women of low socioeconomic status showed no relative improvement in the rate of low birthweight during 1986–1993. For white women with less than 12 years of schooling, improvements were found in the rate of low birthweight; the same was not found in other groups.

Uninsured infants were almost twice as likely to be transferred as privately insured infants even with adjustments for prematurity, severity of illness, and level of the neonatal intensive care unit in the referring hospital (adj. RR = 1.96; 95% CI = 1.67–2.31). Infants with Medicaid were more likely to be transferred than similar privately insured neonates (adj. RR = 1.20; 95% CI = 1.01–1.43). Uninsured and publicly insured infants were more likely to be born prematurely (adj. RR = 1.49; 95% CI = 1.39–1.60) and to have both moderate (adj. RR = 1.11; 95% CI = 1.04–1.23) and high (adj. RR = 1.21; 95% CI= 1.11–1.32) illness severity compared to privately insured infants. Neonates with no insurance or those on Medicaid were more likely to be transferred than those with private insurance.

Medicaid eligibility expansions and improved enrollment procedures for pregnant women during the late 1980s were examined, and it was found that more women enrolled in Medicaid and they enrolled earlier in pregnancy. The percentage of deliveries covered by Medicaid grew from 48 to 116% (depending on the state). However, there are still substantial numbers of women who are enrolling too late, and therefore the expansion may not promote significantly earlier use of prenatal care (39 to 54% joined Medicaid after the first trimester of pregnancy).

	Sample Size/ Data Source	Outcome Measures
Foster et al. (1992) The Impact of Prenatal Care on Fetal and Neonatal Death Rates for Uninsured Patients: A "Natural Experiment" in West Virginia. *Obstet Gynecol*	4,534 patients delivered in one Level 2 hospital between Jan. 1984 and Dec. 1986 in three counties of West Virginia	Fetal death ratio
Glied and Gnanasekaran (1996) Hospital Financing and Neonatal Intensive Care. *Health Serv Res*	1991 data from Greater New York Hospital Association and New York State Department of Health (45 hospitals, $n = 139{,}076$ births)	Number of neonatal intensive care beds in a hospital
Haas et al. (1993b) The Effect of Providing Health Coverage to Poor Uninsured Pregnant Women in Massachusetts. *JAMA*	Massachusetts in-hospital, single-gestation live births in 1984 ($n = 57{,}257$) and 1987 ($n = 64{,}346$)	Satisfaction rates, care initiated before the third trimester, and adverse infant outcomes
Haas et al. (1993) The Effect of Health Coverage for Uninsured Pregnant Women on Maternal Health and the Use of Cesarean Section. *JAMA*	All in-hospital, single-gestation births in 1984 ($n = 57{,}257$) and 1987 ($n = 64{,}346$)	Rates of adverse maternal outcome and cesarean section for uninsured women and for two concurrent control groups: women with Medicaid and women with private insurance
Homan and Korenbrot (1998) Explaining Variation in Birth Outcomes of Medicaid-Eligible Women with Variation in the Adequacy of Prenatal Support Services. *Medi Care*	Medical record data on maternal risks and use of prenatal visits for more than 3,485 women receiving care at 27 ambulatory sites in four regions of California	Birth outcomes

Findings

A program was developed to give prenatal care to a population of uninsured patients. The overall fetal death ratio declined from 11.8 to 7.2 per 1,000 live births ($p = .02$) during the years of clinic operation. Uninsured patients experienced a reduction in fetal deaths during the program, from 35.4 to 7.0 per 1,000 live births ($p = .02$), whereas those covered by medical assistance did not experience a reduction. Privately insured patients also had a significant decrease, from 10.0 to 3.1 per 1,000 live births ($p < .001$). After suspension of the program the death ratio returned to 10.3 deaths per 1,000 live births in 1987. Over the same time period and for the same population, overall neonatal deaths declined.

After adjusting for low birthweight and other measures of patient need and for hospital affiliation, the study found that hospitals with more privately insured patients—especially those with more privately insured, low-birthweight newborns—have statistically significantly more neonatal intensive care beds than those with fewer such patients. These findings remain within hospital affiliation categories as well.

Between 1984 and 1987, the satisfaction rate for prenatal care declined from 96.4% to 93.8% for all women in the state. There was no statewide change in overall incidence of adverse birth outcomes. In 1984, uninsured women were less likely to receive satisfactory prenatal care and to initiate care before the third trimester. They were also more likely to suffer an adverse outcome. There was no statistically significant change between 1984 and 1987.

In 1984, uninsured women had higher rates of adverse maternal health outcome than privately insured women (5.5% and 5.1%, respectively) and received fewer cesarean sections (17.2% and 23.0%, respectively). Between 1984 and 1987, there was no statistically significant change in the interpayer difference in adverse outcome relative to women with private insurance. Theinterpayer difference in cesarean sections between the uninsured and the privately insured was reduced by 2.3% (95% CI = 0.4%–4.2%), although the uninsured continued to undergo fewer cesarean section (22.4% vs. 25.9%); similar results were observed when the uninsured women were compared to women with Medicaid. The provision of health insurance alone to low-income pregnant women may not be associated with . improvement in maternal health An expansion of coverage was associated with an increase in the rate of cesarean sections.

Providing at least one nutrition, psychosocial, and health education service session each trimester of care contributes significantly to explaining better birth outcomes when compared with providing fewer sessions. However, even with these services, outcomes differ among sites and types of settings. Although repeated support service sessions during prenatal care improve the chances of avoiding poor birth outcomes in low-income women, variations in outcomes at different sites and practice settings remain to be explained by other factors.

	Sample Size/ Data Source	Outcome Measures
Howell (2001) The Impact of Medicaid Expansions for Pregnant Women: A Synthesis of the Evidence. *Med Care Res Rev*	Review of published literature and data from the NCHS for 1985–1991 (n = 3.8 million births in 1985 and 4.1 million in 1991)	Prenatal care and birth outcomes
Keeler and Brodie (1993) Economic Incentives in the Choice Between Vaginal Delivery and Cesarean Section. *Milbank Q*	Literature review (225 journal articles, 3 dissertations, and 9 books between 1970 and 1992)	Obstetric decisions
Kenney and Dubay (1995) *A National Study of the Impacts of Medicaid Expansions for Pregnant Women*	County-level aggregate birth certificates for all states (1986–1990)	Prenatal care use
Long and Marquis (1998) Effects of Florida's Medicaid Eligibility Expansion for Pregnant Women. *Am J Pub Health*	Birth and death certificates, linked to hospital discharge abstracts, Medicaid enrollment and claims files, and county health department records from July 1988 to June 1989 (to 100% of poverty), (n = 56,101) and in calendar year 1991 (to 150% of poverty), (n = 78,421)	Use (amount and timing) of prenatal care, low-birthweight rates, and infant death rates
Oberg et al. (1991) Prenatal Care Use and Health Insurance Status. *J Health Care Poor Underserved*	149 women at six hospitals in Minneapolis, MN	Source, use, and quality of prenatal care

Findings

14 studies were used to look at the impact of Medicaid expansion. There was evidence that new groups of pregnant women were receiving coverage and that some women received improved prenatal care services. The improvements in prenatal care vary among states, and patterns were found in national studies showing a greater impact in the South and Midwest. The evidence stating that the expansion led to an improvement in birth outcomes is much weaker. When looking at the data from the NCHS, the results were similar to previous studies. However, an alternative explanation was offered for the decrease that did occur in infant mortality after the expansion. About half of the decline in infant mortality for unmarried women (those with the highest rates of very low birthweight) is due to declines in very low birthweight infant mortality from 1985 to 1991. Medicaid expansion did not result in a reduction in the rate of low birthweight; however, other factors were affected. Due to the expansion and additional resources, hospitals may have been able to expand or improve their neonatal ICUs, providing better care for these infants.

There has been a dramatic increase in cesarean section rates; the cost is high, and there is wide variation in its use. The economic incentives for physicians, hospitals, payers, and mothers all come into play. Providers who encounter higher opportunity costs while attending to mothers in prolonged labor can reduce these costs by operating or restricting their practices. When physician and hospital charges for C-sections ($7,186) and for vaginal births ($4,334) were compared, the C-section cost was 66% more. Private insurance pays more, and there are higher rates of C-sections in populations with private coverage. Not only are physicians, hospitals, and payers influenced by financial incentives, so are the mothers. The mainly indirect evidence on financial incentives shows that insured mothers have low marginal cost sharing when they undergo C-sections. Mothers who have private FFS insurance have higher rates of C-sections than mothers who are covered by staff-model HMOs, are uninsured, or are on public insurance.

Medicaid expansions were associated with a reduced percentage (from 20.8% to 19.2%) of white women receiving late or no prenatal care in the South and Midwest.

The number of deliveries covered by Medicaid increased by 47% after expansion. Access to prenatal care for the target population (low-income women without private insurance) improved: prior to the expansion, 2.3% had no prenatal care, and after the expansion, 1.6% had no prenatal care. Among those receiving care, fewer delayed care after the expansion (4.8% vs. 6.8%), and they had more prenatal visits (11.1 vs. 10.5). The rate of low birthweights declined after the expansion (61.8 vs. 67.9 per 1,000). The number of infant deaths also declined from 7.3 per 1,000 to 5.9 per 1,000.

In this study, insurance status was significantly related to the source of prenatal care (p <.0001). Private physicians cared for 52% of privately insured, 23% of those insured by Medicaid, and 2% of uninsured women. Medicaid and uninsured women, when compared to privately insured women, used public clinics as their primary source of care, experienced longer waiting times, and were more likely to lack continuity of care with a provider.

	Sample Size/ Data Source	Outcome Measures
Phibbs et al. (1993) Choice of Hospital for Delivery: A Comparison of High-Risk and Low-Risk Women. *Health Serv Res*	Data from 1985 California Office of Statewide Health Planning and Development discharge abstracts and hospital financial data	Delivery where there was a newborn intensive care unit
Piper et al. (1990) Effects of Medicaid Eligibility Expansion on Prenatal Care and Pregnancy Outcome in Tennessee. *JAMA*	Linked birth, death certificate, and Medicaid enrollment files	Pregnant women eligible for Medicaid or deliveries covered by Medicaid
Ray et al. (1997) Effect of Medicaid Expansion on Pre-term Births. *Am J Prev Med*	610,056 singleton births to African-American or Caucasian women	Pregnant women eligible for Medicaid or deliveries covered by Medicaid and prenatal care use
Salganicoff and Wyn (1999) Access to Care for Low-Income Women: The Impact of Medicaid. *J Health Care Poor Underserved*	Telephone interview survey of a representative cross-sectional sample of 5,200 low-income women in MN, OR, TN, FL, and TX	Health insurance coverage, health status, access to care, use of care, and satisfaction
Singh et al. (1994) Impact of the Medicaid Eligibility Expansions on Coverage of Deliveries. *Fam Plan Perspect*	Alan Gutmacher Institute Survey of States (national study comparison of states [50 states and District of Columbia, 5 states did not respond]), 1991	Women covered by Medicaid and/or deliveries covered by Medicaid
Stafford (1990) Cesarean Section Use and Sources of Payment: An Analysis of California Hospital Discharge Abstracts. *Am J Pub Health*	California data on hospital deliveries (461,066 deliveries) in 1986	Cesarean section
Stafford et al. (1993) Trends in Cesarean Section Use in California, 1983–1990. *Am J Obstet Gynecol*	Data from CA discharge abstracts on hospital deliveries in 1983–1990 (379,759–587,508 annual deliveries)	Cesarean section

Findings

Results show that high-risk and low-risk women do not have the same choice process. Hospital quality was more important for high-risk women. Results also show that factors influencing choice of hospital are different for those who are privately insured and those who are on Medicaid. High-risk women who were covered by Medicaid were less likely to deliver in a hospital with a newborn intensive care unit than high-risk women who were privately insured.

An expansion to all married women meeting income requirements increased the percentage of births covered by Medicaid from 22 to 29%. The year before Medicaid was compared to the year after; there were no improvements in the use of prenatal care in the first trimester, no changes in the rates of very low and moderately low birthweight and neonatal mortality. There were no improvements in these outcomes for the groups where coverage change was the greatest.

The percentage of deliveries covered by Medicaid increased from 21 to 51%; however Medicaid coverage increased only from 10 to 37% in the first trimester. The rate of inadequate prenatal care went down for all low-income groups and low-education groups (18.5% to 13.7% for unmarried women). Medicaid expansion increased enrollment and use of prenatal care in high-risk women; however it did not decrease the likelihood of preterm birth.

Low-income women were found to experience considerable barriers to care. Uninsured low-income women have significantly more trouble obtaining care, receive fewer recommended services, and are more dissatisfied with the care they receive than their insured counterparts. Women on Medicaid had access to care that was comparable to their low-income privately insured counterparts but, in general, had significantly lower satisfaction with their providers and their plans.

The number of deliveries covered by Medicaid rose from 0.5 million (14.5% of deliveries) in 1985 to 1.2 million (32.0% of deliveries) in 1991. The rise in Medicaid-covered births was due in part to greater coverage among women who previously had received uncompensated care, but about half of the increase was from new coverage of women who in the mid-1980s were covered by private insurance.

Cesarean sections were performed for 24.4% of deliveries; women with private insurance had the highest rates of cesarean section (29.1%). Lower rates were seen for women covered by non-Kaiser HMOs (26.8%), Medi-Cal (22.9%), Kaiser (19.7%), self-pay (19.3%), and indigent services (15.6%). Vaginal birth after cesarean occurred more often in women covered by Kaiser (19.9%) and indigent services (24.8%) compared to those with private coverage (8.1%). There was a sizable, although less pronounced, association between payment source and cesarean sections for breech presentation, dystocia, and fetal distress. Accounting for maternal age and race or ethnicity did not alter the findings.

California C-section rates increased from 21.8% in 1983 to 25% in 1987 and then decreased to 22.7% in 1990. Patterns were similar for all ages, races, and/or ethnicities. Differences in C-section use among patients with different insurance status increased from 1983 to 1990. Privately insured women consistently had higher rates of C-sections.

	Sample Size/ Data Source	Outcome Measures
Weis (1992) Uninsured Maternity Clients: A Concern for Quality. *Appl Nursing Res*	Chart review of inpatient maternity client medical records; 500 cases: half uninsured and half insured (public and private)	Length of stay, maternal complications

Findings

Compared with the privately insured, the uninsured had more life-style risks. Uninsured women had a shorter hospital stay with more maternal complications. Insurance coverage and prenatal care were positive predictors of birthweight, while life-style risk factors detracted. Length of stay was not influenced by insurance coverage but rather by health problems before delivery.

D

Data Tables

TABLE D.1 Federal Poverty Guidelines, 2000 and 2001

Family Size in 48 Contiguous States	Federal Poverty Level (FPL)					
	FPL for 2000			FPL for 2001		
	100% FPL	200% FPL	300% FPL	100% FPL	200% FPL	300% FPL
1 person	$8,350	$16,700	$25,050	$8,590	$17,180	$25,770
2 persons	$11,250	$22,500	$33,750	$11,610	$23,220	$34,830
3 persons	$14,150	$28,300	$42,450	$14,630	$29,260	$43,890
4 persons	$17,050	$34,100	$51,150	$17,650	$35,300	$52,950

SOURCE: DHHS, 2002.

TABLE D.2 Medicaid Income Eligibility Limits and Upper Federal Poverty
Level by Program by State, 2001

States	Medicaid Annual Income-Eligibility Threshold (2 Child Family)[a]	Medicaid Poverty-level Children[b,c]
U.S. total	$9,672	
Alabama	$3,048	0-6 from 15 to 133% 6-17 from 15 to 100%
Alaska	$14,496	0-6 from 71 to 200% 6-17 from 71 to 200%
Arizona	$5,244	Infants from 38 to 140% 1-6 from 38 to 133% 6-17 from 38 to 100%
Arkansas	$4,380	Infants up to 200% 1-14 up to 200%
California	$15,708	Infants from 86 to 200% 1-6 from 86 to 133% 6-17 from 86 to 100%
Colorado	$6,132	0-6 from 39 to 133% 6-17 from 39 to 100%
Connecticut	$10,392	0-17 from 0 to 185%
Delaware	$15,708	Infants from 0 to 185% 1-6 from 0 to 133% 6-18 from 0 to 100%
District of Columbia	$29,256	Infants from 0 to 200% 1-5 from 0 to 200% 6-17 from 0 to 200%
Florida	$9,672	Infants from 28 to 200% 1-6 from 28 to 133% 6-17 from 28 to 100%

Upper FPL by Program	
Medicaid SCHIP (Title XXI)[b,c]	Separate SCHIP (Title XXI)[b]
17-18 from 15 to 100	0-6 from 133 to 200% 6-17 from 100 to 200% 17-18 from 100 to 200%
0-6 from 133 to 200% 6-17 from 100 to 200% 17-18 from 71 to 200%	No program
No program	Infants from 140 to 200% 1-6 from 133 to 200% 6-17 from 100 to 200% 17-18 from 38 to 200%
Children aged 17 up to 100%	No program
17-18 from 86 to 100%	Infants 200 to 250% 1-6 from 133 to 250% 6-17 from 100 to 250% 17-18 from 100 to 250% AIM program, 0-2 from 250 to 300%
No program	0-6 from 133 to 185% 6-17 from 100 to 185% 17-18 from 39 to 185%
17-18 from 0 to 185%	0 to 18 from 185 to 300%
No program	Infants from 185 to 200% 1-6 from 133 to 200% 6-18 from 100 to 200%
Infants from 185 to 200% 1-5 from 133 to 200% 6-14 from 100 to 200% 17-18 from 50 to 200%	No program
Infants from 185 to 200% 17-18 from 28 to 100%	Infants up to 200% 1-6 from 133 to 200% 6-18 from 100 to 200%

continued

TABLE D.2 Continued

States	Medicaid Annual Income-Eligibility Threshold (2 Child Family)[a]	Medicaid Poverty-level Children[b,c]
Georgia	$6,168	Infants up to 185% 1-6 up to 133% 6-18 up to 100%
Hawaii	$16,836	Infants from 0 to 185% 1-6 from 0 to 100% 6-16 from 0 to 100% 17-19 up to 200%
Idaho	$4,884	0-6 up to 150% 6-19 up to 150%
Illinois	$10,584	Infants up to 200% 1-5 from 42 to 133% 6-17 from 42 to 133%
Indiana	$4,536	Infants up to 150% 1-6 up to 150% 6-18 up to 150%
Iowa	$12,780	Infants up to 200% 1-6 up to 133% 6-18 up to 133%
Kansas	$5,916	Infants up to 150% 1-6 up to 133% 6-18 up to 100%
Kentucky	$10,908	Infants from 33 to 185% 1-6 from 33 to 150% 6-17 from 33 to 150%
Louisiana	$3,876	0-6 up to 150% 6-18 up to 150%
Maine	$15,708	Infants up to 150% 1-6 up to 150% 6-16 up to 150% 17-19 up to 100%
Maryland	$6,288	Infants up to 200% 1-17 up to 200% 17-18 up to 200%
Massachusetts	$19,452	Infants up to 200% 1-18 up to 150%

Upper FPL by Program

Medicaid SCHIP (Title XXI)[b,c]	Separate SCHIP (Title XXI)[b]
No program	Infants from 185 to 235% 1-6 from 133 to 235% 6-18 from 100 to 235%
No program	No program
0-3 from 133 to 150% 6-19 from 100 to 150%	No program
6-17 from 100 to 133% 17-18 from 42 to 133%	0-18 from 133 to 185%
1-6 from 133 to 150% 6-17 from 100 to 150% 17-18 up to 150%	0-18 from 150 to 200%
6-18 from 100 to 133%	Infants from 185 to 200% 1-18 from 133 to 200%
No program	Infants from 150 to 200% 1-6 from 133 to 200% 6-18 from 100 to 200%
17-18 from 33 to 150%	Infants from 185 to 200% 1-6 from 133 to 200% 6-18 from 100 to 200%
0-6 from 133 to 150% 6-18 from 100 to 150%	No program
0-6 from 133 to 150% 6-18 from 125 to 150%	Infants from 185 to 200% 1-18 from 150 to 200%
Infants from 185 to 200% 1-17 from 133 to 200% 17-18 from 100 to 200%	No program
Infants from 185 to 200% 1-18 from 133 to 150%	1-18 from 200 to 400%

continued

TABLE D.2 Continued

States	Medicaid Annual Income-Eligibility Threshold (2 Child Family)[a]	Medicaid Poverty-level Children[b,c]
Michigan	$7,464	Infants up to 185% 1-17 up to 150%
Minnesota	$40,224	0-2 from 60 to 280% 2-5 from 60 to 275% 6-17 from 60 to 275%
Mississippi	$5,496	Infants up to 185% 1-6 up to 133% 6-17 up to 100%
Missouri	$15,708	Infants up to 300% 1-6 up to 300% 6-18 up to 300%
Montana	$10,032	0-6 from 40.5 to 133% 6-16 from 40.5 to 100% 17-19 from 40.5 to 71%
Nebraska	$6,420	Infants up to 185% 1-6 up to 185% 6-18 up to 185%
Nevada	$12,660	0-6 from 42 to 133% 6-16 from 42 to 100% 17-19 from 42 to 89%
New Hampshire	$9,780	Infants up to 300% 1-18 up to 185%
New Jersey	$6,396	Infants from 45 to 185% 1-6 from 45 to 133% 6-19 from 45 to 133%
New Mexico	$8,448	0-19 up to 235%
New York	$11,688	Infants up to 185% 1-6 up to 133% 7-19 up to 100%
North Carolina	$9,000	Infants up to 185% 1-6 up to 133% 6-18 up to 100%
North Dakota	$11,856	0-6 from 65 to 133% 6-17 from 65 to 100%

Upper FPL by Program	
Medicaid SCHIP (Title XXI)[b,c]	Separate SCHIP (Title XXI)[b]
17-19 up to 150%	Infants from 185 to 200% 1-18 from 150 to 200%
0-2 from 275 to 280%	No program
17-18 up to 100%	Infants from 185 to 200% 1-6 from 133 to 200% 6-18 from 100 to 200%
Infants from 185 to 300% 1-6 from 133 to 300% 6-18 from 100 to 300%	No program
No program	0-6 from 133 to 150% 6-17 from 100 to 150% 17-18 from 40.5 to 150%
Infants from 150 to 185% 1-6 from 133 to 185% 6-18 from 100 to 185%	No program
No program	0-6 from 133 to 200% 6-17 from 100 to 200% 17-18 from 42 to 200%
Infants 185 to 300%	1-18 from 185 to 300%
6-17 from 100 to 133% 17-18 from 45 to 133%	Infants from 185 to 350% 1-6 from 133 to 350% 6-18 from 133 to 350%
0-18 from 185 to 235%	No program
17-18 medically needy up to 100%	Infants from 185 to 250% 1-6 from 133 to 250% 7-18 from 100 to 250%
No program	Infants from 185 to 200% 1-6 from 133 to 200% 6-18 from 100 to 200%
17-19 from 65 to 100%	0-6 from 133 to 140% 6-18 from 100 to 140%

continued

TABLE D.2 Continued

States	Medicaid Annual Income-Eligibility Threshold (2 Child Family)[a]	Medicaid Poverty-level Children[b,c]
Ohio	$14,628	0-18 up to 200%
Oklahoma	$7,092	Infants up to 185% 1-6 up to 185% 6-17 up to 185%
Oregon	$14,628	Infants up to 133% 1-6 up to 133% 6-18 up to 100%
Pennsylvania	$6,684	Infants from 41 to 185% 1-6 from 41 to 133% 6-17 from 41 to 100% 17-19 up to 71%
Rhode Island	$28,140	0-8 up to 250% 8-15 up to 250%
South Carolina	$8,016	Infants from 50 to 185% 1-6 from 50 to 150% 6-17 from 50 to 150%
South Dakota	$9,552	0-6 up to 140% 6-19 up to 140%
Tennessee	$11,160	Infants up to 185% 1-6 up to 133% 6-17 up to 100%
Texas	$4,740	Infants up to 185% 1-6 up to 133% 6-18 up to 100%
Utah	$8,076	0-6 up to 133% 6-19 up to 100%
Vermont	$28,140	0-18 up to 300%
Virginia	$5,376	0-6 up to 133% 6-18 up to 100%
Washington	$29,256	0-18 up to 200%
West Virginia	$4,560	Infants up to 150% 1-6 up to 150% 6-18 up to 100%

Upper FPL by Program

Medicaid SCHIP (Title XXI)[b,c]	Separate SCHIP (Title XXI)[b]
0-18 from 150 to 200%	No program
Infants from 150 to 185% 1-6 from 133 to 185% 15-17 from 100 to 185%	No program
No program	1-6 from 133 to 170% 6-18 from 100 to 170%
0-8 up to 250%	Infants from 185 to 200% 1-6 from 133 to 200% 6-17 from 100 to 200% 17-18 from 41 to 200%
8-15 from 100 to 250% 15-18 up to 250%	No program
1-6 from 133 to 150% 6-17 from 100 to 150% 17-18 from 50 to 150%	No program
0-6 from 133 to 140% 6-19 from 100 to 140%	No program
17-18 up to 100%	0-19 up to 400%
17-18 up to 100%	Infants from 185 to 200% 1-6 from 133 to 200% 6-18 from 100 to 200%
No program	0-6 from 133 to 200% 6-18 from 100 to 200%
No program	0-18 from 235 to 300%
No program	0-6 from 133 to 185% 6-18 from 100 to 185%
No program	0-18 from 200 to 250%
No program	1-6 from 133 to 150% 6-18 from 100 to 150%

continued

TABLE D.2 Continued

States	Medicaid Annual Income-Eligibility Threshold (2 Child Family)[a]	Medicaid Poverty-level Children[b,c]
Wisconsin	$27,060	0-6 up to 185% 6-19 up to 185%
Wyoming	$9,480	0-5 up to 133% 6-17 up to 100% 17-19 up to 67%

NOTE: AIM = Access for Infants and Mothers; SCHIP = State Children's Health Insurance Program.
[a]Broaddus et al., 2002.
[b]Kaye and Flowers, 2002.
[c]Maloy et al., 2002.

Upper FPL by Program	
Medicaid SCHIP (Title XXI)[b,c]	Separate SCHIP (Title XXI)[b]
6–19 up to 185%	No program
No program	6–17 from 101 to 133%

TABLE D.3 Median Income and Health Insurance Coverage of Family Heads, and Their Spouses and Children by Type of Family, 2000[a]

Family type	Families			Individuals		Children Under 18	
	Number (thousands)	Share (%)	Median Income	Number (thousands)	Share (%)	Number (thousands)	Share
Unmarried, childless persons living alone in home	17,937	17%	$28,000	17,937	7%	N/A	N/A
Unmarried, childless persons living with someone in home but not in same family[b]	16,799	16%	$21,016	16,799	7%	N/A	N/A
Unmarried, childless persons living with someone in household in the same family[c]	5,837	6%	$36,020	14,270	6%	N/A	N/A
Families with child as householder/ reference person[d]	953	1%	$ 0	1,085	0%	N/A	N/A
Married, childless couples	23,683	23%	$62,000	56,206	22%	N/A	N/A
Two parents, median income							
One child	10,243	10%	$63,537	34,713	14%	10,534	15%
Two children	10,563	10%	$63,500	44,284	18%	21,369	30%
Three or more children	5,635	5%	$56,123	31,798	13%	19,413	27%
Single parent, median income							
One child	6,747	7%	$20,658	14,961	6%	6,766	9%
Two children	3,591	3%	$20,112	11,296	4%	7,177	10%
Three or more children	1,779	2%	$15,730	8,308	3%	6,150	9%
Total	103,767	100%	$45,000	251,657	100%	71,409	100%

NOTE: N/A = not available.

[a] The analysis excludes those families living in a group household and those families comprised entirely of adults over age 64.

[b] Living situations of individuals in this category may be vastly different compared to one another. Potentially included in this category are individuals engaged in a rental contract, friends that live together, an unmarried couple, etc. In each instance, the individuals are considered as members of different families.

[c] It will be noted that despite being categorized as families of childless, unmarried adults, the total number of people in these families far exceeds the total number of families. These families are made up of a single adult without a child under 18 and also another adult related to the single adult either as

Both Adults Covered (thousands)			One Adult Covered (thousands)			No Adults Covered (thousands)		
N/A			15,252			2,688		
N/A			11,964			4,835		
N/A			4,646			1,191		
N/A			608			351		
20,008			2,198			1,475		
All children covered	Some children covered	No children covered	All children covered	Some children covered	No children covered	All children covered	Some children covered	No children covered
$67,000			$32,858			$30,000		
8,751	N/A	211	283	N/A	142	258	N/A	597
9,182	87	35	209	18	102	329	36	564
4,493	84	31	185	16	64	227	74	461
			$22,415			$14,280		
N/A	N/A	N/A	4,669	N/A	311	730	N/A	1,037
N/A	N/A	N/A	2,644	46	77	416	67	341
N/A	N/A	N/A	1,323	34	27	182	38	175

a child, grandchild, or other relative. For reasons that cannot be determined through available Census Bureau data, these secondary individuals are not declared as part of a separate subfamily.

d An analysis of Census Bureau data indicates that in a small but notable number of instances, an individual younger than 18 but unmarried and childless is identified as the household or reference person of a subfamily. The Center on Budget and Policy Priorities analysis separates these individuals into an individual family type category.

SOURCE: Tabulations of the Census Bureau's 2001 Current Population Survey public use file were prepared for the IOM Committee by Matthew Broaddus, Center on Budget and Policy Priorities.

TABLE D.4 Health Insurance Coverage of Families Based on the Health
Insurance Coverage of Family Members and the Family's Poverty Status, 2000[a]

| Status | No Children[b] | | | | |
	Category 1	Category 2	Category 3	Category 4	Category 5
Under 50% of Poverty	1,065	2,081	191	830	408
Both adults covered	X	X	X	X	196
All children covered	X	X	X	X	X
Some children covered	X	X	X	X	X
No children covered	X	X	X	X	X
One adult covered	653	923	82	524	72
All children covered	X	X	X	X	X
Some children covered	X	X	X	X	X
No children covered	X	X	X	X	X
No adult covered	412	1,158	109	306	140
All children covered	X	X	X	X	X
Some children covered	X	X	X	X	X
No children covered	X	X	X	X	X
50% to 99% of Poverty	1,645	1,450	315	39	494
Both adults covered	X	X	X	X	295
All children covered	X	X	X	X	X
Some children covered	X	X	X	X	X
No children covered	X	X	X	X	X
One adult covered	1,358	838	227	25	96
All children covered	X	X	X	X	X
Some children covered	X	X	X	X	X
No children covered	X	X	X	X	X
No adult covered	287	612	88	14	103
All children covered	X	X	X	X	X
Some children covered	X	X	X	X	X
No children covered	X	X	X	X	X
100% to 149% of Poverty	1,503	1,812	559	17	830
Both adults covered	X	X	X	X	505
All children covered	X	X	X	X	X
Some children covered	X	X	X	X	X
No children covered	X	X	X	X	X
One adult covered	1,088	1,057	402	8	165
All children covered	X	X	X	X	X
Some children covered	X	X	X	X	X
No children covered	X	X	X	X	X
No adult covered	415	755	157	9	160
All children covered	X	X	X	X	X
Some children covered	X	X	X	X	X
No children covered	X	X	X	X	X

Two-Parent Families with Children			Single-Parent Families with Children		
One Child	Two Children	Three or More Children	One Child	Two Children	Three or More Children
132	141	194	998	651	493
59	83	96	X	X	X
55	80	96	X	X	X
X	1	0	X	X	X
4	2	0	X	X	X
21	10	17	567	424	370
18	8	15	544	413	359
X	0	0	X	2	10
3	2	2	23	9	1
52	48	81	431	227	123
16	18	14	161	119	57
X	0	15	X	18	12
36	30	52	270	90	54
316	381	515	962	580	568
154	200	255	X	X	X
149	192	240	X	X	X
X	6	11	X	X	X
5	2	4	X	X	X
46	41	56	618	384	439
40	32	37	561	361	412
X	1	3	X	9	12
6	8	16	57	14	15
116	140	204	344	196	129
39	56	70	147	119	58
X	2	19	X	11	11
77	82	115	197	66	60
459	663	657	984	664	316
255	420	384	X	X	X
243	405	375	X	X	X
X	9	7	X	X	X
12	6	2	X	X	X
65	60	72	630	474	236
48	44	47	588	443	225
X	2	6	X	12	3
17	14	19	42	19	8
139	183	201	354	190	80
50	77	79	173	104	42
X	6	19	X	18	4
89	100	103	181	68	34

continued

TABLE D.4 Continued

| Status | No Children[b] | | | | |
	Category 1	Category 2	Category 3	Category 4	Category 5
150% to 199% of Poverty	1,417	1,531	568	12	1,026
Both adults covered	X	X	X	X	706
All children covered	X	X	X	X	X
Some children covered	X	X	X	X	X
No children covered	X	X	X	X	X
One Adult Covered	1,043	967	413	5	154
All children covered	X	X	X	X	X
Some children covered	X	X	X	X	X
No children covered	X	X	X	X	X
No Adult Covered	374	564	155	7	166
All children covered	X	X	X	X	X
Some children covered	X	X	X	X	X
No children covered	X	X	X	X	X
200% or Higher of Poverty	12,307	9,924	4,204	54	20,923
Both adults covered	X	X	X	X	18,308
All children covered	X	X	X	X	X
Some children covered	X	X	X	X	X
No children covered	X	X	X	X	X
One adult covered	11,108	8,178	3,522	38	1,709
All children covered	X	X	X	X	X
Some children covered	X	X	X	X	X
No children covered	X	X	X	X	X
No adult covered	1,199	1,746	682	16	906
All children covered	X	X	X	X	X
Some children covered	X	X	X	X	X
No children covered	X	X	X	X	X

[a] Analysis excludes those families living in a group household and those families comprised entirely of adults over 64.

[b] Category 1: Unmarried childless persons living alone in home

Category 2: Unmarried childless persons living with someone in the home but not in the same family

Category 3: Unmarried childless persons living with someone in the home in the same family

Category 4: Families with child as householder or reference person

Category 5: Married, childless couples

SOURCE: Tabulations of the Census Bureau's 2001 Current Population Survey public use file were prepared for the IOM Committee by Matthew Broaddus, Center on Budget and Policy Priorities.

Two-Parent Families with Children			Single-Parent Families with Children		
One Child	Two Children	Three or More Children	One Child	Two Children	Three or More Children
563	888	776	914	428	162
381	701	631	X	X	X
359	678	609	X	X	X
X	17	10	X	X	X
22	6	12	X	X	X
78	40	58	680	322	134
52	17	49	636	310	133
X	10	3	X	6	1
26	13	6	44	6	0
104	147	87	234	106	28
37	59	21	100	46	17
X	1	6	X	16	0
67	87	60	134	44	11
8,774	8,490	3,493	2,889	1,269	240
8,113	7,901	3,243	X	X	X
7,945	7,828	3,173	X	X	X
X	54	56	X	X	X
168	19	14	X	X	X
215	178	62	2,486	1,164	205
125	108	36	2,341	1,117	194
X	4	4	X	17	8
90	66	22	145	30	3
446	411	188	403	105	35
117	120	43	148	28	9
X	26	15	X	4	11
329	265	130	255	73	15

TABLE D.5 Adults' and Children's Health Insurance Coverage in Families by Poverty Status, 2000

	Two-Parent Families with Children			Single-Parent Families with Children		
	One Child	Two Children	Three or More Children	One Child	Two Children	Three or More Children
Under 50% of Poverty						
Both adults covered						
Some children uncovered	7%	4%	0%			
All children covered	93%	96%	100%			
One adult covered						
Some children uncovered	14%	20%	12%	4%	3%	3%
All children covered	86%	80%	88%	96%	97%	97%
No adult covered						
Some children uncovered	69%	63%	83%	63%	48%	54%
All children covered	31%	38%	17%	37%	52%	46%
50%–99% of Poverty						
Both adults covered						
Some children uncovered	3%	4%	6%			
All children covered	97%	96%	94%			
One adult covered						
Some children uncovered	13%	22%	34%	9%	6%	6%
All children covered	87%	78%	66%	91%	94%	94%
No adult covered						
Some children uncovered	66%	60%	66%	57%	39%	55%
All children covered	34%	40%	34%	43%	61%	45%
100%–149% of Poverty						
Both adults covered						
Some children uncovered	5%	4%	2%			
All children covered	95%	96%	98%			
One adult covered						
Some children uncovered	26%	27%	35%	7%	7%	5%
All children covered	74%	73%	65%	93%	93%	95%
No adult covered						
Some children uncovered	64%	58%	61%	51%	45%	48%
All children covered	36%	42%	39%	49%	55%	53%

	Two-Parent Families with Children			Single-Parent Families with Children		
	One Child	Two Children	Three or More Children	One Child	Two Children	Three or More Children
150%–199% of Poverty						
Both adults covered						
Some children uncovered	6%	3%	3%			
All children covered	94%	97%	97%			
One adult covered						
Some children uncovered	33%	58%	16%	6%	4%	1%
All children covered	67%	43%	84%	94%	96%	99%
No adult covered						
Some children uncovered	64%	60%	76%	57%	57%	39%
All children covered	36%	40%	24%	43%	43%	61%
200% of Poverty or Higher						
Both adults covered						
Some children uncovered	2%	1%	2%			
All children covered	98%	99%	98%			
One adult covered						
Some children uncovered	42%	39%	42%	6%	4%	5%
All children covered	58%	61%	58%	94%	96%	95%
No adult covered						
Some children uncovered	74%	71%	77%	63%	73%	74%
All children covered	26%	29%	23%	37%	27%	26%

SOURCE: Tabulations of the Census Bureau's 2001 Current Population Survey public use file were prepared for the IOM Committee by Matthew Broaddus, Center on Budget and Policy Priorities.

TABLE D.6 Health Insurance Coverage of Families Based on the Health Insurance Coverage of Family Members and Race/Ethnicity of Family Head, 2000[a]

Race or Ethnicity	No Children[b]				
	Category 1	Category 2	Category 3	Category 4	Category 5
Black, Non-Hispanic	2,869	2,241	1,312	208	1,654
Both adults covered	X	X	X	X	1,373
All children covered	X	X	X	X	X
Some children covered	X	X	X	X	X
No children covered	X	X	X	X	X
One adult covered	2,361	1,536	946	148	168
All children covered	X	X	X	X	X
Some children covered	X	X	X	X	X
No children covered	X	X	X	X	X
No adult covered	508	705	366	60	113
All children covered	X	X	X	X	X
Some children covered	X	X	X	X	X
No children covered	X	X	X	X	X
White, Non-Hispanic	13,415	11,571	3,447	455	19,269
Both adults covered	X	X	X	X	16,710
All children covered	X	X	X	X	X
Some children covered	X	X	X	X	X
No children covered	X	X	X	X	X
One adult covered	11,681	8,922	3,002	322	1,653
All children covered	X	X	X	X	X
Some children covered	X	X	X	X	X
No children covered	X	X	X	X	X
No adult covered	1,734	2,649	445	133	906
All children covered	X	X	X	X	X
Some children covered	X	X	X	X	X
No children covered	X	X	X	X	X
Hispanic	995	2,133	829	251	1,658
Both adults covered	X	X	X	X	1,095
All children covered	X	X	X	X	X
Some children covered	X	X	X	X	X
No children covered	X	X	X	X	X
One adult covered	689	925	515	116	234
All children covered	X	X	X	X	X
Some children covered	X	X	X	X	X
No children covered	X	X	X	X	X
No adult covered	306	1,208	314	135	329
All children covered	X	X	X	X	X
Some children covered	X	X	X	X	X
No children covered	X	X	X	X	X

Two-Parent Families with Children			Single-Parent Families with Children		
One Child	Two Children	Three or More Children	One Child	Two Children	Three or More Children
903	837	484	1,792	1,032	659
799	726	400	X	X	X
759	704	375	X	X	X
X	17	18	X	X	X
40	5	7	X	X	X
39	36	30	1,326	815	542
15	14	28	1,231	794	515
X	0	0	X	10	15
24	22	2	95	11	12
65	75	54	466	217	117
17	23	11	166	112	55
X	3	8	X	9	14
48	49	35	300	96	48
7,439	7,789	3,775	3,725	1,868	651
6,815	7,174	3,370	X	X	X
6,685	7,109	3,319	X	X	X
X	46	40	X	X	X
130	19	11	X	X	X
234	177	107	2,885	1,498	523
170	127	78	2,734	1,453	509
X	6	4	X	13	10
64	44	25	151	32	4
390	438	298	840	370	128
125	179	101	395	216	67
X	14	14	X	43	6
265	245	183	445	111	55
1,201	1,360	1,125	1,006	570	393
759	914	646	X	X	X
727	883	613	X	X	X
X	21	21	X	X	X
32	10	12	X	X	X
129	104	112	619	367	270
84	58	69	575	320	253
X	12	12	X	16	6
45	34	31	44	31	11
313	342	367	387	203	123
99	103	101	141	82	50
X	15	52	X	16	14
214	224	214	246	105	59

continued

TABLE D.6 Continued

Race or Ethnicity	No Children[b]				
	Category 1	Category 2	Category 3	Category 4	Category 5
Asian and Other	659	853	248	41	1,104
Both adults covered	X	X	X	X	833
All children covered	X	X	X	X	X
Some children covered	X	X	X	X	X
No children covered	X	X	X	X	X
One adult covered	518	581	182	15	143
All children covered	X	X	X	X	X
Some children covered	X	X	X	X	X
No children covered	X	X	X	X	X
No adult covered	141	272	66	26	128
All children covered	X	X	X	X	X
Some children covered	X	X	X	X	X
No children covered	X	X	X	X	X

[a] Analysis excludes those families living in a group household and those families comprised entirely of adults over 64.

[b] Category 1: Unmarried childless persons living alone in home

Category 2: Unmarried childless persons living with someone in the home but not in the same family

Category 3: Unmarried childless persons living with someone in the home in the same family

Category 4: Families with child as householder or reference person

Category 5: Married, childless couples

SOURCE: Tabulations of the Census Bureau's 2001 Current Population Survey public use file were prepared for the IOM Committee by Matthew Broaddus, Center on Budget and Policy Priorities.

Two-Parent Families with Children			Single-Parent Families with Children		
One Child	Two Children	Three or More Children	One Child	Two Children	Three or More Children
699	575	249	226	123	78
588	489	191	X	X	X
579	485	186	X	X	X
X	3	5	X	X	X
9	1	0	X	X	X
24	12	15	151	86	50
15	10	10	130	76	46
X	0	0	0	7	4
9	2	5	21	3	0
87	74	43	75	37	28
17	25	14	29	6	11
X	4	0	0	1	4
70	45	29	46	30	13

TABLE D.7 Adult Health Insurance Coverage in Families with Children by Race, 2000

	Two-Parent Families with Children		Single-Parent Families with Children	
Race	Number	Percentage of Total	Number	Percentage of Total
Black, Non-Hispanic				
Both adults covered	1,925	87%		
One adult covered	105	5%	2,683	77%
No adults covered	194	9%	800	23%
Total	2,224		3,483	
White, Non-Hispanic				
Both adults covered	17,359	91%		
One adult covered	518	3%	4,906	79%
No adults covered	1,126	6%	1,338	21%
Total	19,003		6,244	
Hispanic				
Both adults covered	2,319	63%		
One adult covered	345	9%	1,256	64%
No adults covered	1,022	28%	713	36%
Total	3,686		1,969	
Asian and Other				
Both adults covered	1,268	83%		
One adult covered	51	3%	287	67%
No adults covered	204	13%	140	33%
Total	1,523		427	

SOURCE: Tabulations of the Census Bureau's 2001 Current Population Survey public use file were prepared for the IOM Committee by Matthew Broaddus, Center on Budget and Policy Priorities.

TABLE D.8 Adults' and Children's Health Insurance Coverage in Families by Race, 2000.

Race	Two-Parent Families with Children			Single-Parent Families with Children		
	One Child	Two Children	Three or More Children	One Child	Two Children	Three or More Children
Black, Non-Hispanic						
Both adults covered						
Some children uncovered	5%	3%	6%			
All children covered	95%	97%	94%			
One adult covered						
Some children uncovered	62%	61%	7%	7%	3%	5%
All children covered	38%	39%	93%	93%	97%	95%
No adults covered						
Some children uncovered	74%	69%	80%	64%	48%	53%
All children covered	26%	31%	20%	36%	52%	47%
White, Non-Hispanic						
Both adults covered						
Some children uncovered	2%	1%	2%			
All children covered	98%	99%	98%			
One adult covered						
Some children uncovered	27%	28%	27%	5%	3%	3%
All children covered	73%	72%	73%	95%	97%	97%
No adults covered						
Some children uncovered	68%	59%	66%	53%	42%	48%
All children covered	32%	41%	34%	47%	58%	52%
Hispanic						
Both adults covered						
Some children uncovered	4%	3%	5%			
All children covered	96%	97%	95%			
One adult covered						
Some children uncovered	35%	44%	38%	7%	13%	6%
All children covered	65%	56%	62%	93%	87%	94%
No adults covered						
Some children uncovered	68%	70%	72%	64%	60%	59%
All children covered	32%	30%	28%	36%	40%	41%
Asian and Other						
Both adults covered						
Some children uncovered	2%	1%	3%			
All children covered	98%	99%	97%			
One adult covered						
Some children uncovered	38%	17%	33%	14%	12%	8%
All children covered	63%	83%	67%	86%	88%	92%
No adults covered						
Some children uncovered	80%	66%	67%	61%	84%	61%
All children covered	20%	34%	33%	39%	16%	39%

SOURCE: Tabulations of the Census Bureau's 2001 Current Population Survey public use file were prepared for the IOM Committee by Matthew Broaddus, Center on Budget and Policy Priorities.

TABLE D.9 Citizenship and Health Insurance Coverage of Family Heads and Their Spouses and Children by Type of Family, 2000[a]

Family Type	No Children[b]				
	Category 1	Category 2	Category 3	Category 4	Category 5
Citizen Head of Family	16,990	14,838	5,357	855	22,377
Both adults covered	X	X	X	X	19,226
All children covered	X	X	X	X	X
Some children covered	X	X	X	X	X
No children covered	X	X	X	X	X
One adult covered	14,633	11,129	4,443	564	2,021
All children covered	X	X	X	X	X
Some children covered	X	X	X	X	X
No children covered	X	X	X	X	X
No adult covered	2,357	3,709	914	291	1,130
All children covered	X	X	X	X	X
Some children covered	X	X	X	X	X
No children covered	X	X	X	X	X
Non-citizen Head of Family	947	1,960	481	98	1,306
Both adults covered	X	X	X	X	785
All children covered	X	X	X	X	X
Some children covered	X	X	X	X	X
No children covered	X	X	X	X	X
One adult covered	616	835	203	36	176
All children covered	X	X	X	X	X
Some children covered	X	X	X	X	X
No children covered	X	X	X	X	X
No Adult Covered	331	1,125	278	62	345
All children covered	X	X	X	X	X
Some children covered	X	X	X	X	X
No children covered	X	X	X	X	X

[a] The analysis excludes those families living in a group household and those families comprised entirely of adults over 64.

[b] Category 1: Unmarried childless persons living alone in home

Category 2: Unmarried childless persons living with someone in the home but not in the same family

Category 3: Unmarried childless persons living with someone in the home in the same family

Category 4: Families with child as householder or reference person

Category 5: Married, childless couples

SOURCE: Tabulations of the Census Bureau's 2001 Current Population Survey public use file were prepared for the IOM Committee by Matthew Broaddus, Center on Budget and Policy Priorities.

Two-Parent Families with Children			Single-Parent Families with Children		
One Child	Two Children	Three or More Children	One Child	Two Children	Three or More Children
9,291	9,587	4,971	6,286	3,323	1,576
8,362	8,675	4,303	X	X	X
8,171	8,570	4,201	X	X	X
X	71	78	X	X	X
191	34	24	X	X	X
338	267	189	4,754	2,628	1,253
220	173	137	4,473	2,528	1,201
X	10	9	X	39	30
118	84	43	281	61	22
591	645	479	1,532	695	323
179	244	145	651	369	152
X	26	30	X	57	28
412	375	304	881	269	143
950	976	664	462	267	204
599	629	305	X	X	X
579	612	292	X	X	X
X	16	6	X	X	X
20	1	7	X	X	X
87	63	76	227	138	133
63	36	48	197	115	122
X	8	7	X	7	5
24	19	21	30	16	6
264	284	283	235	129	71
79	85	82	79	47	30
X	10	44	X	10	9
185	189	157	156	72	32

TABLE D.10 Health Insurance Coverage of Family Heads and Their Spouses by Citizenship Status and Family Type, 2000

Family Type	Two-Parent Families with Children		Single-Parent Families with Children	
	Number	Percent	Number	Percent
Citizen Head of Family				
Both parents covered	21,340	89%		
One parent covered	794	3%	8,635	77%
No parents covered	1,715	7%	2,550	23%
Total	23,849		11,185	
Non-citizen Head of Family				
Both parents covered	1,533	59%		
One parent covered	226	9%	498	53%
No parents covered	831	32%	435	47%
Total	2,590		933	

SOURCE: Tabulations of the Census Bureau's 2001 Current Population Survey public use file were prepared for the IOM Committee by Matthew Broaddus, Center on Budget and Policy Priorities.

E

Glossary

Adjusted, adjustment In a statistical analysis, the process of manipulating or stratifying the values of independent variables so as to minimize their confounding influence on the relationship or association between an independent variable of interest and the dependent variable.

Ambulatory-care-sensitive condition (ACSC) A preventable or avoidable hospitalization; a research construct used as an indicator of barriers to access to ambulatory care. Certain diagnoses for inpatient episodes are defined as preventable or avoidable if they are responsive to timely and appropriate ambulatory care. Rates of hospitalization above a specified baseline are construed as indicative of inadequate ambulatory care.

Association A correlation or relationship that may or may not be causal—for example, when events occur more frequently together than one would expect by chance alone.★

Bias Any systematic error in the design, conduct or, analysis of a study that results in a mistaken estimate of an exposure's effect on the risk of disease (Gordis, 1996).

Causality A relationship that may exist between an exposure or treatment (cause) and an outcome (effect), depending in part on the strength of the association between exposure or treatment and outcome.

★Adapted from the Academy for Health Services Research and Health Care Policy glossary at http://www.academyhealth.org/publications.glossary.pdf. Accessed February 4, 2002.

Chronic disease A disease that has one or more of the following characteristics: is permanent; leaves residual disability; is caused by nonreversible physiological damage; requires special training of the patient for rehabilitation; or may be expected to require a long period of supervision, observation, or care.★

Confidence interval (CI) A numeric range estimated with a specific degree of confidence or probability to include a value. Conventionally reported confidence intervals are ranges in which the actual value of the estimated variable can be expected to fall 95 or 99 percent of the time, corresponding to probabilities that a difference or significant result is due to chance of less than 5 percent and 1 percent, respectively ($p < .05$; $p < .01$). In reporting quantified results throughout this report (e.g., odds ratios, relative risks), if the confidence interval is *not* given, point estimates have *at least* a 95 percent probability of being statistically significant. Confidence intervals are given for findings reported with lesser levels of statistical significance.

Confounder A variable that is associated with an exposure or treatment of interest and, as a result, influences the relationship between the exposure or treatment and an outcome. The ability to adjust or analytically control for the presence of a confounder depends on how well this variable is measured.

Cost sharing Any provision of a health insurance policy that requires the insured individual to pay some portion of medical expenses. The general term includes deductibles, copayments, and coinsurance.★

Covariate A variable that is related to or associated with the study variable(s) of interest.

Cross-sectional Describes a research study in which measurements are collected and comparisons made among populations at one point in time.

Dependent variable A factor, indicator, construct, or other measure of an outcome or effect of interest that is influenced by or dependent on independent variables of interest.

Experimental Describes a study design—for example, a randomized clinical trial—where researchers use a defined study population, randomly assign members of the population to exposure or treatment and control groups, control the timing of the exposure or treatment, and influence the timing of measurements.

★Adapted from the Academy for Health Services Research and Health Care Policy glossary at http://www.academyhealth.org/publications.glossary.pdf. Accessed February 4, 2002.

Family coherence and hardiness Based on family systems theory, two research constructs that measure resilience to stress, used to analyze the influence of individual and family-level psychosocial resources on the relationship between stress and adverse health and other outcomes. An individual's sense of coherence (in a family context, often a parent's) and a family's hardiness each influence how families respond to stressful circumstances (Svavarsdottir et al., 2000).

Incidence A measure of the probability of a disease or an outcome's occurrence, defined as the number of new cases within a defined time period for a specific population divided by the total number in the population (Gordis, 1996).

Independent variable A factor, indicator, construct, or other measure that influences a dependent variable of interest or the relationship between an exposure or treatment and the dependent variable.

Longitudinal Describes a research study in which measurements are collected and comparisons made among populations over time.

Medical home An approach to the organization and delivery of health services for children that is associated with quality health care. It is defined as a means to ensure that health services are accessible, family-centered, continuous, comprehensive, coordinated, compassionate, and culturally effective (American Academy of Pediatrics, 2002).

Medically indigent Persons who cannot afford needed health care because of insufficient income and/or lack of adequate health insurance. Indigent care consists of health services provided to the poor or those unable to pay. Since many indigent patients are not eligible for federal or state programs, the costs that are covered by Medicaid are generally recorded separately from indigent care costs.★

Multivariable or multivariate analysis A statistical method to characterize the relationship among at least two independent variables that measure exposures or treatments (e.g., potential causes) and a dependent variable that measures an outcome or effect.

Neonate A newly born infant.

Nongroup market The insurance market for products sold to individuals rather than to members of groups. Typically each state regulates its own nongroup market.

★Adapted from the Academy for Health Services Research and Health Care Policy glossary at http://www.academyhealth.org/publications.glossary.pdf. Accessed February 4, 2002.

Observational Describes a research study with a nonexperimental design, in which researchers gather observations or measurements while not intentionally affecting the conditions of exposure, the treatment of the study population, or the timing of measurements.

Odds ratio (OR) A comparative measure of the strength of a relationship or association between an exposure or treatment and an outcome for two populations, where the baseline incidence of the outcome in these groups may not be known. For example, if the odds of receiving an immunization are 2:1 in a group of uninsured children (i.e., two of every three children, or 67 percent, receive the immunization) and the odds are 4:1 in a group of children who have insurance (i.e., four of every five insured children, or 80 percent, receive it), the odds ratio of uninsured compared to insured children is 0.5 (2:1/4:1). The OR is not a good estimate of the relative risk (the probability of been immunized in the uninsured group divided by the probability of being immunized in the insured group) because immunization is not a rare event.

Perinatal care Health services delivered to a woman and her newborn in the periods immediately before and after birth, ranging from approximately the twentieth to twenty-eighth week of gestation to the first week or month following birth.

Predictor, independent predictor In a statistical analysis, an independent variable (e.g., that measures an exposure or treatment) that is shown to be likely to influence or predict the value of a dependent variable (e.g., an outcome).

Prevalence A measure of how common a disease or condition is within a population, defined as the number of cases in the population at a specified time divided by the number of persons in the population at that same time (Gordis, 1996).

Quasi-experimental Describes a research study—for example, a natural experiment—whose design combines experimental and nonexperimental aspects. Typically, researchers cannot control the timing of the intervention or exposure whose effects are being measured or the random assignment of a defined group of study subjects, but they can influence the timing of measurements.

Randomized trial A research study in which the members of a defined group of subjects are randomly assigned to at least two groups for the purpose of analysis: a treatment or intervention group and a control group.

Relative risk (RR) A comparative measure of the strength of a relationship or association between an exposure, intervention, or treatment and an outcome for a defined study population, where the baseline incidence of the outcome is known. It is expressed as the ratio of two risks, namely, the rate of a disease or condition of interest in the treated portion of the population divided by the rate in an untreated or control portion of the population. A value of one means that the rates in both portions are the same.

Retrospective study A type of study, usually a cohort design, in which historical data are used and outcome data are collected at the time the study begins (Gordis, 1996).

Safety net Those providers that organize and deliver a significant level of health care and other related services to uninsured, Medicaid, and other at-risk, lower-income patients (Institute of Medicine, 2000).

Section 1115 waiver (Medicaid) Section 1115 of the Social Security Act grants the secretary of the Department of Health and Human Services broad authority to waive certain laws relating to Medicaid for the purpose of conducting pilot, experimental or demonstration projects that are "likely to promote the objectives" of the program. Section 1115 demonstration waivers allow states to change provisions of the Medicaid programs, including: eligibility requirements, the scope of services available, the freedom to choose a provider, a provider's choice to participate in a plan, the method of reimbursing providers, and the statewide application of the program (AHSRHP, 2002).

Selection bias In research studies, a systematic error in analysis that results when study subjects are not assigned randomly among treatment and control groups.

Small-group market The insurance market for products sold to groups that are smaller than a specified size, typically employer groups. The size of groups included usually depends on state insurance laws and thus varies from state to state, with 50 employees the most common size (AHSRHP, 2002).

Special health needs Children who have or are at increased risk for a chronic physical, developmental, behavioral, or emotional condition and who also require health and related services of a type or amount beyond that required by children generally (DHHS, 2001).

Statistically significant See definition of *Confidence interval*.

Stress Demands made by an individual's internal environment, or an individual's or family's external environment, that upset the functioning balance or homeostasis of the individual or family, potentially affecting physical or psychological well-being. Stressors may have negative or positive effects, in part depending on how the affected individual or family member perceives the stress and the responses made to stressful circumstances, for example, in the case of economic hardship (Glanz et al., 1997).

Turbulence A research construct to measure the synergistic effect of multiple changes on children. It is defined as the presence of at least two of the following circumstances: moving from one state to another; moving to a different home; moving in with another family; at least two changes in employment by a parent or parent's spouse, at least two changes of school, or a significant decline in the health of the child, its parent, or the parent's spouse (Moore et al., 2000a).

Women, Infants, and Children (WIC) program The Special Supplemental Nutrition Program for Women, Infants, and Children, administered by the U.S. Department of Agriculture's Food and Nutrition Service and operated by the states. WIC programs provide vouchers for purchasing certain types of food and nutrition screening and counseling for eligible persons, usually pregnant and post-partum women, infants, and children under the age of 5 who have been deter-mined to be at risk for inadequate nutrition due to health or dietary problems and who are members of families that earn less than 185 percent of the federal poverty level or who receive other benefits (e.g., food stamps, Medicaid, Temporary Assistance for Needy Families) (USDA, 2002).

F

Biographical Sketches

COMMITTEE ON THE CONSEQUENCES OF UNINSURANCE

SUBCOMMITTEE ON THE FAMILY IMPACTS OF UNINSURANCE

Mary Sue Coleman, Ph.D., *Co-chair*

Dr. Coleman is president of the University of Michigan. She is professor of biological chemistry in the University of Michigan Medical School and professor of chemistry in the College of Literature, Science and the Arts. She previously was president of the University of Iowa and president of the University of Iowa Health Systems (1995–2002). Dr. Coleman served as provost and vice president for academic affairs at the University of New Mexico (1993–1995) and dean of research and vice chancellor at the University of North Carolina at Chapel Hill (1990–1992). She was both faculty member and Cancer Center administrator at the University of Kentucky in Lexington for 19 years, where her research focused on the immune system and malignancies. Dr. Coleman is a member of the Institute of Medicine (IOM) and a fellow of the American Association for the Advancement of Science. She serves on the Iowa Governor's Strategic Planning Council, the Board of Trustees of the Universities Research Association, the Board of Governors of the Warren G. Magnuson Clinical Center at the National Institutes of Health, and other voluntary advisory bodies and corporate boards.

Arthur L. Kellermann, M.D., M.P.H., *Co-chair*

Arthur Kellermann, is professor and director, Center for Injury Control, Rollins School of Public Health, Emory University, and professor and chairman, Department of Emergency Medicine, School of Medicine, Emory University. Dr. Kellerman has served as principal investigator or co-investigator on several research grants, including federally funded studies of handgun-related violence and injury, emergency cardiac care, and the use of emergency room services. Among his many awards and distinctions, he is a fellow of the American College of Emergency Physicians (1992); is the recipient of a meritorious service award from the Tennessee State Legislature (1993); and the Hal Jayne Academic Excellence Award from the Society for Academic Emergency Medicine (1997); and was elected to membership in the Institute of Medicine (1999). In addition, Dr. Kellermann is a member of the Editorial Board of the journal *Annals of Emergency Medicine* and has served as a reviewer for the *New England Journal of Medicine*, the *Journal of the American Medical Association*, and the *American Journal of Public Health*.

Ronald M. Andersen, Ph.D.

Ronald Andersen is the Fred W. and Pamela K. Wasserman Professor of Health Services and professor of sociology at the University of California, Los Angeles (UCLA), School of Public Health. He teaches courses in health services organization, research methods, evaluation, and leadership. Dr. Andersen received his Ph.D. in sociology at Purdue University. He has studied access to medical care for his entire professional career of 30 years. Dr. Andersen developed the Behavioral Model of Health Services Use that has been used extensively both nationally and internationally as a framework for utilization and cost studies of general populations, as well as special studies of minorities, low income, children, women, the elderly, oral health, the homeless, and the HIV-positive population. He has directed three national surveys of access to care and has led numerous evaluations of local and regional populations and programs designed to promote access to medical care. Dr. Andersen's other research interests include international comparisons of health services systems, graduate medical education curricula, physician health services organization integration, and evaluations of geriatric and primary care delivery. He is a member of the IOM and was on the founding board of the Association for Health Services Research. He has been chair of the Medical Sociology Section of the American Sociological Association. In 1994 he received the association's Leo G. Reeder Award for Distinguished Service to Medical Sociology; in 1996 he received the Distinguished Investigator Award from the Association for Health Services Research; and in 1999 he received the Baxter Allegiance Health Services Research Prize.

John Z. Ayanian, M.D., M.P.P.

Dr. Ayanian is an associate professor of medicine and health care policy at Harvard Medical School and Brigham and Women's Hospital, where he practices general internal medicine. His research focuses on quality of care and access to care for major medical conditions, including colorectal cancer and myocardial infarction. He has extensive experience in the use of cancer registries to assess outcomes and evaluate the quality of cancer care. In addition, he has studied the effects of race and gender on access to kidney transplants and on quality of care for other medical conditions. Dr. Ayanian is deputy editor of the journal *Medical Care*, a Robert Wood Johnson Foundation Generalist Physician Faculty Scholar, and a fellow of the American College of Physicians.

Robert J. Blendon, M.B.A., Sc.D.

Dr. Blendon is currently professor of health policy and political analysis at both the Harvard School of Public Health and the John F. Kennedy School of Government; he has received awards for outstanding teaching from both institutions. He also directs the Harvard Opinion Research Program and the Henry J. Kaiser National Program on the Public, Health, and Social Policy, which focuses on the better understanding of public knowledge, attitudes, and beliefs about major domestic public policy issues. Dr. Blendon also codirects the Washington Post–Kaiser Family Foundation (KFF) survey project, which was nominated for a Pulitzer Prize, and a new project for National Public Radio and KFF on American attitudes toward health and social policy, which was cited by the *National Journal* as setting a new standard for public opinion surveys in broadcast journalism. From 1987 to 1996, Dr. Blendon served as chair of the Department of Health Policy and Management at the Harvard School of Public Health and as deputy director of the Harvard University Division of Health Policy Research and Education. Prior to his Harvard appointments, Dr. Blendon was senior vice president at the Robert Wood Johnson Foundation. He was senior editor of a three-volume series The Future of American Health Care and is a member of the Institute of Medicine, the advisory committee to the director of the Centers for Disease Control and Prevention, and the editorial board of the *Journal of the American Medical Association*. Dr. Blendon is a graduate of Marietta College and received his master of business administration and doctoral degrees from the University of Chicago and the Johns Hopkins School of Public Health, respectively.

Sheila P. Davis, B.S.N., M.S.N., Ph.D.★

Dr. Davis is associate professor, Department of Adult Health, in the School of Nursing at the University of Mississippi Medical Center. She is also vice president of Davis, Davis & Associates, a health management consultant company. Her research focuses on minority health issues, especially cardiovascular risk among ethnic populations. Dr. Davis is the founder and chair of the Cardiovascular Risk Reduction in Children Committee at the University of Mississippi. This is a multidisciplinary committee (physicians, nurses, dietician, health educator, college administrator, nurse practitioners, etc.) committed to reducing cardiovascular risks in children. Dr. Davis is a member of the American Nurses Association and has written numerous publications on the profession and the experiences of ethnic minorities in the health professions. She is author of a faith-based program,

---

★Member of the Subcommittee on the Family Impacts of Uninsurance.

Healthy Kids Seminar, that is used to promote the adoption of healthy life-style choices by children.

George C. Eads, Ph.D.★

Dr. Eads is vice president and director of the Charles River Associates (CRA) Washington, D.C. office and is an internationally known expert in the economics of the automotive and airlines industries. Prior to joining CRA, Dr. Eads was vice president and chief economist at General Motors Corporation. He represented the corporation frequently before congressional committees and federal regulatory agencies. He has served as a member of the President's Council of Economic Advisers and as a special assistant to the assistant attorney general in the Antitrust Division of the U.S. Department of Justice. Dr. Eads has published numerous books and articles on the impact of government on business and has taught at several major universities, including Harvard and Princeton.

Sandra R. Hernández, M.D.

Sandra R. Hernández is chief executive officer (CEO) of the San Francisco Foundation, a community foundation serving the five Bay Area counties. It is one of the largest community foundations in the country. Dr. Hernández is a primary care internist who previously held a number of positions within the San Francisco Department of Public Health, including director of the AIDS Office, director of Community Public Health, county health officer, and finally director of health for the City and County of San Francisco. She was appointed to and served on President Clinton's Advisory Commission on Consumer Protection and Quality in the Health Care Industry. Among the many honors and awards bestowed on her, Dr. Hernández was named by *Modern Healthcare* magazine as one of the top 10 health care leaders for the next century. Dr. Hernández is a graduate of Yale University, Tufts School of Medicine, and the John F. Kennedy School of Government at Harvard University. She is on the faculty of the University of California, San Francisco (UCSF), School of Medicine and maintains an active clinical practice at San Francisco General Hospital in the AIDS Clinic.

Willard G. Manning, Ph.D.

Dr. Manning is professor in the Department of Health Studies, Pritzker School of Medicine, and in the Harris School of Public Policy, at the University of Chicago. His primary research focus has been the effects of health insurance and alternative delivery systems on the use of health services and health status. He is an expert in statistical issues in cost-effectiveness analysis and small-area variations. His recent work has included examination of mental health services use and outcomes in a Medicaid population and cost-effectiveness analysis of screening and treating depression in primary care. Dr. Manning is a member of the IOM.

★Chair of the Subcommittee on the Family Impacts of Uninsurance.

James J. Mongan, M.D.

Dr. Mongan is president of the Massachusetts General Hospital Corporation and of the General Hospital. He was previously executive director, Truman Medical Center, and dean, University of Missouri-Kansas City School of Medicine. Dr. Mongan served as assistant surgeon general in the Department of Health and Human Services (DHHS); as former associate director for health and human resources, Domestic Policy Staff, the White House; and as former deputy assistant secretary for Health Policy, Department of Health, Education and Welfare. Dr. Mongan is chair of the Task Force on the Future of Health Insurance for Working Americans, a nonpartisan effort of the Commonwealth Fund to address the implications of the changing U.S. work force and economy for the availability and affordability of health insurance, a member of the KFF Board and the Kaiser Commission on the Underserved and the Uninsured, and a member of the IOM and its governing council.

Christopher Queram, M.A.

Mr. Queram has been CEO of the Employer Health Care Alliance Cooperative (The Alliance) of Madison, Wisconsin, since 1993. The Alliance is a purchasing cooperative owned by more than 175 member companies that contracts with providers, manages and reports data, performs consumer education, and designs employer and provider quality initiatives. Prior to his current position, Mr. Queram served as vice president for programs at Meriter Hospital, a 475-bed hospital in Madison. Mr. Queram is a member of the Board of the National Business Coalition on Health and served as board chair for the past two years. He was a member of the President's Advisory Commission on Consumer Protection and Quality in the Health Care Industry. Mr. Queram served as a member of the Planning Committee for the National Quality Forum and continues as convenor of the Purchaser Council of the Forum. He is a member of the Wisconsin Board on Health Information and the Board of the Wisconsin Private Employer Health Care Coverage program. He holds a master's degree in health services administration from the University of Wisconsin at Madison and is a fellow in the American College of Healthcare Executives.

Cathy Schoen, M.A.*

Cathy Schoen joined the Commonwealth Fund in September 1995 as director of research and evaluation. Prior to joining the Fund, she was director of special projects at the University of Massachusetts Labor Relations and Research Center. She also serves as program director of the Fund's Health Care Coverage and Quality Program, a policy and research grant program established to help inform national and state health insurance and delivery system policy decisions. During the 1980s, Ms. Schoen directed the Service Employees International Union's

---

*Member of the Subcommittee on the Family Impacts of Uninsurance.

(SEIU) Research and Policy Department in Washington, D.C. She went to SEIU after serving as a member of President Carter's national health insurance task force where she was responsible for national reform issues and research and policy related to Medicaid and ambulatory care payment policies. Ms. Schoen also served as a senior health adviser during the 1988 presidential campaign. Prior to federal government service, she was a research associate at the Brookings Institution. Her research interests include health care coverage and quality issues, Medicaid and children's programs, and worker's issues. Ms. Schoen formerly served on the IOM Committee on Immunization Finance Policies and Practices.

Shoshanna Sofaer, Dr.P.H.*

Shoshanna Sofaer is the Robert P. Luciano Professor of Health Care Policy at the School of Public Affairs, Baruch College, in New York City. She completed her master's and doctoral degrees in public health at the University of California, Berkeley; taught for six years at the University of California, Los Angeles, School of Public Health; and served on the faculty of George Washington University Medical Center, where she was professor and associate dean for research of the School of Public Health and Health Services and director of the Center for Health Outcomes Improvement Research. Dr. Sofaer's research interests include providing information to individual consumers on the performance of the health care system; assessing the impact of information on both consumers and the system; developing consumer-relevant performance measures; and improving the responsiveness of the Medicare program to the needs of current and future cohorts of older persons and persons with disabilities. In addition, Dr. Sofaer studies the role of community coalitions in pursuing public health and health care system reform objectives and has extensive experience in the evaluation of community health improvement interventions. She has studied the determinants of health insurance status among the near-elderly, including early retirees. Dr. Sofaer served as co-chair of the Working Group on Coverage for Low Income and Non-Working Families for the White House Task Force on Health Care Reform in 1993. Currently, she is co-chair of the Task Force on Medicare of the Century Foundation in New York City, a member of the Board of Health Care Services, IOM and a member of the Agency for Healthcare Research and Quality (AHRQ) Health Systems Study Section.

Peter Szilagyi, M.D., M.P.H.*

Dr. Szilagyi is professor of pediatrics, division chief of the general pediatric division, and chief of pediatric ambulatory services at the University of Rochester School of Medicine and Dentistry. He is an active member of the Ambulatory Pediatric Association (APA), at which he has just received the lifetime APA

---

*Member of the Subcommittee on the Family Impacts of Uninsurance.

research award, and is a member of the Society for Pediatric Research and the American Pediatric Society. Dr. Szilagyi is a health services researcher with interests in optimizing the health care and functional outcomes of vulnerable children. He has led a number of studies on health care financing for children, focusing on managed care and on uninsured children. Dr. Szilagyi's research team studies on health insurance for uninsured or underinsured children have contributed to state and national health insurance reform, which culminated in the State Children's Health Insurance Program (SCHIP), and he is currently conducting several evaluations of the SCHIP program.

Stephen J. Trejo, Ph.D.

Dr. Trejo is associate professor in the Department of Economics at the University of Texas at Austin. His primary research focus has been in the field of labor economics. He has examined the response of labor market participants to incentives created by market opportunities, government policies, and the institutional environment. Specific research topics include the economic effects of overtime pay regulation; immigrant labor market outcomes and welfare recipiency; the impact of labor unions on compensation, employment, and work schedules; the importance of sector-specific skills; and the relative economic status of Mexican Americans.

Reed V. Tuckson, M.D.

Dr. Tuckson is senior vice president of consumer health and medical care enhancement at United Health Group. Formerly, he was senior vice president, professional standards, at the American Medical Association. Dr. Tuckson was president of Charles R. Drew University School of Medicine and Science from 1991 to 1997. From 1986 to 1990, he was commissioner of public health for the District of Columbia. Dr. Tuckson serves on a number of health care, academic, and federal boards and committees and is a nationally known lecturer on topics concerning community-based medicine, the moral responsibilities of health professionals, and physician leadership. He currently serves on the IOM Roundtable on Research and Development of Drugs, Biologics, and Medical Devices and is a member of the Institute of Medicine.

Edward H. Wagner, M.D., M.P.H., F.A.C.P.

Dr. Wagner is a general internist–epidemiologist and director of the W.A. MacColl Institute for Healthcare Innovation at the Center for Health Studies, Group Health Cooperative. He is also professor of health services at the University of Washington School of Public Health and Community Medicine. Current research interests include development and testing of population-based care models for diabetes, frail elderly, and chronic illnesses; evaluation of the health and cost impacts of chronic disease and cancer interventions; and interventions to prevent disability and reduce depressive symptoms in older adults. Dr. Wagner has written two books and more than 200 journal articles. He serves on the editorial boards of

Health Services Research and the *Journal of Clinical Epidemiology* and acts as a consultant to multiple federal agencies and private foundations. He recently completed a stint as senior adviser on managed care initiatives in the Director's Office of the National Institutes of Health. Since June 1998, he has directed Improving Chronic Illness Care (ICIC), a national program of The Robert Wood Johnson Foundation. The overall goal of ICIC is to assist health systems to improve their care of chronic illness through quality improvement and evaluation, research, and dissemination. Dr. Wagner is also principal investigator of the Cancer Research Network, a National Cancer Institute-funded consortium of 10 health maintenance organizations (HMOs) conducting collaborative cancer effectiveness research.

Lawrence Wallack, Dr.P.H.
Dr. Wallack is professor of public health and director, School of Community Health at Portland State University. He is also professor emeritus of public health, University of California, Berkeley. Dr. Wallack's primary interest is in the role of mass communication, particularly the news media, in shaping public health issues. His current research is on how public health issues are framed in print and broadcast news. He is principal author of *Media Advocacy and Public Health: Power for Prevention and News for a Change: An Advocate's Guide to Working with the Media.* He is also co-editor of *Mass Communications and Public Health: Complexities and Conflicts.* Dr. Wallack has published extensively on topics related to prevention, health promotion, and community interventions. Specific content areas of his research and intervention work have included alcohol, tobacco, violence, handguns, sexually transmitted diseases, cervical and breast cancer, affirmative action, suicide, and childhood lead poisoning. Dr. Wallack is a member of the IOM Committee on Communication for Behavior Change in the 21st Century: Improving the Health of Diverse Populations.

Barbara Wolfe, Ph.D.★
Barbara Wolfe is professor of economics, public affairs, and preventive medicine at the University of Wisconsin, Madison, and the former director of its Institute for Research on Poverty. She teaches health and public economics. She has been a fellow at the Netherlands Institute for Advanced Study, a research associate for the National Bureau of Economic Research, a member of the Board for International Health of the Institute of Medicine, and a scholar at the Russell Sage Foundation. Dr. Wolfe's research interests include determinants of children's attainments, effects of investments in children, health insurance and the labor market, and methodological issues. She received her B.A. degree in economics from Cornell University and an M.A. and Ph.D. in economics from the University of Pennsylvania. Dr. Wolfe previously served on the IOM Committee on Immunization Finance Policies and Practices.

★Member of the Subcommittee on the Family Impacts of Uninsurance.

Institute of Medicine Staff

Wilhelmine Miller, M.S., Ph.D.

Wilhelmine Miller is a senior program officer in the Division of Health Care Services. She served as staff to the Committee on Immunization Finance Policy and Practices, conducting and directing case studies of health care financing and public health services. Prior to joining IOM, Dr. Miller was an adjunct faculty member in the Departments of Philosophy at Georgetown University and Trinity College, teaching political philosophy, ethics, and public policy. She received her doctorate from Georgetown, with studies and research in bioethics and issues of social justice. In 1994–1995, Dr. Miller was a consultant to the President's Advisory Committee on Human Radiation Experiments. Dr. Miller was a program analyst in the Department of Health and Human Services for 14 years, responsible for policy development and regulatory review in areas including hospital and HMO payment, prescription drug benefits, and child health. Her M.S. from Harvard University is in health policy and management.

Dianne Miller Wolman, M.G.A.

Dianne Wolman joined the Health Care Services Division of the IOM in 1999 as a senior program officer. She directed the study that resulted in the IOM report *Medicare Laboratory Payment Policy: Now and in the Future,* released in 2000. Her previous work experience in the health field has been varied and extensive, focused on finance and reimbursement in insurance programs. She came from the General Accounting Office, where she was a senior evaluator on studies of the Health Care Financing Administration, its management capacity, and its oversight of Medicare contractors. Prior to that, she was a reimbursement policy specialist at a national association representing nonprofit providers of long-term care services. Her earlier positions included policy analysis and management in the Office of the Secretary in the Department of Health and Human Services and work with a peer review organization, a governor's task force on access to health care, and a third-party administrator for very large health plans. In addition, she was policy director for a state Medicaid rate-setting commission. She has a bachelor's degree in sociology from Brandeis University and a master's degree in government administration from Wharton Graduate School, University of Pennsylvania.

Lynne Page Snyder, Ph.D., M.P.H.

Lynne Snyder is a program officer in the IOM's Division of Health Care Services. She came to IOM from DHHS, where she worked as a public historian, documenting and writing about past federal activities in medicine, health care, and public health. In addition, she has worked for the Social Science Research Council's Committee on the Urban Underclass and served as a graduate fellow at the Smithsonian Institution's National Museum of American History. She has published on twentieth century health policy, occupational and environmental health, and minority health. Current research interests include health literacy and access to care by low-income seniors. She earned her doctorate in the history and sociology of science from the University of Pennsylvania (1994), working under Rosemary Stevens, and received her M.P.H. from the Johns Hopkins School of Hygiene and Public Health (2000).

Tracy McKay, B.A.

Tracy McKay is a research associate in the IOM Division of Health Care Services. She has worked on several projects, including the National Roundtable on Health Care Quality; Children, Health Insurance, and Access to Care; Quality of Health Care in America; and a study on non-heart-beating organ donors. She has assisted in the research for the National Quality Report on Health Care Delivery, Immunization Finance Policies and Practices, and Extending Medicare Coverage for Preventive and Other Services and helped develop this project on the consequences of uninsurance from its inception. Ms. McKay received her B.A. in sociology from Vassar College in 1996.

Ryan Palugod, B.S.

Ryan Palugod is a senior program assistant in the IOM Division of Health Care Services. Prior to joining the project staff in 2001, he worked as an administrative assistant with the American Association of Homes, Services for the Aging. He graduated with honors from Towson University with a degree in health care management in 1999.

Consultants to the Committee on the Consequences of Uninsurance

Matthew Broaddus, M.A.

Matthew Broaddus joined the Center on Budget and Policy Priorities in December 1999 as a research assistant in the Health Division. His policy, research, and analytical work is conducted in the areas of Medicaid and child health insurance programs. He graduated from Stanford University with an M.A. in sociology and a B.A. in comparative literature.

Gerry Fairbrother, Ph.D.

Gerry Fairbrother is a senior scientist in the division of health and science policy and research director for the New York forum for child health at the New York Academy of Medicine. She also holds a faculty appointment as associate professor of epidemiology and social medicine at Albert Einstein College of Medicine/ Montefiore Medical Center, where she continues to maintain an appointment. Dr. Fairbrother's research areas include access and barriers to care, particularly for low-income children. She has led investigations of barriers to enrollment in child health insurance, cost to enroll in these programs, impact of Medicaid managed care on preventive screening for children, and impact of financial incentives on physician behavior. She has served as a consultant to the Institute of Medicine on projects dealing with immunization financing and the consequences of uninsurance. She also works extensively with the Centers for Disease Control and Prevention on a project to assist states meet their requirement to monitor immunization rates for children in Medicaid. Dr. Fairbrother holds a Ph.D. from the Johns Hopkins University.

Hanns Kuttner, M.A.

Hanns Kuttner is a senior research associate with the Economic Research Initiative on the Uninsured, a research program on the causes and consequences of uninsurance funded by The Robert Wood Johnson Foundation and located at the University of Michigan. Mr. Kuttner is a Ph.D. candidate in the Irving B. Harris Graduate School of Public Policy Studies at the University of Chicago, from which he already holds an M.A. degree. Prior to his graduate studies, Mr. Kuttner was a research affiliate of the Governor's Task Force on Human Services Reform in Illinois, a member of the domestic policy staff in the Office of Policy Development at the White House during the presidency of George H.W. Bush, and special assistant to the administrator of what was then called the Health Care Financing Administration.

References

Acs, George, Richard Shulman, Man Wai Ng, and Steven Chussid. 1999. The Effect of Dental Rehabilitation on the Body Weight of Children with Early Childhood Caries. *Pediatric Dentistry* 21(2):109-113.

Acs, Gregory, and John Sabelhaus. 1995. Trends in Out-of-Pocket Spending on Health Care, 1980–1992. *Monthly Labor Review* 118(12):35-45.

Aday, Lu Ann. 1992. Health Insurance and Utilization of Medical Care for Chronically Ill Children with Special Needs. Health of Our Nation's Children, United States, 1988. *Advance Data* (215): 1-8.

Aday, Lu Ann, Eun Sul Lee, Bill Spears, Chih-Wen Chung, et al. 1993. Health Insurance and Utilization of Medical Care for Children with Special Health Care Needs. *Medical Care* 31(11): 1013-1026.

Administrative Office of the U.S. Courts. 2002. Record Breaking Bankruptcy Filings Reported in Calendar Year 2001. Available at: http://www.uscourts.gov/ttb/mar02ttb/breaking.html. Accessed June 24, 2002.

Agency for Healthcare Research and Quality (AHRQ). 2001a. Health Care Expenses in the U.S. Civilian Non-institutional Population, 1997. Available at: http://www.meps.ahrq.gov/Papers/ RF_01-R035/Tables/Table1_8.pdf. Accessed April 16, 2002.

Agency for Healthcare Research and Quality (AHRQ). 2001b. *Health Care Expenses in the United States, 1996.* Washington, DC: Agency for Healthcare Research and Quality.

American Academy of Pediatrics. 2002. The Medical Home. *Pediatrics* 110(1):184-186.

American College of Obstetricians and Gynecologists (ACOG). 1989. *Standards for Obstetric-Gynecologic Services.* 7th ed. Washington, DC: American College of Obstetricians and Gynecologist.

American College of Obstetricians and Gynecologists (ACOG). 2000. Ob-Gyns Issue Recommendations on Cesarean Delivery Rates. Press Release, August 9. Available at: http://www.acop.org/ from_home/publications/press_releases/nr08-09-00.htm. Accessed May 13, 2002.

Amini, Saied B., Patrick M. Catalano, and Leon I. Mann. 1996. Effect of Prenatal Care on Obstetrical Outcome. *Journal of Maternal-Fetal Medicine* 5(3):142-150.

Andersen, Ronald M. 1995. Revisiting the Behavioral Model and Access to Medical Care: Does It Matter? *Journal of Health and Social Behavior* 36(3):1-10.

259

Andersen, Ronald, and Pamela Davidson. 2001. Improving Access to Care in America: Individual and Contextual Indictators. In: *Changing the U.S. Health Care System: Key Issues in Health Services, Policy and Management.* Ronald Andersen, Thomas Rice, and Gerald Kominski (eds.). San Francisco, CA: Jossey-Bass. Pp. 3-30.

Anderson, Carolyn A., and Constance L. Hammen. 1993. Psychosocial Outcomes of Children of Unipolar Depressed, Bipolar, Medically Ill, and Normal Women: A Longitudinal Study. *Journal of Consulting & Clinical Psychology* 61(3):448-454.

Aron, David C., Howard S. Gordon, David L. DiGiuseppe, Dwain L. Harper, et al. 2000. Variations in Risk-Adjusted Cesarean Delivery Rates According to Race and Health Insurance. *Medical Care* 38(1):35-44.

Bachrach, Deborah, R. Belfort, and Karen Lipson. 2000. *Closing Coverage Gaps: Improving Retention Rates in New York's Medicaid and Child Health Plus Program.* New York: Kalkines, Arky, Zall & Bernstein. LLP.

Baldwin, Laura-Mae, Eric H. Larson, Frederick A. Connell, Daniel Nordlund, et al. 1998. The Effect of Expanding Medicaid Prenatal Services on Birth Outcomes. *American Journal of Public Health* 88(11):1623-1629.

Banthin, Jessica, Thesia Garner, and Kathleen Short. 2000. Medical Care Needs in Poverty Thresholds: Problems Posed by the Uninsured. Available at: http://www.census.gov/hhes/poverty/povmeas/ papers/medneeds7.pdf. Accessed July 14, 2002.

Bates, Ann S., John F. Fitzgerald, Robert S. Dittus, and Fredric D. Wolinsky. 1994. Risk Factors for Underimmunization in Poor Urban Infants. *Journal of the American Medical Association* 272(14):1105-1110.

Beardslee, William R., Martin B. Keller, Philip W. Lavori, Janet E. Staley, et al. 1993. The Impact of Parental Affective Disorder on Depression in Offspring: A Longitudinal Follow-up in a Non-referred Sample. *Journal of the American Academy of Child & Adolescent Psychiatry* 32(4):723-730.

Belle, Deborah. 1990. Poverty and Women's Mental Health. *American Psychologist* 45(3):385-389.

Berk, Marc L., and Amy K. Taylor. 1983. *Women and Divorce: Health Insurance Coverage, Utilization, and Health Care Expenditures.* Rockville, MD: National Center for Health Services Research.

Bernstein, Amy B. 1999. *Insurance Status and Use of Health Services by Pregnant Women.* Washington, DC: March of Dimes.

Bernstein, Jared, Chauna Brocht, and Maggie Spade-Aguilar. 2000. *How Much Is Enough? Basic Family Budgets for Working Families.* Washington, DC: Economic Policy Institute.

Bethell, Christine, Colleen Peck, Marc Abrams, Neal Halfon, et al. 2002. *Partnering with Parents to Promote the Healthy Development of Young Children Enrolled in Medicaid: Results from a Survey Assessing the Quality of Preventive and Developmental Services for Young Children Enrolled in Medicaid in Three States.* New York: Commonwealth Fund.

Bindman, Andrew B., Kevin Grumbach, Dennis Osmand, Miriam Komaromy, et al. 1995. Preventable Hospitalizations and Access to Care. *Journal of the American Medical Association* 274(4):305-311.

Bouma, Ruth, and Robert Schweitzer. 1990. The Impact of Chronic Childhood Illness on Family Stress. A Comparison Between Autism and Cystic Fibrosis. *Journal of Clinical Psychology* 46(6):722-730.

Boyle, Michael H., and Andrew Pickles. 1997. Maternal Depressive Symptoms and Ratings of Emotional Disorder Symptoms in Children and Adolescents. *Journal of Child Psychology & Psychiatry & Allied Disciplines* 38(8):981-992.

Brady, Henry E., Marcia Meyers, and Samantha Luks. 1998. *The Impact of Child Adult Disabilities on the Duration of Welfare Spells.* San Francisco: Public Policy Institute of California.

Braveman, Paula, Geraldine Olivia, Marie Grisham Miller, Randy Reiter, et al. 1989. Adverse Outcomes and Lack of Health Insurance Among Newborns in an Eight-County Area of California, 1982-1986. *New England Journal of Medicine* 321(8):508-513.

Braveman, Paula, Susan Egerter, Trude Bennett, and Jonathan Showstack. 1991. Differences in Hospital Resource Allocation Among Sick Newborns According to Insurance Coverage. *Journal of the American Medical Association* 266(23):3300-3308.

Braveman, Paula, Trude Bennett, Charlotte Lewis, Susan Egerter, et al. 1993. Access to Prenatal Care Following Major Medicaid Eligibility Expansions. *Journal of the American Medical Association* 269(10):1285-1289.

Braveman, Paula, Kristin Marchi, Susan Egerter, Michelle Pearl, et al. 2000. Barriers to Timely Prenatal Care Among Women in Insurance: The Importance of Prepregnancy Factors. *Obstetrics and Gynecology* 95(6 Pt 1):874-880.

Broaddus, Matthew, and Leighton Ku. 2000. *Nearly 95 Percent of Low-Income Uninsured Children Now Are Eligible for Medicaid or SCHIP.* Washington, DC: Center on Budget and Policy Priorities.

Broaddus, Matthew, Shannon Blaney, Annie Dude, Jocelyn Guyer, et al. 2002. *Expanding Family Coverage: States' Medicaid Eligibility Policies for Working Families in the Year 2000.* Washington, DC: Center on Budget and Policy Priorities.

Bronstein, Janet M., Eli Capilouto, Wally A. Carlo, James L. Haywood, et al. 1995. Access to Neonatal Intensive Care for Low-Birthweight Infants: The Role of Maternal Characteristics. *American Journal of Public Health* 85(3):357-361.

Brown, E. Richard, Roberta Wyn, Hongjian Yu, Abel Valenzuela, et al. 1999. Access to Health Insurance and Care for Children in Immigrant Families. In: *Children of Immigrants: Health Adjustment, and Public Assistance,* Donald J. Hernandez and Evan Charney (eds.). Washington, DC: National Academy Press. Pp. 126-186.

Brown, E. Richard, Roberta Wyn, and Stephanie Teleki. 2000. *Disparities in Health Insurance and Access to Care for Residents Across U.S. Cities.* Los Angeles: Regents of the University of California.

Bruen, Brian K., and John Holahan. 2002. *Acceleration of Medicaid Spending Reflects Mounting Pressures.* Washington, DC: Kaiser Commission on Medicaid and the Uninsured.

Brunelle, Janet A. 1989. *Oral Health of United States Children: The National Survey of Dental Caries in U.S. Schoolchildren, 1986-1987.* NIH Pub No. 89-2247. Bethesda, MD: National Institutes of Dental Research.

Buchmueller, Thomas C., and Robert G. Valletta. 1996. The Effects of Employer-Provided Insurance on Worker Mobility. *Industrial and Labor Relations Review* 49(3):439-455.

Buchmueller, Thomas C., and Robert G. Valletta. 1999. The Effect of Health Insurance on Married Female Labor Supply. *Journal of Human Resources* 34(1):42-70.

Bumpass, Larry L., and James A. Sweet. 1989. Children's Experience in Single-Parent Families: Implications of Cohabitation and Marital Transitions. *Family Planning Perspectives* 21(6):256-260.

Bumpass, Larry L., James A. Sweet, and Andrew Cherlin. 1991. The Role of Cohabitation in Declining Rates of Marriage. *Journal of Marriage and the Family* 53(4):913-927.

Bumpass, Larry L., R. Kelly Raley, and James A. Sweet. 1995. The Changing Character of Stepfamilies: Implications of Cohabitation and Nonmarital Childbearing. *Demography* 32(3):425-436.

Burkhauser, Richard V., Kenneth A. Couch, and John W. Phillips. 1996. Who Takes Early Social Security Benefits? The Economic and Health Status of Early Beneficiaries. *Gerontologist* 36(6):789-799.

Byck, Gayle R. 2000. A Comparison of the Socioeconomic and Health Status Characteristics of Uninsured, State Children's Health Insurance Program-Eligible Children in the United States with Those of Other Groups of Insured Children: Implications for Policy. *Pediatrics* 106(1):14-21.

Carr, Willine, Lisa Zeitel, and Kevin B. Weiss. 1992. Variations in Asthma Hospitalizations and Deaths in New York City. *American Journal of Public Health* 82(1):59-65.

Casby, Michael W. 2001. Otitis Media and Language Development: A Meta-Analysis. *American Journal of Speech-Language Pathology* 10(1):65-80.

Casper, Lynne M., and Paul N. Cohen. 2000. How Does POSSLQ Measure Up? Historical Estimates of Cohabitation. *Demography* 37(2):237-245.

Celano, Marianne P., and Robert J. Geller. 1993. Learning, School Performance, and Children with Asthma: How Much at Risk? *Journal of Learning Disability* 26(1):23-32.

Census Bureau. 2000a. *Current Population Survey. Design and Methodology.* Technical Paper 63. Washington, DC: Census Bureau.

Census Bureau. 2000b. Table HIO1. Health Insurance Coverage Status and Type of Coverage by Selected Characteristics: 2000. Available at: http://ferret.bls.census.gov/macro/032001/health/h01_001.htm. Accessed June 16, 2002.

Census Bureau. 2000c. Table A. People Without Health Insurance for the Entire Year by Selected Characteristics. Available at: http://www.census.gov/hhes/hlthins/hlthins00/hi00ta.html. Accessed March 11, 2002.

Census Bureau. 2001a. Health Insurance Coverage: 2000. Publication P60-215. On-line supplemental table HI01. Washington, DC: Bureau of the Census. Available at: http://ferret.bls.census.gov/macro/032001/heatlh/h01_001.htm. Accessed May 13, 2002.

Census Bureau. 2001b. *Statistical Abstract of the United States.* Washington, DC: U.S. Government Printing Office.

Centers for Disease Control and Prevention (CDC). 1996a. Asthma Mortality and Hospitalization Among Children and Young Adults_United States, 1980-1993. *Morbidity and Mortality Weekly Report* 45(17):350-353.

Centers for Disease Control and Prevention (CDC). 1996b. Asthma Surveillance Program in Public Health Departments_United States. Available at: http://www.cdc.gov/mmwr/preview/mwrhtml/00043767.htm. Accessed April 15, 2002.

Centers for Medicare and Medicaid Services (CMS). 2001. *Continuing to Progress: Enrolling & Retaining Low-Income Families and Children in Health Care Coverage.* CMS Publication 11000. Washington, DC: U.S. Department of Health and Human Services.

Centers for Medicare and Medicaid Services (CMS). 2002a. Medicare Basics. Available at: http://www.medicare.gov/Basics/WhatIs.asp?PrinterFriendly=true. Accessed March 25, 2002.

Centers for Medicare and Medicaid Services (CMS). 2002b. *The State Children's Health Insurance Program Annual Enrollment Report. Federal Fiscal Year 2001: October 1, 2000-September 30, 2001.* Washington, DC: U.S. Department of Health and Human Services.

Century Foundation. 2001. *Medicare Reform: A Century Foundation Guide to the Issues.* New York: Century Foundation Press.

Chevan, Albert. 1996. As Cheaply as One: Cohabitation in the Older Population. *Journal of Marriage and the Family* 58(3):656-667.

Citro, Constance F., and Robert T. Michael (eds.). 1995. *Measuring Poverty. A New Approach.* Washington, DC: National Academy Press.

Coate, Stephen. 1995. Altruism, the Samaritan's Dilemma, and Government Transfer Policy. *American Economic Review* 85(1):46-57.

Cohen, Joel W., Steven R. Machlin, Samuel Zuvekas, Marie N. Stagnitti, et al. 2000. *Health Care Expenses in the United States, 1996.* MEPS Research Findings #12. AHRQ Publication 01-0009. Rockville, MD: Agency for Health Care Research and Quality.

Cohen, Rima, and Taida Wolfe. 2001. Implementing New York's Family Health Plan Plus Program Lessons from Other States. New York: Commonwealth Fund. Available at: http://www.cmwf.org/programs/newyork/cohen_nyfhp_485.pdf. Accessed May 15, 2002.

Cole, Michael, and Sheila R. Cole. 1993. *The Development of Children.* New York: Scientific American.

Cole, Nancy. 1995. *Increasing Access to Health Care: The Effects of Medicaid Expansion for Pregnant Women.* Cambridge, MA: Abt Associates.

Collins, Karen Scott, Katie Tenney, and Dora L. Hughes. 2002. *Quality of Health Care for African Americans: Findings from Commonwealth Fund 2001 Health Care Quality Survey.* New York: Commonwealth Fund.

Committee on Ways and Means. *1996 Green Book: Background Material and Data on Programs Within the Jurisdiction of the Committee on Ways and Means.* Washington, DC: U.S. Government Printing Office.

Compas, Bruce E. 1987. Coping with Stress During Childhood Adolescence. *Psychological Bulletin* 101(3):393-403.

Congressional Budget Office (CBO). 2002. *CBO March 2002 Baseline: Medicaid and State Children's Health Insurance Program Fact Sheet.* Washington, DC: Congressional Budget Office.

Cooper, Philip F., and Barbara Steinberg Schone. 1997. More Offers, Fewer Takers for Employment Based Health Insurance: 1987 and 1996. *Health Affairs* 16(6):142-149.

Corman, Hope, and Robert Kaestner. 1992. The Effects of Child Health on Marital Status and Family Structure. *Demography* 29(3):389-408.

Coulam, Robert, Thomas R. Cole, et al. 1995. *Final Report of the Evaluation of the Medicare Catastrophic Coverage Act: Impacts on Maternal and Child Health Programs and Beneficiaries.* Cambridge, MA: Abt Associates.

Cunningham, Peter J., Joy M. Grossman, Robert F. St. Peter, and Cara S. Lesser. 1999. Managed Care and Physicians' Provision of Charity Care. *Journal of the American Medical Association* 281(12):1087-1092.

Currie, Janet. 2000. Do Children of Immigrants Make Differential Use of Public Health Insurance? In *Issues in the Economics of Immigration*, George Borjas (ed.). Chicago, IL: University of Chicago Press.

Currie, Janet, and Thomas Duncan. 1995. Medical Care for Children: Public Insurance, Private Insurance, and Racial Differences in Utilization. *Journal of Human Resources* 30(1):135-162.

Currie, Janet, and Jeffrey Grogger. 2002. Medicaid Expansions and Welfare Contractions: Offsetting Effects on Prenatal Care and Infant Health? *Journal of Health Economics* 21(2):313-335.

Currie, Janet, and Jonathan Gruber. 1996a. Saving Babies: The Efficacy and Cost of Recent Changes in the Medicaid Eligibility of Pregnant Women. *Journal of Political Economy* 104(6):1263-1296.

Currie, Janet, and Jonathan Gruber. 1996b. Health Insurance Eligibility, Utilization of Medical Care, and Child Health. *Quarterly Journal of Economics* 111(2):431-466.

Currie, Janet, and Jonathan Gruber. 2001. Public Health Insurance and Medical Treatment: The Equalizing Impact of the Medicaid Expansions. *Journal of Public Economics* 82(1):63-89.

Dafny, Leemore, and Jonathan Gruber. 2000. Does Public Insurance Improve the Efficiency of Medical Care? In: *Medicaid Expansions and Child Hospitalizations.* Cambridge, MA: National Bureau of Economic Research.

Dallman, Peter R., Ray Yip, and Clifford L. Johnson. 1984. Prevalence and Causes of Anemia in the United States. *American Journal of Clinical Nutrition* 39(3):437-445.

Davidoff, Amy J., Bowen Garrett, Diane M. Makuc, and Matthew Schirmer. 2000a. *Children Eligible for Medicaid but Not Enrolled: How Great a Policy Concern?* New Federalism Issues and Options for States. Series A, A-41. Washington, DC: Urban Institute.

Davidoff, Amy J., A. Bowen Garrett, Diane M. Makuc, and Matthew Schirmer. 2000b. Medicaid-Eligible Children Who Don't Enroll: Health Status, Access to Care, and Implications for Medicaid Enrollment. *Inquiry* 37(2):203-218.

Davidoff, Amy, Garrett Bowen, and Alshadye Yemane. 2001a. *Medicaid-Eligible Adults Who Are Not Enrolled: Who Are They and Do They Get the Care They Need?* New Federalism: Issues and Options for States. Series A, No. A-48. Washington, DC: Urban Institute.

Davidoff, Amy J., Genevieve Kenney, Lisa Dubay, and Alshadye Yemane. 2001b. *Patterns of Child-Parent Insurance Coverage: Implications for Coverage Expansions.* New Federalism National Survey of America's Families. Series B, No. B-39. Washington, DC: Urban Institute.

Davidoff, Amy, Genevieve Kenney, and Alshadye Yemane. 2002 (forthcoming). *The Effect of Parents' Insurance Coverage on Access to Care for Low-Income Children.* Washington, DC: Urban Institute.

Domowitz, Ian, and Robert L. Sartain. 1999. Determinant of the Consumer Bankruptcy Decision. *Journal of Finance* 54(1):403-420.

Doty, Michelle M., and Brett L. Ives. 2002. *Quality of Health Care for Hispanic Populations: Findings from Commonwealth Fund 2001 Health Care Quality Survey*. Commonwealth Fund Publication 526. New York: Commonwealth Fund.

Doty, Michelle M., and Cathy Schoen. 2001. *Maintaining Health Insurance During a Recession: Likely COBRA Eligibility*. New York: Commonwealth Fund.

Downey, Geraldine, and James C. Coyne. 1990. Children of Depressed Parents: An Integrative Review. *Psychological Bulletin* 108(1):50-76.

Dubay, Lisa, and Genevieve M. Kenney. 2001. Health Care Access and Use Among Low-Income Children: Who Fares Best? *Health Affairs* 20(1):112-121.

Dubay, Lisa, and Genevieve M. Kenney. 2002. *Expanding Public Health Insurance to Parents: Effects on Children's Coverage Under Medicaid*. Washington, DC: Urban Institute.

Dubay, Lisa, Genevieve Kenney, and Stephen Zuckerman. 2000. *Extending Medicaid to Parents: An Incremental Strategy for Reducing the Number of Uninsured*. Assessing the New Federalism. Series B, No. B-20. Washington, DC: Urban Institute.

Dubay, Lisa, Ted Joyce, Robert Kaestner, and Genevieve M. Kenney. 2001. Changes in Prenatal Care Timing and Low Birth Weight by Race and Socioeconomic Status: Implications for the Medicaid Expansions for Pregnant Women. *Health Services Research* 36(2):373-398.

Dubay, Lisa, Jennifer Haley, and Genevieve Kenney. 2002a. *Children's Eligibility for Medicaid and SCHIP: A View from 2000*. New Federalism National Survey of America's Families. Series B, No. B-41. Washington, DC: Urban Institute.

Dubay, Lisa, Genevieve Kenney, and Jennifer Haley. 2002b. *Children's Participation in Medicaid and SCHIP: Early in the SCHIP Era*. New Federalism National Survey of America's Families. Series B, No. B-40. Washington, DC: Urban Institute.

Duchon, Lisa, and Cathy Schoen. 2001. *Experiences of Working-Age Adults in the Individual Insurance Market*. Issue Brief. New York: Commonwealth Fund.

Duchon, Lisa, Cathy Schoen, Michelle M. Doty, Karen Davis, et al. 2001. *Security Matters: How Instability in Health Insurance Puts U.S. Workers at Risk. Findings from the 2001 Health Insurance Survey*. Publication 512. New York: Commonwealth Fund.

DuPaul, George J., Kara E. McGoey, Tanya L. Eckert, and John VanBrakle. 2001. Preschool Children with Attention-Deficit/Hyperactivity Disorder: Impairments in Behavioral, Social, and School Functioning. *Journal of the American Academy of Child and Adolescent Psychiatry* 40(5):508-515.

Durbin, Dennis R., Angelo P. Giardino, Kathy N. Shaw, Mary C. Harris, et al. 1997. The Effect of Insurance Status on Likelihood of Neonatal Interhospital Transfer. *Pediatrics* 100(3):381-382.

Edelstein, Burton L., and Chester W. Douglass. 1995. Dispelling the Myth That 50 Percent of U.S. Schoolchildren Have Never Had a Cavity. *Public Health Report* 110(5):522-530.

Edmunds, Margaret, and Molly Joel Coye (eds.). 1998. *America's Children: Health Insurance and Access to Care*. Washington, DC: National Academy Press.

Edmunds, Margaret M., Martha Teitelbaum, and Cassy Gleason. 2000. *All Over the Map. A Progress Report on the State Children's Health Insurance Program*. Washington, DC: Children's Defense Fund.

Ellwood, Marilyn Rymer, and Genevieve Kenney. 1995. Medicaid and Pregnant Women: Who Is Being Enrolled and When. *Health Care Finance Review* 17(2):7-28.

Fairbrother, Gerry, Heidi Park, and Michael Gusmano. 2002. How Community Health Centers Are Coping with Their Uninsured Caseloads. Presented at the National Association of Community Health Centers 27th Policy and Issues Forum. Washington, DC.

Farley, Pamela, and Gail Wilensky. 1984. *Household Wealth and Health Insurance as Protection Against Medical Risk*. Rockville, MD: National Center for Health Services Research.

Farrow, Diana C., Laura-Mae Baldwin, Mary Lawrence Cawthon, and Frederick A. Connell. 1996. The Impact of Extended Maternity Services on Prenatal Care Use Among Medicaid Women. *American Journal of Preventive Medicine* 12(2):103-107.

Federal Trade Commission (FTC). 1999. FTC Facts for Consumers: Fair Credit Reporting. Washington: Federal Trade Commission. Available at: http://www.ftc.gov/bcp/conline/pubs/credit/fcra.pdf. Accessed July 18, 2002.

Ferris, Timothy G., Ellen F. Crain, Emily Oken, Linda Wang, et al. 2001. Insurance and Quality of Care for Children with Acute Asthma. *Ambulatory Pediatrics* 1(5):267-274.

Fischer, Mariellen, Russell A. Barkley, Craig S. Edelbrock, and Lori Smallish. 1990. The Adolescent Outcome of Hyperactive Children Diagnosed by Research Criteria: II. Academic, Attentional, and Neuropsychological Status. *Journal of Consulting and Clinical Psychology* 58(5):580-588.

Fischer, Mariellen, Russell A. Barkley, Kenneth E. Fletcher, and Lori Smallish. 1993. The Adolescent Outcome of Hyperactive Children: Predictors of Psychiatric, Academic, Social, and Emotional Adjustment. *American Academy of Child and Adolescent Psychiatry* 32(2):324-332.

Fishman, Eliot. 2001. Aging Out of Coverage: Young Adults with Special Health Needs. *Health Affairs* 20(6):254-266.

Foster, David C., David S. Guzick, and Robert P. Pulliam. 1992. The Impact of Prenatal Care on Fetal and Neonatal Death Rates for Uninsured Patients: A "Natural Experiment" in West Virginia. *Obstetrics and Gynecology* 79(1):40-45.

Freed, Gary L., Sarah J. Clark, Donald E. Pathman, and Robin Schectman. 1999. Influences on the Receipt of Well-Child Visits in the First Two Years of Life. *Pediatrics* 103(4 Suppl):864-869.

Freudenheim, Milt. 2002. Companies Trim Health Benefits for Many Retirees as Costs Surge. *New York Times*. May 10, p.A:1.

Frick, Paul J., Randy W. Kamphaus, Benjamin B. Lahey, Rolf Loeber, et al. 1991. Academic Underachievement and the Disruptive Behavior Disorders. *Journal of Consulting and Clinical Psychology* 59(2):289-294.

Fronstin, Paul. 2000. Counting the Uninsured: A Comparison of National Surveys. EBRI Issue Brief 225. Washington, DC: Employee Benefit Research Institute.

Fronstin, Paul. 2001. Sources of Health Insurance and Characteristics of the Uninsured: Analysis of the March 2001 Current Population Survey. Issue Brief 240. Washington, DC: Employee Benefit Research Institute.

Gabel, Jon, Larry Levitt, Jeremy Pickreign, Heidi Whitmore, et al. 2001. Job Based Health Insurance in 2001: Inflation Hits Double Digits, Managed Care Retreats. *Health Affairs* 20(5):180-186

Garmezy, Norman, 1983. Stressors in Childhood. In: *Stress, Coping and Development in Children*. New York:McGraw-Hill.

Garrett, Bowen, and John Holahan. 2000a. Health Insurance Coverage After Welfare. *Health Affairs* 19(1):175-184.

Garrett, Bowen, and John Holahan. 2000b. Welfare Leavers, Medicaid Coverage, and Private Health Insurance. Available at: http://newfederalism.urban.org/html/series_b/b13/b13.html. Accessed April 2, 2002.

Gergen, Peter J., and Kevin B. Weiss. 1990. Changing Patterns of Asthma Hospitalization Among Children: 1979 to 1987. *Journal of the American Medical Association* 264(13):1688-1692.

Geronimus, Arline T., and John Bound. 1990. Black/White Differences in Women's Reproductive-Related Health Status: Evidence from Vital Statistics. *Demography* 27(3):457-466.

Geronimus, Arline T., H. Frank Anderson, and John Bound. 1991. Differences in Hypertension Prevalence Among U.S. Black and White Women of Childbearing Age. *Public Health Reports* 106(4):393-399.

Glanz, Karen, Frances M. Lewis, and Barbara K. Rimer (eds.). 1997. *Health Behavior and Health Education. Theory, Research, and Practice.* 2nd edition. San Francisco, CA: Jossey-Bass.

Glied, Sherry A., and Sangeeth Gnanasekaran. 1996. Hospital Financing and Neonatal Intensive Care. *Health Services Research* 31(5):593-605.

Gordis, Leon. 1996. *Epidemiology*. Philadelphia, PA: W.B. Saunders and Co.

Gordon, Michael, Barbara B. Mettelman, and Martin Irwin. 1994. Sustained Attention and Grade Attention. *Perceptual and Motor Skills* 78(2): 555-560.

Grall, Timothy. 2000. *Child Support for Custodial Mothers and Fathers, 1997.* Current Population Reports P60-212. Washington, DC: U.S. Census Bureau.

Grantham-McGregor, Sally, and Cornelius Ani. 2001. A Review of Studies on the Effect of Iron Deficiency on Cognitive Development in Children. *Journal of Nutrition* 131(2S-2):649S-668S.

Gregory, Kimberly D., Sally C. Curtin, Selma M. Taffel, and Francis C. Notzon. 1998. Changes in Indications for Cesarean Delivery: United States, 1985-1994. *American Journal of Public Health* 88(9):1384-1387.

Gregory, Kimberly D., Emily Ramicone, Linda Chan, and Katherine L. Kahn. 1999. Cesarean Deliveries for Medicaid Patients: A Comparison in Public and Private Hospitals in Los Angeles County. *American Journal of Obstetrics* 180(5):177-184.

Gruber, Jonathan. 2000. Health Insurance and the Labor Market. In: *Handbook of Labor Economics*, A.J. Culyer and Joseph P. Newhouse (eds.). New York: North-Holland.

Gruber, Jonathan, and Larry Levitt. 2001. *Rising Unemployment and the Uninsured.* Washington, DC: Henry J. Kaiser Foundation.

Gruber, Jonathan, and Brigitte C. Madrian. 2002. *Health Insurance, Labor Supply, and Job Mobility: A Critical Review of the Literature.* NBER Working Paper 8817. Cambridge, MA: National Bureau of Economic Research.

Guendelman, Sylvia, Helen Halpin Schauffler, and Michelle Pearl. 2001. Unfriendly Shores: How Immigrant Children Fare in the U.S. Health System. *Health Affairs* 20(1):257-266.

Gutstadt, Linda B., Jerry W. Gillette, David A. Mrazek, Joleen T. Fukuhara, et al. 1989. Determinants of School Performance in Children with Chronic Asthma. *American Journal of Diseases of Children* 143(4):471-475.

Guyer, Jocelyn, and Cindy Mann. 1999. *A New Opportunity to Provide Health Care Coverage for New York's Low-Income Families.* Washington, DC: Center on Budget and Policy Priorities.

Guyer, Jocelyn, Matthew Broaddus, and Michelle Cochran. 1999. *Missed Opportunities: Declining Medicaid Enrollment Undermines the Nation's Progress in Insuring Low-Income Children.* Washington, DC: Center on Budget and Policy Priorities.

Guyer, Jocelyn, Matthew Broaddus, and Annie Dude. 2001. *Millions of Mothers Lack Health Insurance Coverage: Most Uninsured Mothers Lack Access Both to Employer-Based Coverage and Publicly-Subsidized Health Insurance.* Washington DC: Center on Budget and Policy Priorities.

Haas, Jennifer S., and Nancy E. Adler. 2001. The Causes of Vulnerability: Disentangling the Effects of Race, Socioeconomic Status and Insurance Coverage on Health. Background paper prepared for the Committee on the Consequences of Uninsurance. Available at: http://www.iom.edu/uninsured.

Haas, Jennifer S., Steven Udvarhelyi, and Arnold M. Epstein. 1993a. The Effect of Health Coverage for Uninsured Pregnant Women on Maternal Health and the Use of Cesarean Section. *Journal of the American Medical Association* 270(1):61-64.

Haas, Jennifer S., I. Steven Udvarhelyi, Carl N. Morris, and Arnold M. Epstein. 1993b. The Effect of Providing Health Coverage to Poor Uninsured Pregnant Women in Massachusetts. *Journal of the American Medical Association* 269(1):87-91.

Hadley, Jack. 2002. *Sicker and Poorer: The Consequences of Being Uninsured. A Review of the Research on the Relationship Between Health Insurance, Health, Work, Income and Education.* Washington, DC: Kaiser Commission on Medicaid and the Uninsured.

Halterman, Jill S., Andrew Aligne, Peggy Auinger, John T. McBride, et al. 2000. Inadequate Therapy for Asthma Among Children in the United States. *Pediatrics* 105(1 Pt 3):272-276.

Halterman, Jill S., Jeffrey M. Kaczorowski, C. Andrew Aligne, Peggy Auinger, et al. 2001. Iron Deficiency and Cognitive Achievement Among School-Aged Children and Adolescents in the United States. *Pediatrics* 107(6):1381-1386.

Hammen, Constance, Cheri Adrian, D. Gordon, Dorli Burge, et al. 1987. Children of Depressed Mothers: Maternal Strain and Symptom Predictors of Dysfunction. *Journal of Abnormal Psychology* 96(3):190-198.

Hanson, Karla L. 1998. Is Insurance for Children Enough? The Link Between Parents' and Children's Health Care Use Revisited. *Inquiry* 35(3):294-302.

Health Care Financing Administration (HCFA). 2002. What is HIPAA? Available at: http://www.hcfa.gov/medicaid/hipaa/content/more.asp. Accessed April 8, 2002.

Heck, Katherine E., and Jennifer D. Parker. 2002. Family Structure, Socioeconomic Status, and Access to Health Care for Children. *Health Services Research* 37(1):173-186.

Henderson Sean O., Philip Bretsky, Brian E. Henderson, and Daniel O. Stram. 2001. Risk factors for Cardiovascular and Cerebrovascular Death Among African Americans and Hispanics in Los Angeles, California. *Academic Emergency Medicine* 8(12):1163-1172.

Herkimer, Jr., Allen G. 1993. *Patient Financial Services: Organizing and Managing a Cost-Effective Patient Financial Services Operation.* Chicago IL: Probus Publishing Company.

Hernandez, Donald J. (ed.). 1999. *Children of Immigrants: Health, Adjustments, and Public Assistance.* Washington, DC: National Academy Press.

Hernandez, Donald J., and Evan Charney, eds. 1998. From Generation to Generation: The Health and Well-Being of Children in Immigrant Families. Washington, DC: National Academy Press.

Herring, Bradley J. 2001. *Does Access to Charity Care for the Uninsured Crowd out Private Health Insurance Coverage?* Unpublished manuscript. New Haven, CT: Yale University.

Hessol, Nancy A., Elena Fuentes-Afflick, and Peter Bacchetti. 1998. Risk of Low Birth Weight Among Black and White Parents. *Obstetrics and Gynecology* 92(5):814-822.

Hoffman, Catherine, and Mary Pohl. 2000. *Health Insurance Coverage in America: 1999 Data Update.* Kaiser Commission on Medicaid and the Uninsured. Washington, DC: Henry J. Kaiser Family Foundation.

Hoffman, Catherine, and Mary Pohl. 2002. *Health Insurance Coverage in America: 2000 Data Update.* Kaiser Commission on Medicaid and the Uninsured. Washington, DC: Henry J. Kaiser Family Foundation.

Hoffman, Saul D,. and Greg J. Duncan. 1988. What Are the Economic Consequences of Divorce? *Demography* 25(4):641-645.

Holahan, John, and Niall Brennan. 2000. *Who Are the Adult Insured?* Assessing the New Federalism Publication No. B-14. Washington, DC: Urban Institute.

Holl, Jane L., Peter G. Szilagyi, Lance E. Rodewald, Robert S. Byrd, et al. 1995. Profile of Uninsured Children in the United States. *Archives of Pediatrics and Adolescent Medicine* 149(4):398-406.

Holl, Jane L., Peter G. Szilagyi, Lance E. Rodewald, Laura Pollard Shone, et al. 2000. Evaluation of New York State's Child Health Plus: Access, Utilization, Quality of Health Care, and Health Status. *Pediatrics* 105(3):711-718.

Homan, Rick K., and Carol C. Korenbrot. 1998. Explaining Variation in Birth Outcomes of Medicaid-Eligible Women with Variation in the Adequacy of Prenatal Support Services. *Medical Care* 36(2):190-201.

Howell, Embry M. 2001. The Impact of the Medicaid Expansions for Pregnant Women: A Synthesis of the Evidence. *Medical Care Research and Review* 58(1):3-30.

Hughes, Dora L. 2002. *Quality of Health Care for Asian Americans: Findings from the Commonwealth Fund 2001 Health Care Quality Survey.* Commonwealth Fund Publication 525. New York: Commonwealth Fund.

Hurtado, Margarita, Elyse Krieger, Angelika Hartl Claussen, and Keith G. Scott. 1999. Early Childhood Anemia and Mild or Moderate Retardation. *American Journal of Clinical Nutrition* 69:115-119.

Institute for Research on Poverty. 2000. What Is the Difference Between Poverty Thresholds and Poverty Guidelines? Available at: http://www.ssc.wisc.edu/irp/faqs/faq7.htm. Accessed February 1, 2002.

Institute of Medicine (IOM). 2000. *America's Health Care Safety Net. Intact but Endangered.* Washington, DC: National Academy Press.

Institute of Medicine (IOM). 2001. *Coverage Matters: Insurance and Health Care.* Washington, DC: National Academy Press.

Institute of Medicine (IOM). 2002a. *Care Without Coverage: Too Little, Too Late.* Washington, DC: National Academy Press.

Institute of Medicine (IOM). 2002b. *Unequal Treatment: Confronting Racial and Ethnic Disparities in Health Care*. Washington, DC: National Academy Press.

Jackson, Aurora P. 1992. Well-Being Among Single, Black, Employed Mothers. *Social Science Review* 66(3):399-409.

Jacoby, Melissa G., Teresa A. Sullivan, and Elizabeth Warren. 2000. *Medical Problems and Bankruptcy Filings*. Rochester, NY: Norton's Bankruptcy Advisor.

Janicke, David M., Jack W. Finney, and Anne W. Riley. 2001. Children's Health Care Use: A Prospective Investigation of Factors Related to Care-Seeking. *Medical Care* 39(9):990-1001.

Johnson, James H. 1986. *Life Events as Stressors in Childhood and Adolescence*. Developmental Clinical Psychology and Psychiatry, Vol. 8. Newbury Park, CA: Sage Publications.

Johnson, Richard W., Amy Davidoff, and Kevin Perese. 1999. *Health Cost and Early Retirement Decisions*. Washington, DC: Urban Institute.

Joyce, Theodore J. 1987. The Demand for Health Inputs and Their Impact on the Black Neonatal Mortality Rate in the U.S. *Social Science and Medicine* 24(11):911-918.

Kaestner, Robert, Ted Joyce, and Andrew Racine. 2001. Medicaid Eligibility and the Incidence of Ambulatory Care Sensitive Hospitalizations for Children. *Social Science and Medicine* 52(2):305-313.

Kahn, Robert S., Paul H. Wise, Bruce P. Kennedy, and Ichiro Kawachi. 2000. State Income Inequality, Household Income, and Maternal Mental and Physical Health: Cross Sectional National Survey. *British Medical Journal* 321(7272):1311-1315.

Kaiser Commission on Medicaid and the Uninsured. 1998. Participation in Welfare and Medicaid Enrollment. Available at: http://www.kff.org/content/archive/1437/enrollment.html. Accessed April 4, 2002.

Kaiser Commission on Medicaid and the Uninsured. 2000. *Medicaid Eligibility and Citizenship Status: Policy and Implications for Immigrant Populations*. Washington, DC: Henry J. Kaiser Family Foundation.

Kaiser Commission on Medicaid and the Uninsured. 2001a. *Medicaid Coverage During a Time of Rising Unemployment*. Washington, DC: Henry J. Kaiser Family Foundation.

Kaiser Commission on Medicaid and the Uninsured. 2001b. *Medicaid "Mandatory" and "Optional" Eligibility and Benefits*. Washington, DC: Henry J. Kaiser Family Foundation.

Kaiser Commission on Medicaid and the Uninsured. 2001c. *The Role of Medicaid in State Budgets*. Washington, DC: Henry J. Kaiser Family Foundation.

Kaiser Commission on Medicaid and the Uninsured. 2002a. *Health Insurance Coverage in America: 2000 Data Update*. Washington, DC: Henry J. Kaiser Family Foundation.

Kaiser Commission on Medicaid and the Uninsured. 2002b. *The New Medicaid and CHIP Waiver Initiatives*. Washington, DC: Henry J. Kaiser Family Foundation.

Kaiser Family Foundation (KFF). 2001. *The Medicare Program*. Washington, DC: Henry J. Kaiser Family Foundation.

Kaiser Family Foundation (KFF)-Health Research and Educational Trust (HRET). 2001. *Employer Health Benefits, 2001. Annual Survey*. Washington, DC: Henry J. Kaiser Family Foundation.

Kaiser Family Foundation (KFF)-Health Research & Educational Trust (HRET) and the Commonwealth Fund. 2002. *Erosion of Private Health Insurance Coverage for Retirees*. Washington, DC: Henry J. Kaiser Family Foundation.

Kalil, Ariel, Catherine E. Born, James Kunz, and Pamela J. Caudill. 2001. Life Stressors, Social Support, and Depressive Symptoms Among First-Time Welfare Recipients. *American Journal of Community Psychology* 29(2):355-369.

Kaye, Neva, and Lynda Flowers. 2002. *How States Have Expanded Medicaid and SCHIP Eligibility*. Portland, ME: National Academy for State Health Policy.

Keeler, Emmett B., and Mollyann Brodie. 1993. Economic Incentives in the Choice Between Vaginal Delivery and Cesarean Section. *Milbank Quarterly* 71(3):365-404.

Keeler, Emmett B., Robert H. Brook, George A. Goldberg, Caren J. Kamberg, et al. 1985. How Free Care Reduced Hypertension in the Health Insurance Experiment. *Journal of the American Medical Association* 254(14):1926-1931.

Kempe, Allison, Brenda L. Renfrew, Jennifer C. Barrow, Debra Cherry, et al. 2001. Barriers to Enrollment in a State Child Health Insurance Program. *Ambulatory Pediatrics* 1(3):169-177.

Kenney, Genevieve, and Lisa Dubay. 1995. *A National Study of the Impact of Medicaid Expansions for Pregnant Women.* Washington, DC: Urban Institute

Kenney, Genevieve, and Jennifer Haley. 2001. *Why Aren't More Uninsured Children Enrolled in Medicaid or SCHIP?* New Federalism National Survey of America's Families. Series B, No. B-35. Washington, DC: Urban Institute.

Kenney, Genevieve. Lisa Dubay, and Jennifer Haley. 2000. *Health Insurance, Access, and Health Status of Children.* Washington, DC: Urban Institute.

Kenney, Genevieve, Jennifer Haley, and Lisa Dubay. 2001. *How Familiar Are Low-Income Parents with Medicaid and SCHIP?* New Federalism National Survey of America's Families. Series B, No. B-34. Washington, DC: Urban Institute.

Kennickell, Arthur B., Martha Starr-McCluer, and Brian J. Surette. 2000. Recent Changes in U.S. Family Finances: Results from the 1998 Survey of Consumer Finances. *Federal Reserve Bulletin* 86:1-29.

Kogan, Michael D., Greg R. Alexander, Martha A. Teitelbaum, Brian W. Jack, et al. 1995. The Effects of Gaps in Health Insurance on Continuity of a Regular Source of Care Among Preschool-Aged Children in the United States. *Journal of the American Medical Association* 274(18):1429-1435.

Kogan, Michael D., Greg R. Alexander, Brian W. Jack, and Marilee C. Allen. 1998a. The Association Between Adequacy of Prenatal Care Utilization and Subsequent Pediatric Care Utilization in the United States. *Pediatrics* 102(1):25-30.

Kogan, Michael D., Joyce A. Martin, Greg R. Alexander, Milton Kotelchuck, et al. 1998b. The Changing Pattern of Prenatal Care Utilization in the United States, 1981-1995, Using Different Prenatal Indices. *Journal of the American Medical Association* 279(20):1623-1628.

Kolata, Gina. 2001. Medical Fees Are Often Higher for Patients Without Insurance. *New York Times.* April 2; p. A:1(1).

KPMG. 1998. *Health Benefits in 1998.* Arlington, VA: KPMG Peat Marwick.

Krebs-Carter, Melora, and John Holahan. 2000. *State Strategies for Covering Uninsured Adults.* Assessing the New Federalism 00-02. Washington, DC: Urban Institute.

Kronebusch, Karl. 2001. Medicaid for Children: Federal Mandates, Welfare Reform, and Policy Backsliding. *Health Affairs* 20(1):97-111.

Ku, Leighton, and Brian Bruen. 1999. *The Continuing Decline in Medicaid Coverage.* Assessing the New Federalism: Policy Brief No. A-37. Washington, DC: Urban Institute.

Ku, Leighton, and Shannon Blaney. 2000. *Health Coverage for Legal Immigrant Children: New Census Data Highlight Importance of Restoring Medicaid and SCHIP Coverage.* Washington, DC: Center on Budget and Policy Priorities.

Ku, Leighton, and Matthew Broaddus. 2000. *The Importance of Family-Based Insurance Expansions: New Research Findings About State Health Reforms.* Washington, DC: Center on Budget and Policy Priorities.

Ku, Leighton, and Alyse Freilich. 2001. *Caring for Immigrants: Health Care Safety Nets in Los Angeles, New York, Miami, and Houston.* Kaiser Commission on Medicaid and the Uninsured. Washington, DC: Henry J. Kaiser Family Foundation.

Ku, Leighton, and Sheetal Matani. 2001. Left Out: Immigrants' Access to Health Care and Insurance. *Health Affairs* 20(1):247-256.

Kuehl, Karen S., Jeanne M. Baffa, and Gary A. Chase. 2000. Insurance and Education Determine Survival in Infantile Coarctation of the Aorta. *Journal of Health Care for the Poor and Underserved* 11(4):400-411.

Lambrew, Jeanne M. 2001a. *Diagnosing Disparities in Health Insurance for Women: A Prescription for Change.* New York: Commonwealth Fund.

Lambrew, Jeanne M. 2001b. *Health Insurance: A Family Affair. A National Profile and State by State Analysis of Uninsured Parents and Their Children.* New York: Commonwealth Fund.

Lang, David M., and Marcia Polansky. 1994. Patterns of Asthma Mortality in Philadelphia from 1969 to 1991. *New England Journal of Medicine* 331(23):1542-1546.

Lanphear, Bruce P., Robert S. Byrd, Peggy Auinger, and Caroline B. Hall. 1997. Increasing Prevalence of Recurrent Otitis Media in the United States. *Pediatrics* 99(3):E1.

Lave, Judith R., Christopher R. Keane, Chyongchiou J.Lin, Edmund M. Ricci, et al. 1998a. Impact of a Children's Health Insurance Program on Newly Enrolled Children. *Journal of the American Medical Association* 279(22):1820-1825.

Lave, Judith R., Christopher R. Keane, Chyongchiou J. Lin, Edmund M. Ricci, et al. 1998b. The Impact of Lack of Health Insurance on Children. *Journal of Health and Social Policy* 10(2):57-73.

Levy, Helen, and Thomas DeLiere. 2002. What Do People Buy When They Don't Buy Health Insurance? Available at: http://www.chas.uchicago.edu/events/wspapers/05302002.pdf. Accessed June 27, 2002.

Lewis, Kimball, Marilyn Ellwood, and John L. Czajka. 1998. *Counting the Uninsured: A Review of the Literature*. Washington, DC: Urban Institute.

Li, Guohua, and Griffin Davis. 2001. Insurance Status and Survival Outcome in Pediatric Trauma. *Academic Emergency Medicine* 8(5):517.

Lieu, Tracy A., Paul W. Newacheck, and Margaret A. McManus. 1993. Race, Ethnicity, and Access to Ambulatory Care Among U.S. Adolescents. *American Journal of Public Health* 83(7):960-965.

Lindgren, Scott, Boris Lokshin, Ann Stromquist, Miles Weinberger, et al. 1992. Does Asthma or Treatment with Theophylline Limit Children's Academic Performance? *New England Journal of Medicine* 327(13):926-930.

Litt, Mark D., Susan Reisine, and Norman Tinanoff. 1995. Multidimensional Causal Model of Dental Caries Development in Low Income Preschool Children. *Public Health Reports* 110(5):607-617

Long, Stephen H., and M. Susan Marquis. 1998. The Effects of Florida's Medicaid Eligibility for Pregnant Women. *American Journal of Public Health* 88(3):371-376.

Looker, Anne C., Peter R. Dallman, Margaret D. Carroll, Elaine W. Gunter, et al. 1997. Prevalence of Iron Deficiency in the United States. *Journal of the American Medical Association* 277(12):973-976.

Lous, Jorgen 1995. Otitis Media and Reading Achievement: A Review. *International Journal of Pediatric Otorhinolaryngology* 32(2):105-121.

Lovejoy, M. Christine, Patricia A. Graczyk, Elizabeth O'Hare, and George Neuman. 2000. Maternal Depression and Parenting Behavior: A Meta-Analytic Review. *Clinical Psychology Review* 20(5):561-592.

Lozoff, Betsy, Elias Jimenez, and Abraham W. Wolf. 1991. Long-Term Developmental Outcome of Infants with Iron Deficiency. *New England Journal of Medicine* 325(10):687-694.

Lozoff, Betsy, Nancy K. Klein, Edward C. Nelson, Donna K. McClish, et al. 1998. Behavior of Infants with Iron-Deficiency Anemia. *Child Development* 69(1):24-36.

Lozoff, Betsy, Elias Jimenez, John Hagen, Eileen Mollen, et al. 2000. Poorer Behavioral and Developmental Outcome More than 10 Years After Treatment for Iron Deficiency. *Pediatrics* 105(4):E51.

Lubker, Bobbie Boyd, Kathleen Y. Bernier, and Andrea D. Vizoso. 1999. Chronic Illnesses of Childhood and the Changing Epidemiology of Language-Learning Disorders. *Topics in Language Disorders* 20(1):59-75.

Lykens, Kristine A., and Paul A. Jargowsky. Forthcoming 2002. Medicaid Matters: Children's Health and Medicaid Eligibility Expansions. *Journal of Policy Analysis and Management* 21(2).

Lyons-Ruth, Karlen, Rebecca Wolfe, and Amy Lyubchik. 2000. Depression and the Parenting of Young Children: Making the Case for Early Preventive Mental Health Services. *Harvard Review of Psychiatry* 8(3):148-153.

Madrian, Brigeitte C., and Nancy Dean Beaulieu. 1998. Does Medicare Eligibility Affect Retirement? In: *Inquiries in the Economics of Aging*, David A. Wise (ed.). Chicago: University of Chicago Press. Pp. 109-131.

Maloy, Kathleen A., Kyle Anne Kenney, Julie Darnell, and Soeurette Cyprien. 2002. *Can Medicaid Work for Low-Income Working Families?* Washington, DC: Kaiser Commission on Medicaid and the Uninsured.

Mannuzza, Salvatore, and Rachel G. Klein. 2000. Long-Term Prognosis in Attention-Deficit/Hyperactivity Disorder. *Child Adolescent Psychiatric Clinics of North America* 93(3):711-726.

Mannuzza, Salvadore, Rachel G. Klein, Abrah Bessler, Patricia Malloy, et al. 1997. Educational and Occupational Outcome of Hyperactive Boys Grown Up. *Journal of the American Academy of Child and Adolescent Psychiatry* 36(9):1222-1227.

Mare, Robert D. 1991. Five Decades of Educational Assortive Mating. *American Sociological Review* 56(1):15-32.

Marshall, Richard M., Vickie A. Schafer, Louise O'Donnell, Jennifer Elliott, et al. 1999. Arithmetic Disabilities and ADD Subtypes: Implications for DSM-IV. *Journal of Learning Disabilities* 32(3):239-247.

Martin, Joyce A., Brady E. Hamilton, Stephanie J. Ventura, Fay Menacker, et al. 2002. *Births: Final Data for 2000.* National Vital Statistics Reports 50(5). Atlanta, GA: Centers for Disease Control and Prevention.

Mason, Joseph R. 1998. Demographics Influences and Personal Bankruptcies. In: *Research in Banking and Finance,* Iftekhar Hasen and William C. Hunter (eds.). Amsterdam: JAI.

McCormick, Marie C., Robin M. Weinick, Anne Elixhauser, Marie N. Stagnitti, et al. 2001. Annual Report on Access to and Utilization of Health Care for Children and Youth in the United States—2000. *Ambulatory Pediatrics* 1(1):3-15.

McCowen, Colin, Fiona P. Bryce, Ronald G. Neville, Iain K. Crombie, et al. 1996. School Absence—A Valid Morbidity Marker for Asthma? *Health Bulletin* 54(4):307-313.

McDuffie, Jr., Robert S., Arne Beck, Kimberly Bischoff, Jean Cross, et al. 1996. Effect of Frequency of Prenatal Care Visits on Perinatal Outcome Among Low-Risk Women: A Randomized Controlled Trial. *Journal of the American Medical Association* 275(11):847-851.

McInerny, Thomas K., Peter G. Szilagyi, George E. Childs, Richard C. Wasserman, et al. 2000. Uninsured Children with Psychosocial Problems: Primary Care Management. *Pediatrics* 106(4 Suppl):930-936.

McLearn, Karen, Karen Davis, Cathy Schoen, and Steven Parker. 1998. Listening to Parents. A National Survey of Parents with Young Children. *Archives of Pediatrics & Adolescent Medicine* 152(3):255-262.

Medical Child Support Working Group. 2000. 21 Million Children's Health: Our Shared Responsibility. The Medical Child Support Working Group's Report to the Honorable Donna E. Shalala and the Honorable Alex M. Herman. Available at: http://www.acf.dhhs.gov/programs/cse/rpt/medrpt. Accessed September 9, 2001.

Merlis, Mark. 2001. *Family Out-of-Pocket Spending for Health Services: A Continuing Source of Financial Insecurity.* Publication 509. New York: Commonwealth Fund.

Merrell, Christine, and Peter B. Tymms. 2001. Inattention, Hyperactivity and Impulsiveness: Their Impact on Academic Achievement and Progress. *British Journal of Educational Psychology* 71(1):43-56.

Meyers, Marcia K., Anna Lukemeyer, and Timothy Smeeding. 1998. The Cost of Caring: Childhood Disability and Poor Families. *Social Service Review* 72(2):209-233.

Miller, Richard D. 1990. *Another Look at the Medically Uninsured Using the 1987 Consumer Expenditure Survey.* Working Paper 206. Washington, DC: Bureau of Labor Statistics.

Mills, Robert J. 2001. *Health Insurance Coverage: 2000.* Current Population Reports. Washington, DC: U.S. Census Bureau.

Minino, Arialdi M., and Betty L. Smith. 2001. *Deaths: Preliminary Data for 2000.* National Vital Statistics Reports 49(12). Atlanta, GA: Centers for Disease Control and Prevention.

Minkovitz, Cynthia S., Patricia J., O'Campo, Yi-Hua Chen, and Holly A. Grason. 2002. Associations Between Maternal and Child Health Status and Patterns of Medical Care Use. *Ambulatory Pediatrics* 2(2):85-92.

Mody, Maria, Richard G. Schwartz, Judith S. Gravel, and Robert J. Ruben. 1999. Speech Perception and Verbal Memory in Children With and Without Histories of Otitis Media. *Journal of Speech, Language and Hearing Research* 42(5):1069-1079.

Monheit, Alan C., Jessica O. Vistnes, and John M. Eisenberg. 2001a. Moving to Medicare: Trends in the Health Insurances Status of Near-Elderly Workers, 1987-1996. *Health Affairs* 20(2):204-213.

Monheit, Alan C., Jessica O. Vistnes, and Samuel H. Zuvekas. 2001b. *Stability and Change in Health Insurance Status: New Estimates from the 1996 MEPS*. Research Findings 18 AHRQ Publication 02-0006. Rockville, MD: U.S. Department of Health and Human Services.

Moore, Kristin Anderson, and Sharon Vandivere. 2000. *Stressful Family Lives: Child and Parent Well-Being*. Assessing the New Federalism. Series B, No. B-17. Washington, DC: Urban Institute.

Moore, Kristin Anderson, Sharon Vandivere, and Jennifer Ehrle. 2000a. *Turbulence and Child Well-Being*. National Survey of America's Families. Series B, No. B-16. Washington, DC: Urban Institute.

Moore, Kristin Anderson, Sharon Vandivere, and Jennifer Ehrle. 2000b. *Sociodemographic Risk and Child Well-Being*. Assessing the New Federalism. Child Trends Series B, No. B-18. Washington, DC: The Urban Institute.

Moss, Nancy, and Karen Carver. 1998. The Effect of WIC and Medicaid on Infant Mortality in the United States. *American Journal of Public Health* 88(9):1354-1361.

Mullahy, John, and Barbara L. Wolfe. 2001. Health Policies for the Non-Elderly Poor. In: *Understanding Poverty*. Shelton H. Danziger and Robert H. Haveman (eds.). New York: Russell Sage Foundation. Pp. 278-313.

Myers, Hector F., Sylvie Taylor, Kerby T. Alvy, Angela Arrington, et al. 1992. Parental and Family Predictors of Behavior Problems in Inner-City Black Children. *American Journal of Community Psychology* 20(5):557-576.

National Academy for State Health Policy and Lake Snell Perry and Associates. 2002. *Why Eligible Children Lose and Leave SCHIP*. Portland, ME.

National Association of State Budget Officers (NASBO). 2002. *Medicaid and Other State Health Care Issues: The Current Situation. A Supplement to the Fiscal Survey of the States*. Washington, DC: NASBO.

National Center for Health Statistics (NCHS). 1996. *Third National Health and Nutrition Examination Survey (NHANES III) Reference Manuals and Reports* [CD ROM], Hyattsville, MD: U.S. Department of Health and Human Services, 2001. Atlanta, GA: Centers for Disease Control and Prevention.

National Center for Health Statistics (NCHS). 1997. *Priority Area 13. Oral Health. Healthy People 2000 Review*. Hyattsville, MD: U.S. Department of Health and Human Services.

National Center for Health Statistics (NCHS). 2000. *Health, United States 2000, with Adolescent Health Chartbook*. Hyattsville, MD: Centers for Disease Control and Prevention.

National Center for Health Statistics (NCHS). 2001. *Urban and Rural Health Chartbook: Health, United States, 2001*. National Center for Health Statistics, Hyattsville, MD.

National Center on Women and Aging, Heller Graduate School, Brandeis University, and Phillis H. Mutschler. 2001. If I Can Just Make It to 65 . . . Measuring the Impact on Women of Increasing the Eligibility Age for Medicare. Available at: www.heller.brandeis.edu/national/shelf.html. Accessed February 6, 2002.

National Institutes of Health (NIH). 2000. National Institutes of Health Consensus Development Conference Statement: Diagnosis and Treatment of Attention-Deficit/Hyperactivity Disorder (ADHD). *Journal of the American Academy of Child and Adolescent Psychiatry* 39(2):182-193.

National Public Radio (NPR), Kaiser Family Foundation, and Kennedy School of Government. 2002. National Survey on Health Care. Washington, DC: Kaiser Family Foundation.

Nelson, David E., Betsy L. Thompson, Shayne D. Bland, and Richard Rubinson. 1999. Trends in Perceived Cost as a Barrier to Medical Care, 1991-1996. *American Journal of Public Health* 89(9):1410-1413.

Newacheck, Paul W. 1992. Characteristics of Children with High and Low Usage of Physician Services. *Medical Care* 30(1):30-42.

Newacheck, Paul W., and Neal Halfon. 1986. The Association Between Mother's and Children's Use of Physician Services. *Medical Care* 24(1):30-38.

Newacheck, Paul W., Dana C. Hughes, and Jeffery J. Stoddard. 1996. Children's Access to Primary Care: Differences by Race, Income, and Insurance. *Pediatrics* 97(1):26-32.

Newacheck, Paul W., Bonnie Strickland, Jack P. Shonkoff, James M. Perrin, et al. 1998a. An Epidemiologic Profile of Children with Special Health Care Needs. *Pediatrics* 102(1):117-123.

Newacheck, Paul W., Jeffery J. Stoddard, Dana C. Hughes, and Michelle Pearl. 1998b. Health Insurance and Access to Primary Care for Children. *New England Journal of Medicine* 338(8):513-518.

Newacheck, Paul W., Claire D. Brindis, Courtney Uhler Cart, Kristin Marchi, et al. 1999. Adolescent Health Insurance Coverage: Recent Changes and Access to Care. *Pediatrics* 104(2):195-202.

Newacheck, Paul W., Dana C. Hughes, Yun-Yi Hung, Sabrina Wong, et al. 2000a. The Unmet Health Needs of America's Children. *Pediatrics* 105(4):989-997.

Newacheck, Paul W., Margaret McManus, Harriette B. Fox, Yun-Yi Hung, et al. 2000b. Access to Health Care for Children with Special Health Care Needs. *Pediatrics* 105(4):760-766.

Newhouse, Joseph P., and The Insurance Experiment Group. 1993. *Free for All? Lessons from the RAND Health Insurance Experiment.* Cambridge, MA: Harvard University Press.

Nolen-Hoeksema, Susan, Amy Wolfson, Donna Mumme, and Karen Guskin. 1995. Helplessness in Children of Depressed and Nondepressed Mothers. *Developmental Psychology* 31(3):377-387.

Oberg, Charles N., Betty Lia-Hoagberg, Catherine Skovholt, E. Hodkinson, et al. 1991. Prenatal Care Use and Health Insurance Status. *Journal of Health Care for the Poor and Underserved* 2(2):270-292.

Office of Personnel Management (OPM). 2001. Federal Employees Health Benefits Program. Available at: http://www.opm.gov/insure/health/fehb facts/index.htm. Accessed April 8, 2002.

Orne, Roberta M., Seja Joyce Fishman, Mary Manka, and Mary Ellen Pagnozzi. 2000. Living on the Edge: A Phenomenological Study of Medically Uninsured Working Americans. *Research in Nursing and Health* 23(3):204-212.

Otero, Gloria A., Dalia M. Aguirre, Rosario Porcayo, and Thalia Fernandez. 1999. Psychological and Electroencephalographic Study in School Children with Iron Deficiency. *International Journal of Neuroscience* 99(1-4):113-121.

O'Toole, Stuart J., Hratch L. Karamanoukian, James E. Allen, Michael G. Caty, et al. 1996. Insurance-Related Differences in the Presentation of Pediatric Appendicitis. *Journal of Pediatric Surgery* 31(8):1032-1034.

Overpeck, Mary D., and Jonathan B. Kotch. 1995. The Effect of U.S. Children's Access to Care on Medical Attention for Injuries. *American Journal of Public Health* 85(3):402-404.

Overpeck, Mary D., Diane H. Jones, Ann C. Trumble, Peter C. Scheidt, et al. 1997. Socioeconomic and Racial/Ethnic Factors Affecting Non-fatal Medically Attended Injury Rates in U.S. Children. *Injury Prevention* 3(4):272-276.

Pappas, Gregory, Wilbur C. Hadden, Lola Jean Kozak, and Gail F. Fisher. 1997. Potentially Avoidable Hospitalizations: Inequalities in Rates Between U.S. Socioeconomic Groups. *American Journal of Public Health* 87(5):811-816.

Parker, Jennifer D., and Kenneth C. Schoendorf. 2000. Variation in Hospital Discharges for Ambulatory Care-Sensitive Conditions Among Children. *Pediatrics* 106(4):942-948.

Paulin, Geoffrey D., and Wolf D. Weber. 1995. The Effect of Health Insurance on Consumer Spending. *Monthly Labor Review* 118(3):34-54.

Phibbs, Ciaran S., David H. Mark, Harold S. Luft, Deborah J. Peltzman-Rennie, et al. 1993. Choice of Hospital for Delivery: A Comparison of High-Risk and Low-Risk Women. *Health Services Research* 28(2):201-222.

Piper, Jeanna M. Wayen A. Ray, and Marie.R. Griffin. 1990. Effects of Medicaid Eligibility Expansion on Prenatal Care and Pregnancy Outcome in Tennessee. *Journal of the American Medical Association* 264(17):2219-2223.

Pollitz, Karen, Richard Sorian, and Kathy Thomas. 2001. *How Accessible Is Individual Health Insurance for Consumers in Less-than-Perfect Health?* Washington, DC: Henry J. Kaiser Family Foundation.

Public Health Service Expert Panel on Prenatal Care. 1989. *Caring for Our Future: The Content of Prenatal Care.* Washington, DC: U.S. Department of Health and Human Services, Public Health Service.

Quinn, Kevin, Cathy Schoen, and Louisa Buatti. 2000. *On Their Own: Young Adults Living Without Health Insurance.* The Commonwealth Task Force on the Future of Health Insurance. New York: Commonwealth Fund.

Rana, Uzma A., Sherri M. Jurgens, Salvatore Mangione, Josephine Elia, et al. 2000. Asthma Prevalence Among High Absentees of Two Philadelphia Middle Schools. *Chest* 118(4):79S.

Ray, Wayne A., Edward F. Mitchel, Jr., and Joyce M. Piper. 1997. Effect of Medicaid Expansion on Pre-term Birth. *American Journal of Preventive Medicine* 13(4):292-297.

Reading, Richard, and Shirley Reynolds. 2001. Debt, Social Disadvantage and Maternal Depression. *Social Science and Medicine* 53(4):441-454.

Resnick, Michael D., Lauren J. Harris, and Robert Wm. Blum. 1993. The Impact of Caring and Connectedness on Adolescent Health and Well-Being. *Journal of Pediatrics and Child Health* 29(Suppl. 1):S3-S9.

Rietveld, Simon, and Vivian T. Colland. 1999. The Impact of Severe Asthma on Schoolchildren. *Journal of Asthma* 36(5):409-417.

Roberts, Joanne E., Margaret R. Burchinal, Sandra C. Jackson, Stephen R. Hooper, et al. 2000. Otitis Media in Early Childhood in Relation to Preschool Language and School Readiness Skills Among Black Children. *Pediatrics* 106(4):725-735.

Rodewald, Lance E., Peter G. Szilagyi, Jane Holl, Laura Stone, et al. 1997. Health Insurance for Low-Income Working Families: Effect on the Provision of Immunizations to Pre-School Age Children. *Archives of Pediatrics & Adolescent Medicine* 151(8):798-803.

Rodriguez, Michael A., Marilyn A. Winkleby, David Ahn, Jan Sundquist, et al. 2002. Identification of Population Subgroups of Children and Adolescents with High Asthma Prevalence: Findings from the Third National Health and Nutritional Examination Survey. *Archives of Pediatric and Adolescent Medicine* 156(3):269-275.

Rosenbach, Margo, Marilyn Ellwood, John Czajka, Carol Irvin, et al. 2001. *Implementation of the State Children's Health Insurance Program: Momentum Is Increasing After a Modest Start.* Cambridge, MA: Mathematica Policy Research, Inc.

Rosenbaum, Sara. 2000. *Medicaid Eligibility and Citizenship Status: Policy Implications for Immigrant Populations.* Policy Brief. Washington, DC: Kaiser Commission on Medicaid and the Uninsured.

Ross, Donna Cohen, and Laura Cox. 2000. *Making It Simple: Medicaid for Children and CHIP Income Eligibility Guidelines and Enrollment Procedures. Findings from a 50-State Survey.* Kaiser Commission on Medicaid and the Uninsured. Pub. No. 2166. Washington, DC: Henry J. Kaiser Family Foundation.

Ross, Donna Cohen, and Laura Cox. 2002. *Enrolling Children and Families in Health Care Coverage: The Promise of Doing More.* Washington, DC: Kaiser Commission on Medicaid and the Uninsured.

Salganicoff, Alina, and Roberta Wyn. 1999. Access to Care for Low-Income Women: The Impact of Medicaid. *Journal of Health Care for the Poor and Underserved* 10(4):453-467.

Schoen, Catherine, and Catherine DesRoches. 2000a. Role of Insurance in Promoting Access to Care. *Health Services Research* 35(1):187-206.

Schoen, Cathy, and Catherine DesRoches. 2000b. Uninsured and Unstable Insured: The Importance of Continuous Insurance Coverage. *Health Services Research* 35(1):187-206.

Schoen, Cathy, and Elaine Puleo. 1998. Low-Income Working Families at Risk: Uninsured and Underserved. *Journal of Urban Health* 75(1):30-49.

Schoen, Cathy, Barbara Lyons, Diane Rowland, Karen Davis, et al. 1997. Insurance Matters for Low Income Adults: Results from the Kaiser/Commonwealth Five State Survey. *Health Affairs* 16(5):163-171.

Selden, Thomas, Jessica S. Banthin, and Joel W. Cohen. 1998. Medicaid's Problem Children: Eligible but Not Enrolled. *Health Affairs* 17(3):192-200.

Shelton, Terri L., Russell A. Barkley, C. Crosswait, Martha J. Moorehouse, et al. 1998. Psychiatric and Psychological Morbidity as a Function of Adaptive Disability in Preschool Children with Aggressive and Hyperactive-Impulsive-Inattentive Behavior. *Journal of Abnormal Child Psychology* 26(6):475-494.

Shi, Leiyu, and Ning Lu. 2000. Individual Sociodemographic Characteristics Associated with Hospitalization for Pediatric Ambulatory Care Sensitive Conditions. *Journal of Health Care for the Poor and Underserved* 11(4):373-384.

Shonkoff, Jack P., and Deborah A. Phillips (eds.). 2000. *From Neurons to Neighborhoods. The Science of Early Childhood Development.* Washington, DC: National Academy Press.

Short, Pamela Farley, Joel C. Cantor, and Alan C. Monheit. 1998. The Dynamics of Medicaid Enrollment. *Inquiry* 25(4):504-516.

Siefert, Kristine, Phillip J. Bowman, Colleen M. Heflin, Sheldon Danziger, et al. 2000. Social and Environmental Predictors of Maternal Depression in Current and Recent Welfare Recipients. *American Journal of Orthopsychiatry* 70(4):510-522.

Silverstein, Marc D., Joanne E. Mair, Slavica K. Katusic, Peter C. Wollan, et al. 2001. School Attendance and School Performance: A Population-Based Study of Children with Asthma. *Journal of Pediatrics* 139(2):278-283.

Simantov, Elizabeth, Cathy Schoen, and Stephanie Bruegman. 2001. Market Failure? Individual Insurance Markets for Older Americans. *Health Affairs* 20(4):139-149.

Singer, Ingrid. 2000. Cost-Sharing and the Uninsured: Trends at Safety Net Institutions. Washington, DC. National Association of Public Hospitals and Health Systems.

Singh, Susheela, Rachel Benson Gold, and Jennifer J. Frost. 1994. Impact of the Medicaid Eligibility Expansions on Coverage of Deliveries. *Family Planning Perspectives* 26(1):31-33.

Smith, James P. 1999. Healthy Bodies and Thick Wallets: The Dual Relation Between Health and Economic Status. *Journal of Economic Perspectives* 13(2):145-166.

Smith, Vernon K., and David M. Rousseau. 2002. *SCHIP Program Enrollment: December 2001 Update.* Washington, DC: Kaiser Commission on Medicaid and the Uninsured.

Sox, Colin M., Helen R. Burstin, Roger A. Edwards, Anne C. O'Neil, et al. 1998. Hospital Admissions Through the Emergency Department: Does Insurance Status Matter? *American Journal of Medicine* 105(6):506-512.

Sox, Colin M., Katherine Swartz, Helen R. Burstin, and Troyen A. Brennan. 1998. Insurance or a Regular Physician: Which Is the Most Powerful Predictor of Health Care? *American Journal of Public Health* 88(3):364-370.

Spivak, William, Robbyn Sockolow, and Anastasia Rigas. 1995. The Relationship Between Insurance Class and Severity of Presentation of Inflammatory Bowel Disease in Children. *American Journal of Gastroenterology* 90(6):982-987.

Stafford, Randall S. 1990. Cesarean Section Use and Source of Payment: An Analysis of California Hospital Discharge Abstracts. *American Journal of Public Health* 80(3):313-315.

Stafford, Randall S., Sean D. Sullivan, and Laura B. Gardner. 1993. Trends in Cesarean Section Use in California, 1983 to 1990. *American Journal of Obstetrics and Gynecology* 168(4):1297-1302.

Stanley, David T., and Marjorie Girth. 1971. *Bankruptcy: Problem, Process, Reform.* Washington, DC: Brookings Institution.

Starfield, Barbara. 1995. Social, Economic, and Medical Care Determinants of Children's Health. In: *Health Care for Children: What's Right, What's Wrong, What's Next.* Ruth E. K. Stein (ed.). New York: United Hospital Fund of New York. Pp. 39-52.

Starr-McCluer, Martha. 1996. Health Insurance and Precautionary Savings. *American Economic Review* 86(1):285-295.

Stevens, Rosemary. 1989. *In Sickness and in Wealth: America's Hospitals in the Twentieth Century.* New York: Basic Books.

Stoddard, Jeffrey J., Robert F. St. Peter, and Paul W. Newacheck. 1994. Health Insurance Status and Ambulatory Care for Children. *New England Journal of Medicine* 330(20):1421-1425.

Straus, Murray A., Richard J. Gelles, and Suzanne Steinmetz. 1980. *Behind Closed Doors: Violence in the American Family.* Garden City, NY: Anchor Press/Doubleday.

Sullivan, Teresa A., Elizabeth Warren, and Jay Lawrence Westbrook. 2000. *The Fragile Middle: Americans in Debt.* New Haven, CT: Yale University Press.

Svavarsdottir, Erla Kolbrum, Marilyn A. McCubbin, and Janet H. Kane. 2000. Well-Being of Parents of Young Children with Asthma. *Research in Nursing and Health* 23(5):346-358.

Szilagyi, Peter G., and Edward L. Schor. 1998. The Health of Children. *Health Services Research* 33(4 Pt 2):1001-1039.

Szilagyi, Peter G., Lance E. Rodewald, Judy Savageau, Lorrie Yoos, et al. 1992. Improving Influenza Vaccination Rates in Children with Asthma: A Test of a Computerized Reminder System and an Analysis of Factors Predicting Vaccination Compliance. *Pediatrics* 90(6):871-875.

Szilagyi, Peter G., Jane L. Holl, Lance E. Rodewald, Lorrie Yoos, et al. 2000a. Evaluation of New York State's Child Health Plus: Children Who Have Asthma. *Pediatrics* 105(3):719-727.

Szilagyi, Peter G., Jane L. Holl, Lance E. Rodewald, Laura Pollard Shone, et al. 2000b. Evaluation of Children's Health Insurance: From New York State's Child Health Plus to SCHIP. *Pediatrics* 105(3):687-691.

Szilagyi, Peter G., Jack Zwanziger, Lance E. Rodewald, Jane L. Holl, et al. 2000c. Evaluation of a State Health Insurance Program for Low-Income Children: Implications for State Child Health Insurance Programs. *Pediatrics* 105(2):363-371.

Taragonski, Paul V., Victoria W. Persky, Peter Orris, and Whitney Addington. 1994. Trends in Asthma Mortality Among African Americans and Whites in Chicago, 1968 Through 1991. *American Journal of Public Health* 84(11):1830-1833.

Taylor, Amy K., Joel W. Cohen, and Steven R. Machlin. 2001a. Being Uninsured in 1996 Compared to 1987: How Has the Experience of the Uninsured Changed over Time? *Health Services Research.* 36(6, Part II):16-31.

Taylor, Amy K., Joel W. Cohen, and Steven R. Machlin. 2001b. Unpublished tables that are an extension of the 2001a article and are tabulations from the 1996 MEPS Survey. Center for Cost and Financing Studies. Rockville, MD: Agency for Healthcare Research and Quality.

Teachman, Jay D., Lucky M. Tedrow, and Kyle D. Crowder. 2000. The Changing Demography of America's Families. *Journal of Marriage and the Family* 62:1234-1246.

Teele, David W., Jerome. O. Klein, Cynthia Chase, Paula Menyuk, et al. 1990. Otitis Media in Infancy and Intellectual Ability, School Achievement, Speech and Language at Age 7 Years. *Journal of Infectious Diseases* 162(3):685-694.

Thorpe, Kenneth E., and Curtis S. Florence. 1999. Why Are Workers Uninsured? Employer-Sponsored Health Insurance in 1997. *Health Affairs* 8(2):213-218.

Trafton, Sarah, Laura Pollard Shone, Jack Zwanziger, Dana B. Mukamel, et al. 2000. Evolution of a Children's Health Insurance Program: Lessons from New York State's Child Health Plus. *Pediatrics* 105(3):692-696.

Urban Institute. 2002a. Urban Institute Model for Uninsured and Enrollment Estimates. Washington, DC. Available at http://www.coveringkids.org/entrypoints/press/UrbanMethodology.pdf. Accessed August 5, 2002.

Urban Institute. 2002b. *Welfare Reform: The Next Act,* Alan Weil and Kenneth Finegold (eds.). Washington, DC: Urban Institute Press.

U.S. Department of Agriculture (USDA). 2002. Food and Nutrition Service. Women, Infants, and Children. Available at: http://www.fns.usda.gov/wic. Accessed May 30, 2002.

U.S. Department of Health and Human Services (DHHS). 2000. *Healthy People 2010: Understanding and Improving Health.* 2nd ed. Washington, DC: U.S. Government Printing Office.

U.S. Department of Health and Human Services (DHHS). 2001. The State Children's Health Insurance Program (SCHIP). Available at http://www.fns.usda.gov/cnd/SCHIP/SCHIP.background.htm. Accessed March 29, 2002.

U.S. Department of Health and Human Services (DHHS). 2002a. Medicaid: A Brief Summary. Available at: http://www.hcfa.gov/pubforms/actuary/ormedmed/DEFAULT4.htm. Accessed April 2, 2002.

U.S. Department of Health and Human Services (DHHS). 2002b. The 2002 HHS Poverty Guidelines. Available at http://aspe.hhs.gov/poverty/02poverty.htm. Accessed March 15, 2002.

U.S. General Accounting Office (GAO). 2000. *Medicaid and SCHIP: Comparisons of Outreach, Enrollment, Practices, and Benefits.* GAO/HEHS-00-86. Washington, DC: U.S. General Accounting Office.

Vargas, Clemencia M., James J. Crall, and Donald A. Schneider. 1998. Sociodemographic Distribution of Pediatric Dental Caries: NHANES III, 1988-1994. *Journal of the American Dental Association* 129(9):1229-1238.

Verhulst, Frank C., and Jan van der Ende. 1997. Factors Associated with Child Mental Health Service Use in the Community. *Journal of the American Academy of Child and Adolescent Psychiatry* 36(7):901-909.

Viner, Russell, Mary McGrath, and Philip Trudinger. 1996. Family Stress and Metabolic Control in Diabetes. *Archives of Disease in Childhood* 74(5):418-421.

Walker, Lynn S., Deborah A.Van Slyke, and J.R. Newbrough. 1992. Family Resources and Stress: A Comparison of Families of Children with Cystic Fibrosis, Diabetes and Mental Retardation. *Journal of Pediatric Psychology* 17(3):327-343.

Weidner, Gerdi, Joanne Hutt, Sonja L. Connor, and Nancy R. Mendell. 1992. Family Stress and Coronary Risk in Children. *Psychosomatic Medicine* 54(4):471-479.

Weil, Alan, and Kenneth Finegold (eds.). 2002. *Welfare Reform: The Next Act.* Washington, DC: Urban Institute Press.

Weinick, Robin M., and Nancy A. Krauss. 2000. Racial/Ethnic Differences in Children's Access to Care. *American Journal of Public Health* 90(11):1771-1774.

Weinick, Robin M., and Alan C. Monheit. 1999. Children's Health Insurance Coverage and Family Structure, 1977-1996. *Medical Care Research and Review* 56(1):55-73.

Weinick, Robin M., Margaret E. Weigers, and Joel W. Cohen. 1998. Children's Health Insurance, Access to Care, and Health Status: New Findings. *Health Affairs* 17(2):127-136.

Weinick, Robin M., Samuel H. Zuvekas, and Joel W. Cohen. 2000. Racial and Ethnic Differences in Access to and Use of Health Care Services, 1977 to 1996. *Medical Care Research and Review* 57 (Suppl 1):36-54.

Weir, David R., and Robert J. Willis. 2000. Prospects for Widow Poverty. In: *Forecasting Retirement Needs and Retirement Wealth.* Olivia S. Mitchell, P. Bret Hammond, and Anna M. Rappaport (eds.). Philadelphia: University of Pennsylvania Press. Pp. 208-234.

Weir, David R., and Robert J. Willis. Forthcoming. *Health Insurance and the Economics of Widowhood.* Working Paper. Ann Arbor, MI: Institute for Survey Research, University of Michigan.

Weis, Darlene. 1992. Uninsured Maternity Clients: A Concern for Quality. *Applied Nursing Research* 5(2):74-82.

Weissman, Joel S., Paul Dryfoos, and Katharine London. 1999. Income Levels of Bad-Debt and Free-Care Patients in Massachusetts Hospitals. *Health Affairs* 18(4):156-166.

Wielawski, Irene. 2000. Gouging the Medically Uninsured: A Tale of Two Bills. *Health Affairs* 19(5):180-185.

Willcutt, Erik G., and Bruce F. Pennington. 1996. Comorbidity of Reading Disability and Attention-Deficit/Hyperactivity Disorder: Differences by Gender and Subtype. *Journal of Learning Disabilities* 33(2):179-191.

Willcutt, Erik G., Bruce F. Pennington, and John C. DeFries. 2000. Etiology of Inattention and Hyperactivity/Impulsivity in a Community Sample of Twins with Learning Difficulties. *Journal of Abnormal Child Psychology* 28(2):149-159.

Wolfe, Barbara L. 1985. The Influence of Health on School Outcomes. A Multivariate Approach. *Medical Care* 23(10):1127-1138.

Yager, Joel. 1982. Family Issues in the Pathogenesis of Anorexia Nervosa. *Psychosomatic Medicine* 44(1):43-60.

Yelowitz, Aaron S. 1995. The Medicaid Notch, Labor Supply, and Welfare Population. *Quarterly Journal of Economics* 110(4):909-940.

Young, Kathryn Taafe, Karen Davis, Cathy Schoen, and Steven Parker. 1998. Listening to Parents with Young Children. *Archives of Pediatrics and Adolescent Medicine* 152(3):255-262.

Yudkowsky, Beth K., and Suk-fong S. Tang. 1997. Children at Risk: Their Health Insurance Status by State. *Pediatrics* 99(5):E2.

Zargi, Miha, and Irena Hocevar Boltezar. 1992. Effects of Recurrent Otitis Media in Infancy on Auditory Perception and Speech. *American Journal of Otolaryngology* 13(6):366-372.

Zuckerman, Stephen, Jennifer Haley, and John Holahan. 2000. *Health Insurance, Access, and Health Status of Nonelderly Adults.* Assessing the New Federalism. Washington, DC: Urban Institute.

Zuckerman, Stephen, Genevieve M. Kenney, Lisa Dubay, Jennifer Haley, et al. 2001. Shifting Health Insurance Coverage 1997-1999. *Health Affairs* 20(1):169-177.

Zwanziger, Jack, Dana B. Mukamel, Peter G. Szilagyi, Sarah Trafton, et al. 2000. Evaluating Child Health Plus in Upstate New York: How Much Does Providing Health Insurance to Uninsured Children Increase Health Care Costs? *Pediatrics* 105(3):728-732.